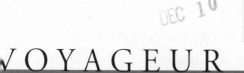

VOYAGEUR CLASSICS

BOOKS THAT EXPLORE CANADA

Michael Gnarowski — Series Editor

The Dundurn Group presents the Voyageur Classics series, b⌐‾ ‾ on the tradition of exploration and rediscovery and bringing ⸢ ⸍‾ tested writing about the Canadian experience in all i⸔

This series of original or translated works in t¹ tory, politics, and biography has been gath⸍ our understanding of a multi-faceted ⸢ ⸏ard, knowledgeable, and reader-friendly i⸏. ⸍lassics series provides context and accessibility ⸍w life into these timeless Canadian masterpieces.

The Voyageur Classics series was designed with tne widest possible readership in mind and sees a place for itself with the interested reader as well as in the classroom. Physically attractive and reset in a contemporary format, these books aim at an enlivened and updated sense of Canada's written heritage.

OTHER VOYAGEUR CLASSICS TITLES

The Blue Castle by Lucy Maud Montgomery,
introduced by Dr. Collett Tracey 978-1-55002-666-5

Canadian Exploration Literature: An Anthology,
edited and introduced by Germaine Warkentin 978-1-55002-661-0

The Donnellys by James Reaney,
introduced by Alan Filewod 978-1-55002-832-4

Empire and Communications by Harold A. Innis,
introduced by Alexander John Watson 978-1-55002-662-7

The Firebrand: William Lyon Mackenzie and the Rebellion in Upper Canada
by William Kilbourn, introduced by Ronald Stagg 978-1-55002-800-3

In This Poem I Am: Selected Poetry of Robin Skelton,
edited and introduced by Harold Rhenisch 978-1-55002-769-3

The Letters and Journals of Simon Fraser 1806–1808,
edited and introduced by W. Kaye Lamb, foreword by Michael Gnarowski
978-1-55002-713-6

Maria Chapdelaine: A Tale of French Canada by Louis Hémon,
translated by W.H. Blake, introduction and notes by Michael Gnarowski
978-1-55002-712-9

Mrs. Simcoe's Diary by Elizabeth Posthuma Simcoe,
edited and introduced by Mary Quayle Innis, foreword by Michael Gnarowski
978-1-55002-768-6

The Refugee: Narratives of Fugitive Slaves in Canada by Benjamin Drew, introduced by George Elliott Clarke 978-1-55002-801-0

Selected Writings by A.J.M. Smith,
edited and introduced by Michael Gnarowski 978-1-55002-665-8

A Tangled Web by Lucy Maud Montgomery, introduced by Benjamin Lefebvre
978-1-55488-403-2

The Yellow Briar: A Story of the Irish on the Canadian Countryside by Patrick Slater,
introduced by Michael Gnarowski 978-1-55002-848-5

VOYAGEUR CLASSICS

BOOKS THAT EXPLORE CANADA

THE SCALPEL, THE SWORD

THE STORY OF DOCTOR NORMAN BETHUNE

TED ALLAN & SYDNEY GORDON

INTRODUCTION BY
JULIE ALLAN, DR. NORMAN ALLAN & SUSAN OSTROVSKY

DUNDURN PRESS
TORONTO

Editor: Michael Carroll
Copy Editors: Jason Karp and Kelvin Kong
Design: Erin Mallory
Printer: Marquis

Library and Archives Canada Cataloguing in Publication

Allan, Ted
    The scalpel, the sword : the story of Doctor Norman Bethune / by Ted Allan and Sydney Gordon ; introduction by Julie Allan, Dr. Norman Allan, and Susan Ostrovsky.

First ed. published 1952.
ISBN 978-1-55488-402-5

    1. Bethune, Norman, 1890-1939. 2. Surgeons--Canada--Biography.
I. Gordon, Sydney II. Title.

R464.B4 A6 2009   617.092   C2009-900103-9

1   2   3   4   5   13   12   11   10   09

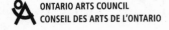

Conseil des Arts du Canada   Canada Council for the Arts

ONTARIO ARTS COUNCIL
CONSEIL DES ARTS DE L'ONTARIO

Canadä

We acknowledge the support of the Canada Council for the Arts and the Ontario Arts Council for our publishing program. We also acknowledge the financial support of the Government of Canada through the Book Publishing Industry Development Program and The Association for the Export of Canadian Books, and the Government of Ontario through the Ontario Book Publishers Tax Credit program, and the Ontario Media Development Corporation.

Care has been taken to trace the ownership of copyright material used in this book. The author and the publisher welcome any information enabling them to rectify any references or credits in subsequent editions.

J. Kirk Howard, President

Printed and bound in Canada.
Printed on recycled paper

www.dundurn.com

Dundurn Press
3 Church Street, Suite 500
Toronto, Ontario, Canada
M5E 1M2

Gazelle Book Services Limited
White Cross Mills
High Town, Lancaster, England
LA1 4XS

Dundurn Press
2250 Military Road
Tonawanda, NY
U.S.A. 14150

To those for whom he worked and died;
and more personally, to Julie, Norman and Susan

CONTENTS

FOREWORD

BY MADAME SUN YAT-SEN

In comparison with the human world of past times, our world is highly complex. Because of its highly developed communications, events in every part of the globe and of human society are closely interconnected. There are no isolated disasters and there is no progress that does not help the progress of all.

This situation is reflected in the minds of men. The contents of men's minds have also become worldwide in scope and complexity. It is not enough for a man, seeking the welfare of his own people and country, to consider his domestic situation in relation to his immediate neighbours. World trends encompass every one of us, and it is by participating in them and contributing to them that we influence our own future. The highest task before men's minds today is to understand, to fight against the forces of regression and death, to strengthen and convert into reality the possibilities which our world offers, as no previous world has offered, for a fuller life for all men.

The hero in any age is one who carries out with a surpassing degree of devotion, determination, courage and skill the main tasks with which his times challenge every man. Today these tasks are world-wide, and the contemporary hero — whether he works at home or in a foreign land — is a world hero, not only in historical retrospect but now.

Norman Bethune was such a hero. He lived, worked and fought in three countries — in Canada, which was his native land; in Spain, where forward-looking men of all nations flocked to fight in the first great people's resistance to the darkness of Nazism and fascism; and in China, where he helped our guerilla armies to capture and build new bases of national freedom and democracy in territory which the military fascists of Japan fondly hoped they had conquered, and where he helped us forge the mighty peoples' army which finally liberated all China. In a special sense he belongs to the peoples of these three countries. In a larger sense he belongs to all who fight against oppression of nations and of peoples.

Norman Bethune was a doctor, and he fought with and within his profession with the weapons he knew best. He was an expert and a pioneer in his own science — he kept his weapons sharp and fresh. And he devoted his great skill, consciously and consistently, to the vanguards of the struggle against fascism and imperialism. To him fascism was the disease holding a greater evil for mankind than any other, a plague that destroys minds and bodies by tens of millions, and by denying the value of man also denies the value of all the sciences which have arisen to minister to men's health, vigour and growth.

The value of the techniques Norman Bethune taught his Chinese students under Japanese gunfire was determined by the purpose for which they were used. Germany and Japan were countries of high technical development, but because they were led by enemies of human progress their science and their skills brought only misfortune to mankind. Fighters for the people have the duty of attaining the highest technical skill, because only in their hands can technique really serve man.

Dr. Bethune was the first medical man to bring blood banks to the battlefields, and his transfusions saved the lives of hundreds of fighters for the Spanish Republic. In China he launched and practised the slogan, "Doctors! Go to the wounded! Do not wait for them to come to you." In an environment totally different, and far more backward than that of Spain, he organized a procedure of guerilla medical service which saved tens of thousands of our best and bravest. His plans and practice were based not only on medical science and experience, but also on military and political study and experience on the fronts of the people's war. Bethune in Spain and China was a pioneer in the battlefield of medicine.

He understood thoroughly the conditions, strategy, tactics and terrain of the struggle, and he knew what could be expected of medical workers who were free men, fighting beside other free men for their homes and their future. The doctors, nurses and orderlies whom he trained learned to regard themselves not only as technical auxiliaries but as front-line soldiers, with tasks as responsible and important as those of the fighting branches.

These things Dr. Bethune accomplished amid conditions such as no medical man without a broad understanding of his tasks could possibly have coped with. He accomplished them in mountain villages in the most primitive parts of China, almost without any previous knowledge of the language, of the people among whom he worked, and without any strength in his own tuberculosis-ravaged body apart from his burning conviction and iron will.

His broad world understanding, the sources of power that he drew from it, were the things that give his work more universal meaning for our time than that of other medical heroes who laboured against similar heart-breaking conditions, such as Father Damien or Dr. Grenfell in Labrador.

What killed Dr. Bethune? Dr. Bethune fell in the fight against fascism and reaction to which he had given his passion, skill and strength. The region in which he worked was not only block-aded by the Japanese enemy. It was blockaded also by Chiang Kai-shek's reactionary government which had always been ready to compromise victory rather than fight a people's war. The men whom Bethune fought for were adjudged unworthy not only of arms and ammunition but even of medical supplies to heal their wounded. They died of infections because they could not receive modern antidotes.

Bethune died of septicemia, the result of operating without rubber gloves and having no sulfa drugs for treatment.

The International Peace Hospitals which Dr. Bethune founded now work under new conditions — China, at last, is free. But after Bethune died his appointed successor, Dr. Kisch, who worked beside him in Spain, was prevented by Chiang Kai-shek's blockade from assuming his post. Dr. Kotnis of the Indian Medical Units, who finally took up the directorship of one of Dr. Bethune's hospitals and valiantly carried on his work, also died at his post — again because there were no drugs on hand to treat him. Dr. Bethune and Dr. Kotnis were two among many victims, who, were it not for the blockade, might still be living and fighting in the cause of the world's free peoples.

I am very happy to introduce the life of Dr. Norman Bethune to greater numbers of people than have hitherto been able to acquaint themselves with the life of this hero of our time, who symbolizes so nobly the common stake of all people in the fight for freedom. His life, death and heritage have been particularly close to me, not only because of the great service he performed in our peoples' war of national liberation, but also because of my own activity in the China Welfare League, of which I am chairman. The League has been directed toward securing support for the Bethune Peace Hospital and Bethune Medical School network that carries on his work and his memory.

The new China will never forget Dr. Bethune. He was one of those who helped us become free. His work and memory will remain with us forever.

INTRODUCTION

BY JULIE ALLAN,
DR. NORMAN ALLAN,
AND SUSAN OSTROVSKY

The Scalpel, the Sword tells the story of a man whose life was shaped by his ideals. It came into being because its two authors shared those basic values. Both Alan Herman, later to become Ted Allan, and Sydney Ostrovsky, later to become Sydney Gordon, were the sons of Jewish immigrants in Montreal and grew up in a country of promise during the Great Depression. As the poor became poorer and Spain's Francisco Franco and Germany's Adolf Hitler gathered strength, many young Jews gravitated toward the political left, the Communist Party, the only voice that seemed to realize the dangers posed by fascism. Ted and Sydney were among these ardent young "politicos."

Sydney was the methodical rationalist — the reader, the thinker, the wordsmith. The charismatic Ted, a year younger, was full of youthful passion and a thirst for adventure that he maintained throughout his life.

The events that culminated in this book began in March 1934, about a couple of months after Ted's eighteenth birthday. The telephone rang, and his mother, Annie, answered. "Alan," she called, "it's a Dr. Bethune. He wants to speak to some Ted Allan."

Young Alan had gotten a job as a reporter for the communist newspaper *The Daily Clarion*, covering the political and labour scene. He had received a tip that Adrian Arcand's local National Social Christian Party was being bankrolled by the Nazis in Berlin. Arcand was a Quebec anti-communist demagogue who promoted the forcible removal of all Canadian Jews to Hudson Bay.

To reveal Arcand's activities, Ted decided to go undercover and join the homegrown fascists. His name, Alan Herman, was considered "Jewish," so he became "Ted Allan, Nazi" for five weeks and gathered evidence that Germany was financing hate groups all over North America. He wrote the exposé under his pseudonym, and the name stuck. Coincidentally, at the same time, Sydney Ostrovsky, also working for the communist press, changed his last name to Gordon, seeking to protect his parents from the eyes of the establishment who were covertly watching his political activities.

Ted's first short story had been published in a left-wing literary magazine. One afternoon, while visiting his family, the life-changing call came.

Dr. Norman Bethune, "Beth" to his friends, was chief of thoracic surgery at Sacré Coeur Hospital in Cartierville, just north of Montreal. He was one of the most popular figures in liberal and left-wing circles. To young Ted Allan he was a superstar.

Ted's mother handed her son the telephone receiver. "Norman Bethune here. Miriam Kennedy gave me your phone number. I loved your story in *New Frontier*. I'm having a party this coming Saturday evening to celebrate my forty-fourth birthday, and I'd love you to come."

Bethune's Beaver Hall Hill apartment was up three flights of stairs. The first things one noticed on entering the room were the children's paintings on the walls. Bookshelves lined the other walls from floor to ceiling.

Escorting Ted along the hallway, Bethune brought him into the bathroom. On one wall hung all of Bethune's diplomas, while the wall facing the door was covered with handprints. By each handprint was a signature. Bethune led Ted to a bowl of blue paint, took his left hand and placed it in the bowl. Then he grasped Ted's hand and pressed it against the wall with the other handprints and said, "Now sign your name."

Dr. Norman Bethune posing for the documentary film Heart of Spain, *Madrid, 1937.*

Photo by Geza Korvin. Courtesy Julie and Norman Allan.

14

Ted wrote "Ted Allan."

"You are now numbered among my special friends," Beth said.

By virtue of Bethune's friendship and sponsorship, Ted joined the city's intelligentsia. The warmth of this relationship gave him confidence and opened many doors.

Two years later, in 1936, the Spanish army, controlled by fascist officers led by General Francisco Franco, staged an insurrection against the elected government, and the Spanish Civil War between the fascist "Nationalists" and the democratic "Loyalists" began. Bethune set out to help the Loyalists. The battle against fascism came first before other imperatives. Bethune eventually developed a mobile transfusion unit to deliver blood to the front lines.

Ted planned to follow Beth to Spain. He intended to go over as a reporter and work with the doctor. That was the idea. The Canadian Communist Party, in the person of Fred Rose, agreed to send Ted to Spain as a correspondent for *The Daily Clarion*, but in the end another journalist got the job.

So Ted decided to volunteer for the International Brigades. If he wasn't needed as a reporter, he would fight in the trenches. He was going to participate directly in the war one way or another to fight fascism. It was a heady time for a young man not yet twenty-one.

Great Britain, France, the United States and Canada stayed "neutral" regarding Spain as Hitler and Italy's Benito Mussolini used the country as a dress rehearsal for the Second World War. They stood silent, convinced that Germany would attack the Soviet Union and rid the world of Joseph Stalin. They turned a blind eye to the concentration camps where political prisoners were being incarcerated and to the new racial laws against German Jews. Only the Soviet Union was alarmed and only it helped the democratically elected government of Spain against Franco.

By January 1937, Ted was on his way to Spain by ship, embarking from New York City with a group of North American volunteers. While in New York, Ted called in at the office of Federated Press, a wire service for the trade union movement, and convinced it to accredit him as a Spanish correspondent.

On the ship Ted befriended John Lenthier, a young actor. John had recently married Kate Schwartz, a beautiful Bostonian he had met when he was touring with the left-wing Group

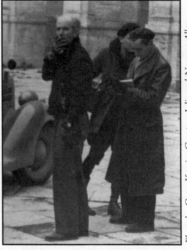

Norman Bethune and Ted Allan in Madrid, 1937.

Photo by Geza Korvin. Courtesy Julie and Norman Allan.

Theater in New England. He gave Ted a letter to be delivered to Kate in New York in case he was killed in the trenches.

Arriving in Albacete, Spain, the volunteers were taught to handle the few rifles they had. These guns were a mixed bag of new, old and ancient. Then, in the night, the planes came — German Heinkels. The barracks were hit and some recruits were hurt, but miraculously no one was killed. Albacete itself, though, was bombed into a smouldering ruin.

Ted got a transfer to work as a correspondent for the International Brigades. He broadcast radio reports from Madrid to North America. Ted found himself in the Telefónica building in Madrid every night at midnight so that his broadcasts could reach the East Coast of North America in the afternoon.

The siege of Madrid lasted two years. During that time, the centre of Madrid was shelled regularly by the Nationalists. The Telefónica building, a modest skyscraper twelve stories high, became a primary target.

Before leaving for Madrid, Ted had dinner with Peter Kerrigan, a colonel in the Brigades and the political commissar of the British Battalion. Discovering that Ted was from Montreal and knew Norman Bethune, Kerrigan spoke of the rumours that had been circulating in Madrid concerning the doctor's Blood Transfusion Unit. Bethune was drinking heavily and fighting with the Spanish doctors. The morale in the unit was said to be low. Maybe Ted could find out what was going on.

Later, when Ted told Beth that he had been asked to investigate the stories of discontent in the doctor's unit, Bethune laughed and said the Spanish physicians were driving him crazy. He was delighted that Ted was going to help and appointed him the "political commissar of the Spanish-Canadian Blood Transfusion Unit" to give him more authority.

Ted was haunted by the memory of a dead child he had pulled out of the ruins in Albacete — the town in flames, the noise, the nightmare of it. He remembered holding the child and weeping and screaming and then having a peculiar sensation that something terrible had happened to him once, as if *he* were the child. Ted told Beth about it. Bethune said, "Write it quickly before you forget." So Ted began to make notes that eventually led to the writing of his first novel, *This Time a Better Earth*, about his days in Spain.

One morning Ted woke up to discover a brand-new typewriter beside his bed. He had been using the unit's typewriter. Beth had commented, "How in hell can you call yourself a writer and not have a typewriter?"

In February 1937, the Nationalist fascists renewed their Madrid offensive with a flanking attack on the southeastern approaches to the city. The Loyalists and the International Brigades halted the enemy advance on the Jarama River but paid a terrible price. Ted, Hungarian photographer Geza Karpathi and American documentarian Herbert Kline went to the scene of the battle. John Lenthier was dead, as was everyone else who had come over with Ted on the ship.

Ted was sending cables to Federated Press and broadcasting his regular radio reports to North America. He split his time between working with Bethune at the Blood Transfusion Unit and living the life of a war correspondent in the besieged city. Madrid seemed like the centre of the world. He rubbed shoulders with writers Ernest Hemingway and John Dos Passos and met American photographer Robert Capa and his German Jewish photojournalist partner Gerda Taro.

During this period, Kline and Karpathi were making a film documentary, *Heart of Spain*, about Bethune's work, but the antagonism between Beth and the Spanish Dr. Culebras, who worked at the unit, was becoming impossible. Culebras thought, as a Spaniard, he should be in charge. Beth felt Culebras was incompetent and couldn't forgive him for insisting on an afternoon siesta no matter what was happening. Ted couldn't blame Bethune for being angry, but Beth was drinking too much and he screamed at the Spaniard in front of everyone. In Spain Bethune was in danger of

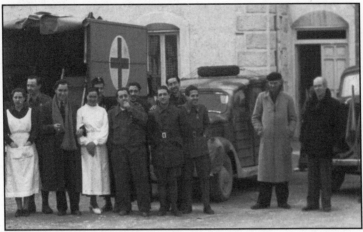

Photo by Hazen Sise. Courtesy Julie and Norman Allan.

*Scottish Ambulance Unit, Spain, April 1937. Ted Allan is on the left be-
tween the two nurses; Bethune is at the far right.*

becoming a liability. At home he could be of service by speaking
and raising money for the Spanish Aid Committee.

At the end of May 1937, Bethune was sent back to Canada,
publicly a hero but privately humiliated. "Spain is a scar on my
heart!" Bethune wrote to his ex-wife, Frances. He would soon
go to China.

Meanwhile Ted returned to New York. He had a letter to
deliver to John Lenthier's widow. Again destiny stepped in. Within
a year Ted and Kate were married, and two years after that their
daughter, Julie, was born. Ted went to work for the Office of War
Information and wrote for *Life*, *Collier's* and *The New Yorker*. But
Bethune wasn't far from his thoughts. When Ted's son was born
in 1943, he named him Norman Bethune Allan.

Bethune had died in China in November 1939 of blood
poisoning after joining Mao Zedong to fight the Japanese invaders and was already a hero to the Chinese. Ted started to write
a treatment for a movie about this incredible man who had
meant so much to him and to so many people. It would be an
epic, encompassing Bethune's life in Montreal, Spain and China.
Twentieth Century-Fox bought the treatment in 1945, and Ted
moved his family to Hollywood. He purchased a small house and
settled down to write the screenplay.

The next year, using the name Alan Herman to disguise himself, he flew back to Madrid to write about what was happening in postwar Spain and to do research for the movie. It was a dangerous mission. By the time he got back to New York, he had developed typhoid fever and was near death in the hospital for months. But he recovered and went home to California.

There was now a darkening cloud on the horizon. The U.S. House Un-American Activities Committee had raised its ugly head in the late 1940s and turned its sights on unions and Hollywood's left-wing writers, directors and actors. Anyone who had even given money to Loyalist Spain was suspect. Ted was accused of being "prematurely anti-fascist." Not surprisingly, Twentieth Century-Fox decided against making a movie about a Canadian doctor, a communist, who had gone to Spain to fight fascism and then to China to help Mao Zedong.

Ted moved his family back east. In 1949 the Federal Bureau of Investigation visited Ted in New York and told him he wouldn't be deported if he came to Washington to testify that he had seen a person they were investigating at a Communist Party meeting in New York in the early 1940s. Ted said, "Sure, tell me where and when." That night he took a train to Montreal. Kate packed up the house and children and followed him three months later. Not long after, beginning in 1950, Republican Wisconsin Senator Joseph McCarthy started making increasingly vociferous allegations of communist infiltration in the U.S. Army and State Department.

During the early 1950s, Ted found himself thinking more and more about Norman Bethune. The doctor had been written out of the history books in Canada because he had been a communist. People had forgotten that Bethune had been an early proponent of socialized medicine and an inspiration behind Saskatchewan Premier Tommy Douglas's introduction of the first government-supported hospital plan in North America in 1947 (and later, in 1962, the first universal Medicare plan on the continent). Canadians also knew nothing of Bethune's work in Spain and China. Ted felt that Canada didn't have enough heroes, and he wanted to tell Bethune's story. He began to write *The Scalpel, the Sword*.

Now living in Toronto, he turned to a childhood friend, reporter Sydney Gordon, for help with the voluminous material.

Ted Allan upon his return to North America from his surreptitious trip to Spain in 1946.

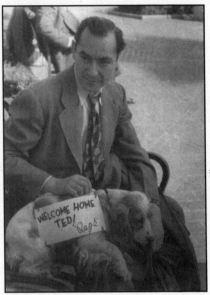

Courtesy Julie and Norman Allan.

They had known each other from the streets of Montreal in the neighbourhood of St. Lawrence Boulevard, or "The Main," as it was known. The opportunity to work on this important story came at just the right time for Sydney, whose marriage to Monica Mugan, a popular radio show host, had just ended. Monica had fled with their daughter, Susan, to England, where she married again.

The two men came together at Daisy Moiston's rooming house in Toronto, a big, warm home overflowing with talk, laughter and occasional tears, a shelter for like-minded men and women who believed that all people were created equal. The great black American singer and actor Paul Robeson was a frequent visitor. Franco's fascism held sway in Spain, but the great experiment of creating a society of equality where workers owned the means of production was still progressing in the Soviet Union and China, and Ted wanted to chronicle Bethune's role.

Ted's personal knowledge of and admiration for Bethune, combined with his experiences in the field in Spain, made it difficult for him to view the story as an objective outsider. And, as sometimes happens in the creative process, the synergy between the two authors allowed a work to be created that was more than the sum of each.

The book was a resounding success and was translated into dozens of languages and published around the world. It was even used as a school textbook in many socialist countries. But the success of *The Scalpel, the Sword* was a mixed blessing for Ted. He became a target of McCarthy-style anti-communism once more. Ted was called into the Toronto office of Andrew Allan, the head of CBC Television. Allan told Ted that CBC would still put on his plays, but he would have to use a pseudonym.

The writing was on the wall. Once more Ted packed up his family, but this time he went to Britain. A small group of expatriates had gathered there, fleeing from Senator McCarthy and men like him. Sydney's ex-wife, Monica, and daughter, Susan, became regular visitors and lifelong friends.

In the late 1950s, the Chinese government invited Ted and Sydney to China to write a film scenario about Bethune. The two authors accepted the offer, but Ted was already busy with many other projects, so finally they decided that Sydney would stay in China to draft the script while Ted returned to England. After spending a thrilling year in China, Sydney's work on the script ground to a halt. The Chinese insisted that the film could focus only on Bethune's life in China. The authors, united on this point, were adamant that the Bethune story was that of a man awakening to injustice and taking action and that his entire life had to be told.

When Joseph Stalin was revealed to be a dictator as ruthless as his fascist counterparts, an enormous wave ripped through the Communist Party, and many ardent followers withdrew, disappointed and dismayed. A rift grew between the two authors — Sydney who could forgive all in the name of the ends justifying the means, and Ted whose idealism couldn't tolerate the darkness.

Sydney accepted an invitation to spend a year in the German Democratic Republic where all his writing would be translated and published. For a communist journalist whose articles could find no outlets in the West, this was an ideal arrangement. His one-year contract extended to two and three years, and finally East Germany became his home. He died there in 1983, still a firm and hopeful believer in Marxist dogma before the collapse of his beloved communist "utopias" in Eastern Europe and the Soviet Union.

Ted found success in London beyond his wildest dreams in television and the theatre. Laurence Olivier produced his play *Gog and Magog*, written with Roger MacDougall and starring Richard Attenborough. It ran for a year in London's West End and then for four years in Paris. Sean Connery directed *I've Seen*

Sydney Gordon in China in the 1950s.

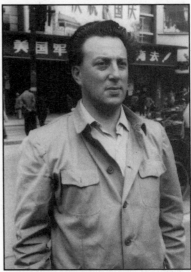

Courtesy Susan Ostrovsky.

You Cut Lemons, about Ted's relationship with his sister, Sadie (Ted later adapted this play for John Cassavetes, who directed and starred in the film *Love Streams*). *The Secret of the World*, about Ted's disillusionment with Stalin after Nikita Khrushchev's revelations in the late 1950s, was staged at Joan Littlewood's Stratford East Theatre to glowing reviews.

With McCarthyism and the House Un-American Activities Committee things of the past, Ted was back in favour with Hollywood. In 1976 the movie version of his iconic tale, *Lies My Father Told Me* (based on a short story he had written in 1949), won a Golden Globe for Best Foreign Film and a 1975 Academy Award nomination for Best Original Screenplay (which Ted penned). In Canada in 1977, his children's book *Willie the Squowse* was published, with subsequent editions printed in Britain and the United States, while his novel *Love Is a Long Shot* received the Steven Leacock Medal for Humour in 1985.

Most important for Ted, his screenplay about Norman Bethune was finally made into a movie. *Bethune: The Making of a Hero* was filmed in 1988–89 in Montreal, Spain and China and starred Donald Sutherland and Helen Mirren. It was the first official co-production between China and the West.

Today, as people in many corners of the world continue to oppress and profit from other humans, Julie, Norman and Susan are proud to know that their fathers' lives and work were inspired by ideals that still hold true.

SERIES EDITOR'S NOTE

BY MICHAEL GNAROWSKI

The year 2009 is the seventieth anniversary of the death of Norman Bethune or, more appropriately, Dr. Norman Bethune, a period of whose remarkable life forms the theme of this narrative being reissued here. He was a complex, tempestuous and unpredictable individual (how else to describe a man who married and divorced the same woman twice) whose life story may well be used to illustrate that saying about a prophet being without honour in his own country. Not only was he a foremost thoracic surgeon in his time who invented surgical instruments that were in use many years after his death, but he also agitated for socialized medicine, lent his apartment for the teaching of disadvantaged children using art as an important prop in the process, and pioneered the use of blood transfusion on the battlefield, helping to save countless combatants' lives.

If he is remembered at all, it is for his having embraced left-wing politics by becoming a communist, and it is his affiliation with the Communist Party in Canada that has helped to preserve any historical sense of the man. His principled activism first took him to Spain in 1936–37 during the Spanish Civil War where he headed the Blood Transfusion Unit. A short time later after his return from that conflict, Bethune left for China to join the communist forces led by Mao Zedong. Contrary to popular myth, Bethune did not participate in the epic Long March of the Red Army, that event having been concluded in October 1935, years before he reached China. Bethune served as a battlefield surgeon in 1938–39 before dying in the night of November 12–13, 1939, from blood poisoning contracted from a cut suffered during an operation on a wounded Chinese soldier.

There is not much in Canada to commemorate this extraordinary individual other than the place of his birth in Gravenhurst, Ontario, and a life-size statue in the typical heroic Marxist pose, erected on the corner of boulevard de Maisonneuve and rue Guy in Montreal by the People's Republic of China, where Bethune is venerated to this day as a great hero of that country's revolution. Mao Zedong was his first eulogist a month after his death, placing Bethune in the pantheon of outstanding men and describing him as "... a man noble-minded and pure, a man of moral integrity and above vulgar interests, a man who is of value to the people." Of value to the people ... No greater accolade could have been bestowed by the man who in later days would be called the Great Helmsman by the most populous communist republic the world is ever likely to see.

The Spanish Civil War (1936–39), which is seen by many as a prelude to the Second World War, was eclipsed and overshadowed by the cataclysmic events of that great conflict, so that the people and the battles that unfolded on the Iberian peninsula have receded from memory and are hardly familiar to the contemporary reader. Yet the war in Spain had a remarkable significance for the history of the twentieth century, since it became a testing ground for the great ideological struggles that characterized that violent and bloody epoch. It should also be remembered that the Spanish war with its hallmark divisions of right against left was fought not only by Spaniards but drew into its vortex strange alignments of idealists, adventurers, pragmatists and mercenaries.

On the right, the fascist forces led by rebellious generals relied on the support of Nazi Germany and fascist Italy while it drew on the manpower of Moroccan colonial troops who became known as the Army of Africa. On the republican left help came from the Soviet Union and well-intentioned idealists who joined the International Brigades. Poets, writers, artists, scientists, defying the expressed neutrality of the Western democracies, organized themselves independently and made their way to Spain, some to fight, some to write, some to carry the wounded. Garment workers were the founding nucleus of the English contingent that would grow to include many of the young members of the creative and artistic community in England — Stephen Spender,

W.H. Auden, George Orwell, John Cornford, Christopher Caudwell (who was killed), to name a few of the intelligentsia.

As a matter of fact, the first one killed was Felicia Browne, an artist. Spain, as Julian Symons observed, became "a battleground of hope and conscience." Having seen the ferocious cauldron, Stephen Spender wrote in 1937: "The final horror of war is the complete isolation of a man dying in a world whose reality is violence." It is the reality of violence, one would like to think, that Norman Bethune endeavoured to assuage, and although his stints in the two war zones to which he gravitated were relatively brief — he spent barely six months in Spain and barely a year in China — he managed to leave an image and a legacy that were nothing short of heroic.

For what is an essentially personal reminiscence such as the introductory remarks that usher in this new edition of *The Scalpel, the Sword*, what matters most is the capture of what was said at the dinner table, and was thus made into family lore without much need of reference or explanation. The reader as stranger, however, is at a loss when names or events arise in the course of the narrative that are obscure or have faded into the shadows of history. Some of these have been enriched in their interest and value to the story with, what is hoped, is the benefit of context.

Adrian Arcand, a graduate in science from McGill University and a Canadian nationalist, was a journalist and publisher of several small newspapers that were inspired by strong right-wing conservatism and propagated fascist ideals. While he was undoubtedly supported by the German Nazi propaganda machine, what is little known and rarely mentioned is that he was richly supported by the conservative prime-minister-to-be of Canada, R.B. Bennett, who provided considerable subsidies that helped to keep Arcand's scurrilously anti-Semitic publications afloat. Bennett hoped that Arcand's backing would assist the Conservative Party in Quebec, which it did, allowing the Tories to win the July 1930 election with some two dozen seats in that province.

Miriam (née Carpin) Kennedy was the first wife of the Canadian poet Leo Kennedy. Born and raised in the same Jewish neighbourhood as Ted Allan, she was an early radical who became a social worker. Her left-leaning views and sensibility obviously attracted her to Bethune.

Fred Rose (né Rosenberg) was a prominent member of the Communist Party in Canada. He was the first and only communist elected to the Canadian Parliament from the constituency in Montreal that included a large Jewish population. He became embroiled in the aftermath of the Igor Gouzenko spy trials, served time in prison, and returned to his native Poland where he died.

The Scalpel, the Sword was first published in Canada and the United States in 1952 and went into several reprints before being issued in a revised edition in 1971. The spellings of Chinese personal names and place names as they appeared in earlier editions have been retained.

Related Reading: Howard, Victor, and Mac Reynolds. *The Mackenzie-Papineau Battalion: The Canadian Contingent in the Spanish Civil War* (Ottawa: Carleton University Press, 1986); Shephard, David A.E., and Andrée Lévesque, eds. *Norman Bethune: His Times and Legacy* (Ottawa: Canadian Public Health Association, 1982); Stewart, Roderick. *Bethune* (Toronto: New Press, 1973).

PREFACE
TO THE FIRST EDITION

The material on which this biography is based was gathered in the course of research that spanned eleven years and followed Dr. Bethune's life from Gravenhurst, Ontario, through most of the cities of Canada, the major cities of the United States, to Britain, France, Spain, Italy, Austria, Switzerland, the Soviet Union and finally China. Both of us had to acquaint ourselves with Bethune's Canadian background, the origins of the Spanish war of 1936–1939, the evolution of modern China, the wide interplay of world events which helped shape Bethune's life and to which he reacted in his own characteristic manner. Though Bethune first won international fame as a thoracic surgeon, he was also in varying degrees a painter, a poet, soldier, critic, teacher, lecturer, inventor, medical writer and theorist. He lived on many levels, had many careers, was involved with many people, and became a stormy petrel of some of the decisive happenings of our era.

One of us knew Bethune intimately and shared with him part of the agony of the Spanish war. The other knew him only casually in Montreal but followed his career closely until his death. We were thus in the fortunate position of being able to combine the subjective insight of a friend with the detached objectivity of an observer. From the beginning, then, we can lay claim to having known Bethune from both the "inside" and the "outside."

He left behind him so many vivid memoirs, diaries, letters and other writings that he exercised a potent posthumous influence on the style of this book and made our task immeasurably simpler. In general, we have avoided using explanatory notes because in compiling our sources for statements, conversations and incidents, we found that our footnotes were so numerous as to constitute almost another book! Therefore, wherever a source is not given we would like the reader to know that all the conversations were either heard by one of us, described in Bethune's letters, or recalled by his intimates.

Often, in the course of the book, we refer to Bethune's thoughts: his innermost feelings. In every case we are paraphrasing his own words, or actually quoting them as they appeared in his letters and diaries, or as he expressed them to one of the authors or to a friend. In the acknowledgments we have listed many people who have helped us to make this book possible. But here, without any invidious comparisons, we feel it necessary to single out a few names for special mention. These include his mother, the late Mrs. Elizabeth Ann Bethune, his brother, the late Malcolm Bethune, and his sister, Mrs. Janet Stiles, who supplied us with all the necessary early family data. Frances Campbell Penney, Bethune's former wife, gave us much valuable information which would have otherwise been unavailable.

To four people we are indebted for the fact that the material on Bethune's life in China is in many respects the most detailed and the most documented. Tung Yueh Chian, his "other self," his interpreter and friend who was with him during most of his life in China, supplied us with invaluable personal notes. Soong Ching-ling (Madame Sun Yat-sen), whose preface opens our book, was instrumental in having all of Bethune's papers and diaries, during his stay in China, made available to us. Israel Epstein, author of perhaps the best book on the background of modern China★ in the English language, deserves special thanks for his untiring efforts to assemble Bethune's papers and diaries. Without his work in China and the additional notes and documents supplied by Madame Sun, it would have been difficult to describe Bethune's last, climactic years.

In addition, we were immeasurably helped by the lengthy published chronicle written by the Chinese writer Chou En Fou on Bethune's work in China. Chou's firsthand account was important corroborative material for Bethune's personal diaries, especially with regard to events nowhere else as yet described in any language. Chou's chronicle, as well as other unpublished Chinese material, was translated for us by Gerald Chen (Chen Wei Shi).

★ *The Unfinished Revolution in China.*

Further, this book received the wholehearted co-operation of Bethune's medical colleagues, many of them now world-famous in their respective fields. We refer particularly to his colleagues in the American Tuberculosis Association, the Council of the American Association of Thoracic Surgery, the University of Toronto, McGill University, Trudeau Sanatorium (Saranac Lake, New York), the Royal Victoria Hospital (Montreal), the Sacré Coeur Hospital, the Federal Department of Health and Pensions, and of the Montreal Medico-Chirurgical Society. While the book has been checked by seven different physicians, we assume all responsibilities for any medical errors.

The Authors
Toronto, 1952

PREFACE
TO THE REVISED EDITION

In the nineteen years since its first appearance in Canada *The Scalpel, the Sword* has made its way round the world. It has been published in nineteen languages, including Serbian, Hebrew and Chinese. It has sold over a million copies, and is still appearing in new editions on three continents. It appears to be the most widely translated, widely published book in Canadian history.

Dr. Norman Bethune, his life and his work, have been accepted as part of their own heritage by North American students, Dutch workers, German medical men, Italian intellectuals, many thousands of dispossessed people in India, African freedom-fighters, and the vast masses on the Chinese mainland.

What is the reason for the tremendous impact Bethune's life story has had all over the world? The answer to this question can best be sought in the book itself. But certain preliminary points should be made.

Bethune was a unique Canadian, a unique human being, yet shaped by both his country and the contemporary world. He was truly a neo-Renaissance figure, driven by the necessity to experience and enrich all of life. To him, encrusted conventions were silly; love, a great hunger and an affirmation of life; medicine and surgery his art, his work, and his commitment; the growing brutality of our world a personal wound. At the end, his confrontation with death as a surgeon-soldier was a natural response to the cry of the starving, the downtrodden, the brave on all the battlefields of freedom.

He was a man who achieved painful consciousness of his weaknesses. But rather than succumbing, he achieved greatness in vanquishing them. Deliberately he abandoned the role of sybarite, roisterer and roué, to become the front-line doctor, the guerilla in straw sandals, the revolutionary, for whom life was no more than a few handfuls of rice for sustenance, and surgery performed in the midst of bloody battles. He knew comradeship with strangers who called him brother, and his indestructible strength lay in his vast dream of remaking the world. At the end, his personal life had become completely merged with the fate of the world's peoples. Today, wherever their cause has succeeded, he is honoured. Wherever they must still fight on, he is a banner, a call to arms.

Such a man brings hope to all who yearn for an end to wars, to bloodshed, to the disintegration of society and personality which torments so much of mankind. But he also disturbs the philistines and the smugly comfortable, inspiring fear and even secret hatred among those who still refuse to admit that the world is changing before our eyes.

It is no accident that he has recently become the central figure in a number of new literary and film activities — projects concerning his life undertaken, and others being planned — all without reference to the present biography. These activities are international in scope, but have been most intensively pursued in Canada. To the extent that such a renewal of interest demonstrates the power and attraction of the man, it can be accepted as an accolade. To the extent that it attempts to distort and falsify his image, it must be instantly dismissed.

One example is sufficient to demonstrate this overt game of plagiarism and distortion. A recent Canadian novel uses Bethune as one of its three central characters. In a sense, he emerges as the most potent of the three. Though he is, of course, given another name, his identity is clear. But it is at this point that the novelist departs from even an approximation of reality. Bethune is deliberately translated into an "anti-Bethune," into the exact opposite of what he was, and what he became. The novel presents him, not as a conscious revolutionary, who died as surgeon-soldier on the battlefield, but as a disillusioned idealist, who winds up broken and defeated, bitterly antagonistic to everything he once believed in. This is not only a pitiful perversion of the truth — it is cynicism at its worst.

It is also proof that Bethune, today, is as alive as any man can be; that he is still a potent challenge to those who fear everything he represents, and everything that he died for.

It is for all these reasons that this new edition of *The Scalpel, the Sword* comes at a particularly appropriate moment. Whatever its merits and its weaknesses, it should help to re-establish facts, confound the cynics, and inspire a new generation. It will remind us again that man need not live, nor end his life, in hopelessness — but *can* experience greatness of thought and of action. We need to be reminded that there *are* men, heroic in stature and action, who bring hope and inspiration to the rest of us. Bethune was such a man.

The Authors, 1971

PART ONE

DEATH AND BIRTH

1

HOPEI, NORTH CHINA

They brought him out of the hills over the twisting, narrow passes where the enemy feared to set foot and where the horses no longer led but followed.

They carried him on one of the litters for the wounded. At first he had waved aside the litter-bearers with an angry toss of his head and mounted his brown mare, sitting in the saddle with his left arm dragging. But before they had gone many *li* from Sky-Kissing Peak he had fallen into a dead faint. When he awoke to find himself on a stretcher suspended from two crossbars, moving rhythmically with the motion of the litter-bearers, he only rolled his eyes to look at them and made no protest.

For a day and a night they crawled up and down the mountain wasteland of West Hopei, a silent, dogged caravan of men, horses, and mules. By day the November sun was like a great, single eye, filmed over as if with tears, staring at them out of furrowed brows of clouds. At night the stars hung low above the cliffs, as if to touch them with a cold warmth and light their way. By day and by night it seemed they need only reach out to touch the sky. With the sound of artillery still echoing like distant thunder behind them, they made their way through dust, through mists spread out over the hollows like silvery lakes, passes cut out of sheer rock, wild brush where every step was a struggle. Then they broke out of the towering mountains, and stocky Tung Yueh Chian, leading now on the brown mare, raised his hand. They halted, gazing at the broad valley below, and Fong spoke:

"It will be Yellow Stone Village there," he said, pointing, and · they began the descent.

For an hour they zigzagged down the mountainside until they could clearly see the brown houses of Yellow Stone Village and the tiny figures racing in from the fields. When they reached the valley a crowd had gathered at the northern gate, and as they approached the village a triumphant cheer echoed through the valley.

"Pai Chu En! Pai Chu En!"

At the edge of the village the people chanted the name, waving their hands and smiling broadly. But as the brown mare reached the gate and the caravan entered, the shouts of welcome died on their lips. With troubled faces they watched Fong, slumped forward in the saddle, his head bowed, pain and defeat in his eyes. They moved apart to let Fong pass, murmuring among themselves. Where was Pai Chu En? Why did the procession enter the village so silently? Why did the litter-bearers walk with their eyes fixed on the ground? Then they saw the stretcher coming slowly through the gate, and their faces grew wrinkled with torment and disbelief.

Tung reined in the mare, the caravan came to a stop, the litter-bearers knelt to lower the stretcher carefully to the ground, hanging their heads as if they felt themselves accountable for their burden.

The villagers slowly assembled about the stretcher. Yes, it was Pai Chu En, the foreign one, White Seek Grace. Only two weeks ago he had passed like a whirlwind through the village, his proud, white head held high as he galloped before the caravan into the hills. Only two weeks ago he had left for the front, and now he lay before them, his head thrown back, his eyes shut, his beard pointing towards the sky. They look on in baffled silence. Yes, it was Pai Chu En, but how could this be — that he should lie here like the dead? In all the liberated areas he had worked his wonders. His face had lit up the villages of Shansi. He had blazed his way across the Middle Plain, across Hopei and Shansi. He had made fools of the invaders even in the occupied territories. His name had been like a sword against the enemy. How could this be?

They looked to Tung for a sign that all would be well, then looked back at Pai Chu En. Surely of all the wonders he had performed he had some still left for himself; surely he would rise up in a moment, straight and erect, with the awe and power of a pillar of fire, his white mane towering above them, his arms outstretched to reassure them, his green eyes smiling as always. But as they watched he twisted suddenly in pain, tearing the blankets from him, and they saw the bandages and the path of hideously discoloured, swollen flesh reaching to the shoulder.

They fell back with a groan, the children clinging to the elders' legs, the litter-bearers wincing.

Pai Chu En opened his eyes as if from a deep sleep, raised himself up on an elbow and looked about till he saw Tung. He spoke for a while in the strange language that only Tung understood, and fell back wearily again.

Tung dismounted and faced the villagers. "We must stop here," he said heavily. "We are a day and a night from the front without pause. He can travel no further. He must have a rest so he can defeat his great sickness."

One of the elders stepped forward. He stood before the stretcher and bowed gravely in the traditional Hopei manner. "At first we thought it might be the enemy coming out of the hills, and we were filled with worry," he said. "Then we recognized the brown mare and the litter-bearers, and we were filled with joy. Now we are filled with grief.... Better that it should have been the enemy, better *Chian Pi Ching Y'eh*,★ better that our homes should now be ashes, and our families scattered in the mountains, than that you should return to us in this suffering."

Pai Chu En turned his head and extended his hand vaguely.

"We must have a suitable place," Tung said, "till we are able to move him again."

The old man rose. "At the house of Yu the landlord. His is the best house in the village."

They followed the stretcher to Yu's courtyard, waiting outside, while the children watched their elders, quick to read the signs on their parents' faces, sensitive to the menace hanging over the valley, the mountains of Hopei, the whole vast world of China, and wondering now at the sorrow more terrible than the enemy had cast its shadow over the village....

Late in the afternoon there was a second alarm. This time it was a messenger hastening through the mountains from Staff Headquarters. He had set out on direct orders from General Nieh as soon as Headquarters had received the wireless message from the front the day before. The news had caused great consternation, and had been relayed to Mao Tse-tung in Yenan immediately. General Nieh had been instructed in urgent messages in Yenan to

---

★ The slogan of "scorched earth."

keep Chu Teh and Mao Tse-tung informed of all developments, and to spare no cost in the effort to get Pai Chu En safely to Staff Headquarters. Though worn and hungry from his journey the messenger refused food impatiently. "Pai Chu En is ill, and in Wu Tai Shan and Yenan they are waiting for word," he said. "Do you know what our men will say if anything goes wrong, and do you offer me food? I want to see him at once."

Fong led Nieh's representative into the house, thinking it would be good for Pai Chu En to know that the vigil was being kept not only here, beside the *k'ang*,★ in the house of Yu, not only here in Yellow Stone Village, not only at Sky-Kissing Peak, where the men had watched him leave with the sickness upon him, but in all territories of Chin-Cha-Chi.

The villagers waited for word, but as the hours passed and the two remained in the house, they slipped away. The men returned to the fields, turning often as they worked to shield their eyes from the sun and look back at the village with a preoccupied air. From their meager stores the women brought baskets of chicken, millet pancakes, eggs, vegetables, leaving them at Yu's door. In the single rutted street the children hushed one another at their play. Shou, the "little devil,"★★ crept to Pai Chu En's door, refusing to leave and asking all who went in or out, "Will he be well enough to leave tomorrow? Shall I bring him some food? Can I ask him if he would like some food?"

All through the night Fong remained in the room. In the morning he came out with a distracted look on his long face and made off rapidly through the village. Tung found him outside the village square, sitting on a rock, gazing vacantly into the distance. Tung squatted silently beside him, tracing patterns in the dusty earth with a stick. The sun was still hidden behind the mountains. The first faint sounds of life came from the village.

"How is he now?" Tung asked the question without looking up.

Fong buried his head in his hands. "My heart was filled with gladness that I was able to attend our teacher. Now it has turned

---

★ A low brick or clay oven which also serves as a bed.

★★ Boys under sixteen who accompanied the Red Army on the "Long March" were nicknamed "little devils."

to stone. He is very sick and I am helpless." He raised his head. "What shall we tell General Nieh and Mao Tse-tung?"

"He called me his 'other self,'"Tung said, "and it seems as if I am dying too. We must go back to him. We must not let him die."

In the courtyard Tung found a rough bench, placed it beneath the window of Pai Chu En's room and took up the vigil.

Night came. A shadow glided through the courtyard. "This is the house where Pai Chu En lies?" a voice whispered.

"Yes." Tung turned to see a young man in the padded blue cotton of the guerillas.

"We are a detachment of the People's Guard," the soldier said. "We are passing through on our way to Sky-Kissing Peak. In the village they have told us the grief-heavy news. In the name of Pai Chu En we have adopted a resolution of self-sacrifice. Our whole unit has pledged that when we reach the front we will offer ourselves for any duty as an example to the others — self-sacrifice till death, if necessary…. You will tell Pai Chu En?"

"Yes," Tung said. "I will tell him."

The soldier saluted and marched silently into the night. Then Fong came to sit beside Tung, asking, "Has he called?"

"No," Tung said. "He lies quietly. Once he rose to sit at the table, writing…."

"It is strange that he should still have strength to rise, or to sit at the table." Fong sat sunk in thought, looking in at the room bathed in the cherry glow of the *k'ang* fire. "What should he write now? What is in his mind, I wonder?"

"Perhaps the bitterness of things he remembers," Tung said. "It is a night of many stars, such as always pleased him, and I have heard from him as many memories as there are stars. In the mountains, when the night sky was like the jeweled ceiling of a Buddhist temple, he would say to me: 'My other self, these Hopei nights are like the nights I knew when I was a boy in my own country….' Always his *other self*…. And now there was a soldier here … from a unit passing through. They go with a resolution of self-sacrifice in the name of Pai Chu En. So they too are his *other selves*…."

"*I — you — they*…. But let us go in … We must not leave him any longer…."

Tung began to weep, quietly, without shame. "I shall come in a moment … forgive my weak tears. They are a spring that will soon run dry. It is more bitter for him than for all the others I have seen. If he dies he will be dying a second time. And he is only 49 years old. Do you understand? Every man dies — so many of our own have died — but all of us have one life and one passing, and he has had many lives and this is his *second* death. Did you know? — This is the second time he is dying, and there are not enough tears in all China to mourn his second passing...."

Fong rose heavily. "Not in all China," he said. "No, Comrade Tung, not in all the world will there be enough tears...."

2

DETROIT, UNITED STATES — 1926

He was thirty-six years old, and according to the medical evidence he was dying.

He lay in his bed, and considered how it had all started and was now ending.

History would pass him by without the merest footnote, he told himself, not knowing that even in 1926 history was already marshalling great lands and obscure men for wars, revolts, mass murder, heroism. Nor did he know that he would yet taste the rushing darkness of death a second time; that some day one quarter of the human race would sing his name as Pai Chu En; that in mountain wildernesses he had never heard of, a man called Tung would watch over him recalling this, his *first* "dying."

There would come a time when he himself would write: "It is not given to many men to face death, to learn the truth of one's life in facing death — and then to live." But now he knew only that he was dying, and that all his years had gone to waste. He told himself he didn't give a damn. But why, he asked himself, had it happened?

During the long Detroit nights, ghostly with the sounds and lights of the streets below his window, he tossed between his tortured dreams and bitter wakings, exploring the chaotic pattern of his life, gritting his teeth against remorse and self-pity, searching endlessly for the clues to his defeat, and counting the search his only valid last will and testament.

He remembered many faces, cities, hurts, vanities. He remembered home, the war, flight to Bohemia, debaucheries and exaltation, work, the thrill of flesh and clay in his hands, love turning mouldy, fierce yearnings, frenzy, despair. Where, in the wilderness called living, had he lost his way? And why?

3

The manse, the frame church, the lakes he loved to swim in, the hills where he had chased butterflies — they were part of Gravenhurst, Ontario, where he was born, and of his childhood.

He remembered them all, and also the legends about the Bethunes who had migrated from northern France to Scotland in the mid-sixteenth century. They had been French Huguenots — nonconformists, he often thought with secret satisfaction, even three hundred years ago. For two centuries they gave Scotland doctors, teachers, and clergymen, some becoming Hereditary Physicians to the Lords of the Isle of Skye. Then, in the eighteenth century, they migrated to Canada, where a Bethune became an Anglican bishop, the first Anglican in a long line of Presbyterians. Another Bethune became a principal of McGill University. Still another, Norman's grandfather, turned to medicine and became one of Toronto's outstanding surgeons.

He remembered the stories told of his grandfather — of his strong views, unorthodoxy and scientific inclinations — and how the memory had served him as a childhood goal. And he remembered, above all, his father, with his passion for the written and spoken word, and his mother, combining tenderness and strength with the quiet faith she had always had that he was destined for great things.

At the age of twenty-one, his father, Malcolm Nicholson Bethune, had turned his back on the family traditions of medicine, pulpit and teaching for the more worldly pursuit of business. In 1880 he took ship for Hawaii with an older brother, Angus, to buy an orange grove and make his fortune. But in Honolulu he met Elizabeth Ann Goodwin, a Presbyterian missionary. The meeting changed his life.

Miss Goodwin was the daughter of an English cabinet-maker.* At the age of ten she had distributed religious pamphlets on the streets of her native London. At twenty-one she left England to become a missionary in Hawaii. She was filled with a vast love for mankind, a vast determination to save the heathen and spread the word of Christ. She turned her persuasiveness loose on Malcolm with such overwhelming effects that he was converted to the church of his fathers, returned to Toronto with her blinding vision, and abandoned all thoughts of orange groves and fortunes in a flow of letters written to Honolulu asking her to marry him.

His persuasiveness was equal to hers. She soon followed him to Canada and married him.

In 1888 their marriage was doubly climaxed: their first child, Janet, was born, and Malcolm entered Knox College to become a minister. The transformation in his life, begun in Hawaii, was now complete. After he had been ordained he moved his small family to the northern Ontario town of Gravenhurst, where he took over the duties of his first congregation. And here, on a blustery March day in 1890, in the Presbyterian manse, a Bethune was born — their first son.**

As a preacher Malcolm Bethune held strongly personal views. Though he was to win more than ordinary recognition for his powerfully delivered sermons, he refused all calls to wealthy congregations. "The rich," he said, "are too worldly." He would only accept pulpits in communities where he considered the people closer to his precepts of Christian living. As a result, his ministry took the family from one small Ontario town to another in relatively quick succession.

---

* Henry Goodwin.

** Their third child, Malcolm, was born three years later.

When Norman was two years old the Reverend Malcolm Bethune was transferred to Beaverton, then to Toronto, then, over a period of years, to Aylmer, Blind River, Sault Sainte Marie, Owen Sound and finally back to Toronto again. But for years Norman spent his summers at Gravenhurst. Here, in the Muskoka Lakes, he developed a passion for swimming. Here, too, he showed his first delight with the forests and the summer skies.

Wherever the Bethune family found itself, home life was stimulating, rich and warm. For years a favourite diversion of the family was a word game. As they assembled for supper, each child who properly pronounced and defined a new word received a prize of five cents. Norman usually ran off with the prize, but shared his wealth with his older sister and younger brother. Another game that was Norman's alone was the moving of furniture. He loved to rearrange every room according to his own notions of form and colour. The family considered him somewhat young to assume the role of interior decorator, but patiently indulged his fancies.

From his earliest years his venturesome spirit and his intention of being a surgeon were taken for granted. By the time he was eight he had begun the messy but scientifically necessary job of dissecting flies and chicken bones. Later his personal investigation of anatomy led his mother to an investigation of her own when a dreadful odour suddenly pervaded the house one afternoon. She traced it to the attic, where she found Norman carefully cutting away the flesh from a cow's leg he had just boiled. "What are you doing?" she asked in amazement. Laconically, he replied, "I'm getting the flesh off so I can examine the bones. They'll make good specimens." She hurriedly left him to his scientific pursuits and later that day he placed the bones along the fence in the back yard to dry. It was also at the age of eight that he ceremoniously announced that he was no longer to be called Henry, but Norman, and hung the brass plate of his surgeon grandfather and namesake on his bedroom door.

When the family first settled in Toronto, he was only seven but he fell in love with the big city. Once, on a shopping tour with his mother, he stole away and was brought back by a policeman hours later. His frantic mother asked him what had happened. He smiled mischievously. "I wanted to see what it would be like to be lost. So I went up and told the policeman I was lost. It was fun."

During the next few years his curiosity and love of adventure took on bolder proportions. He managed to transform the bucolic pursuit of butterflies into a dangerous sport. Once, outside of Gravenhurst, he led his younger brother, Malcolm, up a steep cliff at the top of which he had spied a butterfly. Halfway up, when the going became rough, he told Malcolm to wait for him. Slipping, clutching rocks, roots, bushes, he pulled himself to the summit as Malcolm cried out in fear and warning. When he came down, the butterfly in his hand, he said breathlessly, "There are two things about catching butterflies, Malcolm. First, there's the catching. Then there's the butterfly itself." Twice, on similar sorties, he fell and broke his leg. At the age of ten, when the family was vacationing on Georgian Bay, he watched his father swim across the bay at Honey Harbor. The next day he tried it himself and was saved from drowning by his father, who came up in a boat just in time. But the following year Norman swam the harbor.

His father grew increasingly nervous at his son's disregard for danger but the mother's calmer view prevailed. "He must learn to take chances," she said, "so let him do what he wants and learn that way."

His early education was spread over a number of schools and towns, but he finally graduated from the Jesse Ketchum Public School in Toronto and the Owen Sound Collegiate High School. When he was ready for college, the Bethunes moved back to Toronto so that Norman, and Malcolm soon after, would be able to go to the University of Toronto.

New winds were blowing across the oceans to the Dominion. The very year of Norman's birth saw completion of the first railroad linking the vast expanse of Canada. During Norman's childhood, Sir Wilfrid Laurier emerged to express in increasingly articulate terms the country's maturing nationhood. The steel and smoke of industry spread across the country, drawing billions of dollars in British and American investments. Great waves of immigration from Europe brought farmers to the empty plains of the west and labourers to the factories of the east. Across the Great Lakes steamers carried the prize wheat of the prairies to the St. Lawrence River, and from the St. Lawrence the rich harvest poured out to ports all over the world. With industry, immigration, expansion came technique, the spur of modernity, increasing involvement in the word scene, the germs of new ideas that soon would disturb the Bethunes and challenge their son.

Among the new ideas the young Bethune was absorbing at college was Darwin's theory of evolution. To his parents Darwinism was synonymous with anti-Christ. They were among Ontario's leading followers of the then well-known Chicago evangelist, Dwight Moody, who fought vigorously against the teaching of evolution in the schools of America. When Mrs. Bethune discovered Darwin's *Origin of Species* among Norman's schoolbooks, she was horrified and took to placing religious tracts between the pages of his scientific books to offset its seeming blasphemy.

For a while Norman read the tracts in good humour, then one night he stole into his parents' bedroom while his mother was asleep and slipped a copy of *Origin of Species* under her pillow. His prank put her forbearance to an impossible test: she burned the book in the kitchen stove. He apologized, but she could discern that it was as the loving son he asked her forgiveness, not as the growing man who was announcing his revolt with typical Puckish humour.

Though they lived comfortably, the salary of a Presbyterian minister was hardly adequate to put two sons through a university. Norman, who years before had earned pocket money by delivering newspapers, now went to work to earn his tuition. He paid for his freshman year by working as a waiter in the university restaurant. Then, in the summer, he got a job as a fireman on a Great Lakes steamer. Next came a stint as a reporter in Windsor, during which he found stringing words together not only easy but exhilarating. For a year he stayed away from the university, earning enough money for the next term by teaching school at Edgely, Ontario. Dinning the three R's into his pupils, some of them older than he, netted him $300. On other occasions he taught a Bible class and worked as a lumberjack in the woods of northern Ontario. Working there broadened his frame and hardened his muscles. He always spoke proudly of his stint as a lumberjack, and for years treasured a photo showing him with four "real" lumberjacks, all towering over him, all six feet or more and heavily muscled.

He was now twenty-four. He had his mother's small nose, wide, strong jaw, and blond colouring, his father's large forehead and green-blue eyes. "On my mother's side," he would say, "I'm an evangelist. On my father's side I have a compulsion to do, to act." Somewhere along the way he had developed his passion for drawing, painting and sculpture. He had long, powerful hands which were the source of his greatest conceit.

He had also developed a zest for living. The clay that took form in his fingers, the colours that he put on canvas, whatever pleased his eye, the ever-wider horizons opening up before him in the textbooks and lecture halls — all of it was good, youth was good, life was good.

And then the First World War burst across his dreams and plans, as it did for all the young men who were twenty-four and avid for the future.

He had one year left before getting his M.D., but he joined the armed forces the day Canada declared war, the tenth man in Toronto to enlist. He left for France as a stretcher bearer with the 1st Canadian Division Field Ambulance.

In French-Canada there were mutterings against "*their war.*" In the streets of Quebec City massed crowds were denouncing "*les impérialistes*" and conscription. But for Bethune, as for most young men in Ontario, there were no doubts, no searchings of conscience. He was carried along by the general excitement, and in France there was a thrill of a new land, new people, new sights, and new experiences.

Before long it was no longer *la belle France* but a charnel house. He went among the wounded, carrying maimed men and hulks no longer men, blood on the earth and blood on his hands, apprenticed to death and comrade to those still wanting to live. Away from the politicians' oratory and exhortations of all the home-front patriots, his mind absorbed the picture of ruin, mud, futility and carnage. He started drinking heavily. In a letter to a friend* at home he wrote: "The slaughter has begun to appall me. I've begun to question whether it was worth it. Attached to the medical services, I see little of war's glory, and most of war's waste." And then at Ypres, with Canadians going down in waves before the enemy fire, he fell in a burst of shrapnel, his left thigh ripped to the bone. It was his turn to be carried from the battlefield, weak from loss of blood, the moaning of the wounded and the ear-splitting percussion of battle remaining in his memory to haunt his dreams.

He spent the next six months in French and English hospitals, then was invalided home. The war was over for him.

A few weeks later he re-entered the university to take his degree. At graduation he was offered an internship in a Toronto army hospital, but turned it down. He had come home from the wars wondering whether something lay behind the slaughter and wreckage; but he only wondered. He had no answers, not even any clearly defined questionings. All he knew was that others were over there, and no matter what it was all about, he felt a distaste for sitting on the sidelines and a need to be among them.

He enlisted in the British Navy, serving as lieutenant-surgeon on HMS *Pegasus* until 1918. Six months before the Armistice he asked for, and was granted, a transfer to the Canadian Flying Corps in France, in which he served as medical officer.

He was in France when Germany surrendered. After the victory celebrations were over, he sat in a Paris *bistro* with his friends and wondered with them what would happen now. He was twenty-eight; the first grey hairs had begun prematurely to show at his temples; the locusts had eaten the years of his prime. The war had put a period before Bethune the student; it now put a question mark before Bethune the man. He suddenly felt aged, baffled — with a vague, burgeoning desire for something new.

As a youth he had known only Canada; as a man he knew only Europe. He had been dispossessed, it occurred to him. There

* Letter to A.F.

was nothing to return to, nowhere to go; only lost time to be made up. He was part of the disenchantment with which Western novelists were to feed the Western world for the next quarter century.... He grew a moustache and had himself demobilized in England.

4

"The innocent abroad," he said of himself, later, when remembering the postwar London years.

He had arrived in London with nothing but his air force pay; soon he was living lavishly. "I had no money," he explained, "but love for art. I soon found, to my great amusement, that many people with a lot of money knew nothing about art. I put my critical faculties to work."

He put them to work by combing studios, dealers' stores and dusty warehouses in France and Spain for things to sell in London at a handsome profit. On his first trip he had a total capital of a hundred pounds, all borrowed from friends. He returned with booty and *objets d'art* which he sold to London art dealers at a net profit of 200 pounds. Whenever the treasury became low, he crossed the Channel. For two years he earned enough money this way to buy the best clothes, the best food, the best liquor, enormous quantities of books, to lend money to anyone who asked for it, and to keep himself supplied with clay, paints and canvas.

His fellow interns at the Hospital for Sick Children and later at the Fever Hospital, unaware of his "business trips," put him down as the heir of some wealthy Canadian rancher. He did not try to disabuse them of the illusion because it amused him to think of the simplicity of his home while they imagined he had always been used to a life of opulence. Only the son of a millionaire could show such disdain for money. He was making up for all the long years when he had to save every penny earned to pay his way through college.

He walked the streets, swinging a cane, his moustache and grey temples making him look older than he was, his figure trim in impeccably tailored clothes. He was an impressive sight as he went to and from the Soho flat he shared with an Australian doctor he had met in France. Here, in the heart of Soho, they tried to "out-Bohemia Bohemia."

His flat was littered with strange sculpture — plaster hearts, kidneys, brains, coiled intestines, bones, legs, hands and fingers. Along with the outward forms of the human body, he was also fascinated by its members and inner organs. "My place looked like a bloody butcher shop," he later recalled.

In this "butcher shop" he held court, surrounded by a coterie of young admirers, writers, artists, musicians who gathered nightly to be fascinated by his talk, and his freely dispensed liquor. In the backwash of the war, the controversies of the peace, the fears, complacencies and disillusionments of a dislocated world, he defined his philosophy of life to them.

As he regaled his acquaintances with his glib views, men elsewhere were searching for answers to their vast uncertainty much less glibly. Along with fads, religious cults, jazz, unpunctuated poetry, the names of new prophets had found their way into public consciousness. Some dreamed wistfully of Wilson's Fourteen Points as guides to the new world; some of Fabian socialism; some enthroned the unconscious in the name of Sigmund Freud; some acted under the banner of Karl Marx.

George Bernard Shaw was at the height of his popularity, but his plays and his Fabian views managed to escape Bethune's notice. It was no easy feat in the London of the early twenties, but Bethune accomplished it, much to his embarrassment later when he became a Shawdolator.

Bethune had his own prophet, almost obscure by then but once a potent literary influence in England. He had been spiritual father to Oscar Wilde. His name was Walter Pater: professor, author, critic, prophet of the senses, tastes, pleasures; intellectual hero to many a student in the England of Victoria. He was made to order for Bethune, who now invoked the famous Pater dictum with a vengeance: "Not the fruit of experience, but experience itself is the end....To burn always with a hard, gemlike flame, to maintain this ecstasy, is success in life."

In the London of the early twenties, Bethune worked hard for "success" as defined by Walter Pater.

There was time for the hospital and time for study and time for all-night binges as the young doctor wallowed in the uninhibited atmosphere of postwar London. The idea was to experience everything. The war had taught him that life was cheap and death came fast and there was little time for man to taste everything that life offered.

In the meantime his mother wrote him regularly, urging him to remember the Bible to go to church and to avoid the pitfalls of sin. He answered dutifully, giving her accounts of his progress as an intern.

For three years he busied himself with his surgery, painting, sculpture, meeting new people, interpreting Pater, and accepting the certainty that he would become a great surgeon. It was only a matter of working and waiting. At the end of three years he finished his internship and took a position with a private clinic in London's East End.

"Ah, the fates, the fates," he wrote of this period later, "they assumed the form of two women."

The first was Dr. Eleanor Dell,★ wife of a wealthy British industrialist, wealthy in her own right, and head of the East Side clinic at which Bethune worked. Dr. Dell became his friend, his sponsor and his benefactor. Under her prodding and guidance, he studied hard and prepared for his exams to become a Fellow of the Royal College of Surgeons. To study, a young doctor needed money, more money than he could earn taking trips to France and Spain. Dr. Dell provided the money, and Dr. Bethune listed the amounts, to be repaid in full. He promised Dr. Dell to pursue his studies for two more years in Europe, and then establish himself in London with her help.

In the autumn of 1923 he went to Edinburgh to take his F.R.C.S. exams. There he met the second woman, Frances Campbell Penney. "It was love at first *sound*," he was fond of repeating. Frances spoke with a soft, musical Edinburgh cadence. Her voice,

---

★ This is a pseudonym.

her beauty, and a "remarkable innocence, a remarkable unworld-
liness, plus a remarkable intelligence," all combined to sweep him
off his feet. His dynamic wooing, in turn, swept her off her feet,
and they were married in London a few months after his exams.

She was 22 at the time, the only daughter of a prominent
Edinburgh family, an upper-class product of the best finishing
schools of England and Europe.

The day after their marriage he announced he was penni-
less and that he had better prepare to set up in private practice.
In Edinburgh, he had mentioned to her that he planned to
study in Europe. Why, she inquired, had he abandoned the plan?
The answer seemed simple. He was now a married man, ready
to assume the responsibilities of a husband. He would have to
postpone some of his plans. But Frances couldn't understand
why. She had, she announced, a small inheritance, and saw no
reason why he couldn't continue his studies. The small inheritance was news, good news, and he wondered if it wouldn't be
a better idea to use part of it to establish an office in London.
But Frances wouldn't hear of it. She did not want their marriage interfering with his medical career. So off to Europe they
went in the spring of 1924 on a combined honeymoon and
study course.

Frances, at 22, was an inordinately shy and retiring personality. Bethune, at 34, was inordinately outspoken and flamboyant in
manner. They loved each other, but their backgrounds clashed.
Like so many young upper-class women of the period, Frances
had what amounted to a pathological fear of the intimacies of
marriage. Before long a pattern of frustration, antagonism, and
misunderstanding was established between them, threatening the
regard and love they had for each other. Bethune's marriage soon
became a symbol to him of failure, and the chaotic atmosphere
of postwar Europe contributed to his confusion.

His personal frustrations led him to irrational behaviour
which frightened Frances and led to more withdrawal on her
part. It became an unhappy circle of argument and reconciliation,
anger and tenderness, of recriminations and remorse. They left
each other unremembered times, and always ended up vowing
they couldn't live apart. Always impetuous, his unhappy relationship motivated new impetuousness, childish testing of her love,

brooding over misunderstandings, real and imagined. Once he plunged into the English Channel during a raging storm and was almost drowned. He explained to her sheepishly that he had always wanted to swim in the Channel during a storm. To her it seemed he was bent on destroying himself.

Another time, he dared her to jump across a wide ravine which might have meant serious injury or death if she slipped. She jumped, and then ran back to her hotel and took the first boat to London. He wrote her, begging for forgiveness, expressing his dismay at his strange behaviour which he himself couldn't understand. When she returned there was a week of mutual tenderness, but it exploded in the conflict of daily frustrations and antagonisms.

Again, in Italy, while looking at Giotto's "Life of St. Francis," he experienced something as akin to a revelation and decided he wanted to become a monk. The mood left him in Vienna, where he studied under some of the leading surgeons. There he was sure he could be nothing but a surgeon.

A few weeks later he felt the need for action and excitement, and they went skiing in Switzerland. He was an excellent skier but his need for excitement and action overreached itself and he strained his heart. This necessitated a three weeks' rest in bed. They were the quietest three weeks spent in Europe.

He drank hard, studied hard, lived hard, and within a year helped Frances go through most of her inheritance.

The year wasn't wasted, since he had observed the work of the great European surgeons in Paris, Vienna and Berlin, but he always hated to remember it. "I was like some butterfly batting its crazy wings against a light, blinded and stupid, going around in circles, with no purpose in life and no purpose in death."*

The honeymoon was a mockery. His marriage was a mockery. His life was a mockery. So it seemed to him when they came to the end of their madcap cavortings about Europe.

---

* Letter to Frances.

5

Two hundred pounds was what remained of Frances's inheritance at the end of a year. It took them to London, from London to Canada, and from Canada to Detroit, Michigan.

Why Detroit? Bethune had the answers....

The city just across the Canadian border was bursting with activity. It was already the capital of the automotive industry, a sprawling centre of America's mass production industries, a magnet for those seeking opportunity, a new Mecca for those filled with the prophecies of Henry Ford. America was rich, and a great torrent of its riches washed through Detroit. America was on the road to prosperity never dreamed of before and Detroit was the promise of the limitless future. In Detroit there was money, work, push, endeavour. There, he told himself, he would have to kiss no one's hand, bend the knee to no British upper-class dowager. It was the man-made frontier of America's glittering future. "Detroit," he said, "is where we shall open our first office."

And so, in the late winter of 1924, Dr. and Mrs. Norman Bethune rented a flat at the corner of Cass and Seldon Streets, with exactly twenty-four dollars between them, old pewter and odd antiques picked up in Europe, assorted art objects and Louis Quatorze chairs. For Frances, Detroit was dreary, dirty, mawkish and disturbing. For Bethune it was the twentieth century, a machine-age citadel where opportunity knocked on every door.

He hung out his grandfather's shingle, and waited for opportunity to knock. He waited a year and only the faintest tappings came.

Bethune had selected the corner of Cass and Seldon Streets because it had seemed to be a busy section of the city. It soon turned out to be even busier than he had imagined.

It was then the centre of the red-light district, and when he had borrowed a desk, bought a mattress and opened for business, he found himself a fledgling Hippocrates administering to the age-old Magdalen. In the rest of the city industry and commerce grew by leaps and bounds; around Cass and Seldon Streets, prostitution flourished with the times. Patients slowly began to trickle into his office, but it was mainly the prostitutes who were able to pay.

In his bare office Bethune learned a lesson seldom mentioned in his medical courses at Toronto, London, Vienna and Berlin: those who most needed his services were those who could least pay for them.

By a stroke of luck he was called in by the corner grocer one day to look at his wife. The woman had a repulsively swollen leg, and the grocer explained frantically that a doctor had declared it had to be amputated. Bethune incised the affected area, kept draining the pus under close supervision, and in a matter of days had the patient out of danger. The grocer's cash register was as empty of money as his heart was full of gratitude. "The only way I can pay you, Doctor," he said humbly, "is in trade. For what you did you can have all the groceries you want, free of charge, as long as you want." That settled most of the problem of food. The rest of the problem was settled by a butcher across the street with a fortunate fondness for children.

He came to Bethune's office, tapping the sawdust from his shoes on the stairs, and said hesitantly, "I gotta houseful a kids. You look after the kids an' I give ya all the meat ya kin eat."

"At least," Bethune told Frances, "we shall now have a balanced diet."

When the owner of a hardware and furniture store brought his ailing wife to join the parade, the circle was complete. They got a bed to put under the mattress, pots and pans for the kitchen and Grand Rapids furniture to put in incongruous intimacy with the Louis Quatorze chairs.

He gave it a little time — and more time — and still his fortunes remained at the level of his patients. Gradually more people came to his office, but the poverty of the many yielded him little more income than the poverty of the few. Some of his patients became a source of irritation. They would come to his office, or send someone to take him to their homes, and they would be dangerously ill with ailments that could easily have been handled in the initial stages. Either it was a pain that was left unattended till it was a ruptured appendix, or an unheeded discomfort that was already advanced venereal disease, or a hernia now strangulating, or a hundred and one other illnesses complicated by neglect.

"Why do you wait so long before calling in a doctor?" he would rage. And the patient, a Slav, or a Hungarian, or a native-born auto worker, would be incoherent with the embarrassment of his poverty.

The shabby flats, the unpaid bills, the senseless all-pervading sickness on the boom city of fat America began to depress Bethune. "This isn't medicine," he would say to Frances. "It's like putting a mustard plaster on a wooden leg. When they need treatment they either don't know it or are afraid they can't pay for it. When they finally do come, it's often too late, or their health has become completely undermined. And what can I do for a prostitute, when her problem is not really that she is diseased, but that she is a prostitute?" He passed the blame on to the world, and at such moments told himself that it was not really his concern, that he was a doctor, that the world was what it was, that he could only mend a leg when it was broken, repair hernias, viscera, internals, and send "Mary" to the hospital when she was caught in the net of her "occupational hazards."

As the months dragged by a new fear cut into the unrelieved drabness of his life and work. He found himself tiring more easily and needing more sleep. He worried lest he should be losing the drive and energy which had never failed him before. And with increasing fatigue came more doubts, more moodiness, more bitterness.

Then he would be called out on a case. He would find a patient dying and would pit himself doggedly against the unknown menace that stole the fruits of the body and mind. He immersed himself in cause and cure and won the patient back to health. He would feel triumph and accomplishment flowing through him again, reviving him, re-establishing the old hopes and pride. His knowledge and skill would become a warm glow inside him, with no room for moodiness or doubt. Once again he was the confident surgeon, certain of the future, biding his time and undismayed by poverty.

And suddenly, overnight, before he had time to realize what was happening, he went from failure to success — and money.

He had managed to get himself attached to one of the city hospitals, performing routine surgery. He was coming out of the operating theatre one day when a well-dressed, pleasant-mannered individual stopped him in the corridor, introducing himself as Dr. Grant Martin.* Bethune had heard of him as one of Detroit's most successful practitioners.

"I admire your work," Dr. Martin told him, "and I would like to suggest that I send my surgery cases to you.... Perhaps you and your wife could come up to the house some evening and we could discuss it further."

"That would be fine."

They shook hands. "I think we'll make a good combination," Dr. Martin said cordially.

A brief conversation — and everything was changed.

At Martin's home Bethune and Frances met other eminent doctors and socialites. To the office at Cass and Seldon there now began to come men and women of wealth and social position. Other doctors followed Martin's lead and turned their patients over to the surgeon everybody was suddenly talking about. Sped on its way by Martin, the word spread that Bethune was the "man to see."

Money now began to pour in. Whereas his neighbourhood patients came to him only in their extremity, pleading their poverty, his new patients expected to be billed handsomely for the most trivial services. At the hospital he began to move ahead in surgery, applying the skills and techniques he had learned under the masters in Europe. Within a few months they moved to an expensive home in a fashionable residential area. He refused to move his office, however, though more of his patients now were extremely well-to-do.

Success was welcome but sometimes, as he sat in his newly furnished office, he looked at his hands and thought: what has

* A pseudonym.

changed? They were the same hands. Had they some new magic today that they lacked yesterday? He knew the answer: yesterday they had treated the poor, today they treated the rich.

Money, now, was what he sought. He needed money! But in the making of money he came to hate the very methods by which he made it. With success he was no longer the old Dr. Bethune. He found himself now a prisoner in a rigid system, with its "scratch-my-back-and-I'll-scratch-yours" outlook, and its rake-off for the general practitioners who sent him their patients. The specialist was expected to charge all that the traffic would bear, and the "gravy" would pass down the line, with the patient "taxed" to keep the system going.

Money was the beginning and end. He took as much as he could, and returned to his first patients in the slums to find his lost sense of peace, the tarnished ideals of the doctor serving the sick and the poor.

Money was the goal to which the system shaped all aspirations, and he let himself ride the success that swelled his earnings daily. But life intruded with the reality of suffering men and women who needed his help but couldn't pay for it.

One night he was awakened by a banging at the door. A man was standing in the darkness. He let loose a torrent of words. Bethune finally managed to learn that the stranger's wife was in labour and could find no doctor who would perform the delivery. He soon found out why. The man lived with his wife and two children in an abandoned boxcar on the outskirts of the city.

By the light of a kerosene lamp, with the husband assisting and two children huddling on a mattress in the corner, he delivered an undersized, wrinkled baby. He washed it, wrapped it in some torn blankets the father handed him, and put it beside the mother, for there was no crib.

As he washed up in a basin of water filled from the barrel outside, the father came up nervously, holding a dollar bill in his hand. Bethune took the bill, folded it, and put it back in the man's shirt pocket.

In the morning he returned with a basket of food, diapers for the baby and a nightgown for the mother. He prepared a diet for the undernourished mother and examined the baby. When he left he cut short the father's nervous thanks gruffly. He knew the mother would recover, but the baby would probably be dead within the month. This they called medicine — the hallowed art of healing!

A job at twenty dollars a week, he complained to Frances, would have done more for the husband than all the wonders that could now be performed for his doomed child. Medicine? The fakers even refused to interrupt their comfortable slumber to deliver a boxcar child!

He became outspoken about some of his colleagues. While Frances would sit quietly reading he gave vent to his bitter feelings. "Some of them have as much right to be practising as the medieval barber. I'd weed out half of them to begin with and put them to work behind a counter. And I'd see to it that the remainder understood they were doctors, not men of commerce."

To a new-found friend, Dr. Short, after being called in to repair some bone surgery another man had bungled, he said, "I could make a better mother than he could make a surgeon. The idiots think they've gone into business! I tell you the medical profession should establish a commission of the best men available to pass on the qualifications of doctors and surgeons after they've been in this — this 'business' — for two years. Talk about ethics. A Philadelphia lawyer is a paragon of virtue compared to some of us."

His strong views, openly and everywhere expressed, aroused resentment and criticism among some doctors. "Some of them are so damned sanctimonious," he complained. "that they expect everybody to swallow the fairy tale of their infallibility and devotion to duty. They just can't stomach criticism. They want the public to think they're infallible. And some of them actually end by convincing themselves that they can never be wrong. Their slogan should be 'save the surface and you save all.' That's all they know and are interested in — the surface. In the slums people don't come to me, when they should, because they have no money. Now I charge many times the fees I should, and there are others who do even better. When I saved a man's life for nothing I was a failure. Now when I give a woman a simple tonic where a good, bracing set of exercises would do just as well, I collect a fantastic fee and am a success."

Frances rarely saw him now. He was always in his office, or out on calls, or, she suspected, spending part of the night with drinking companions. She began to notice a change in him that filled her with new fears.

Along with his drinking, his fits of rage, his long moods of bitterness, he was slowly undergoing a strange physical transformation. His colleagues, noticing it, cautioned him to cut down on his work. The suggestion threw him into an irrational fury. He was now a successful surgeon, wasn't he? And success was measured in terms of income, wasn't it? Well, he would make money, and more money and still more money — till he had all he needed so that he could do what he wanted: to turn his back on the world, if it so pleased him; to laugh at the unimportant aches and pains of the useless rich; to see if medicine could be practised the way he had once dreamed, during the idealism of his adolescence.

There came a time when his energy and resilience glimmered away entirely. He was tired in the early hours of the morning, and just as tired when he started painfully on the morning's round of patients, but he turned away no call, during the day or night, especially if the patient was poor.

Frances, watching him with apprehension, urged him to take a holiday. "You're driving yourself into the grave. You can't possibly go on this way."

"I'm perfectly all right," he replied irritably.

He developed a racking cough which, at first, he ignored, then treated with the usual nostrums, but it grew steadily worse, jarring Frances when she heard him come in with it and waking her often in the night.

His cheeks grew flushed as if with fever. He began visibly to shrink. When he weighed himself on his scale one day he found he had lost 50 pounds, and was down to an impossible 115. He mixed himself a tonic and looked at himself in the mirror. His hair was thinner over the high, domed forehead, and turning grey. To Frances, when he caught her once looking at his head, he said: "It's not unusual. My father was prematurely grey also."

As he drove himself to keep up with his practice he found himself suddenly falling into fits of weakness in which everything receded and he felt only an overwhelming desire to crawl into bed.

Then he began waking in the middle of the night, starting up suddenly in terror, not knowing why, his heart pounding madly, his pajamas wet with perspiration. He would pace the floor, sleepless, coughing for hours.

One evening he came in early. Frances went into the hallway and·stopped in her tracks as she saw him. He held a handkerchief over his mouth, soaking with blood. His eyes stared at her above the crimson handkerchief, then he lurched unsteadily upstairs to his room. She stood transfixed for a moment, then rushed to the telephone to call a neighbourhood doctor.

When the doctor came Bethune was lying in bed, his eyes closed, his face white. He had draped a towel about his chin which was stained with blood and sputum. He was gasping for breath, a gargling, bubbling sound rising and falling with the throat.

The doctor grunted, waved Frances away from his bed, bent swiftly and listened to Bethune's chest. "It's fairly clear," he said crisply, "but we'll have to have some X-rays at once."

6

For two weeks he lay on his back. A mist seemed to have wrapped itself about his mind, clogging his thoughts. Sometimes his lips twisted into a brief, bitter smile. The faces of doctors swam into his view, and he heard whisperings in the hallway. Sometimes the mist lifted, and he looked up at Frances. He seemed to study her face then, impersonally, as if she were a stranger, and said nothing. The doctors muttered, "Very bad hemorrhage." He heard them, staring frozenly at the ceiling. Shock, hemorrhage, loss of blood.... *More than that*, he thought to himself; much more than they could label with their poverty-stricken teams or reveal on their X-ray plates.

For days the voices whispered in the hallway, the shadow of Frances hovered over him, the warm, salty bubbling in his throat awakened him sometimes to darkness, sometimes to light. The faces peered at him and receded, the shadows chased each other in a devil's dance on the ceiling....

"Dr. Bethune ..."

It was one of the doctors beside his bed. Why were they still plaguing him?

"Dr. Bethune ..." The well-preserved face, with the well-trimmed beard, the well-cultivated bedside manner. The face of a handsome fee. "How do you feel?" What a restricted vocabulary they all had. "How do I feel?" he mimicked. "As if I'm dying. How do you feel?"

The face withdrew, beard and all.

The old goat ... Would he answer a call in the middle of the night to deliver a woman in a boxcar, with her husband out of work, no food for the children, and two other families sharing the car? It was too tiring even to think of it. He closed his eyes and let himself sink into the half-sleep for which his body yearned.

One day he awoke early. His mind seemed clearer. He watched the sun slant in through the window, relieved that his breathing was a little easier and that the hemorrhaging had stopped completely. He wondered what day of the month it was and listened idly to the sounds of the street. Listening, it struck him as somehow incongruous that his was another day like all days, and the sounds in the street were as familiar as always. Had he forgotten so easily, he wondered, that life would go on outside his room as before?

Morning in Detroit — with birds chirping somewhere, up among the chimney stacks, whistles blowing, children shuffling to school ... In London, it would be noon, and on the Mediterranean coast, time for siesta. On such a day, in Soho, he might dream of boating on the Thames; in Vienna, skiing on the Alps; in Rome, of the hot beaches in the south. Now it all seemed far away. He marveled at the disinterest with which the thought left him. Gravenhurst, London, Europe, memories of the war, his marriage to Frances, poverty and fortune in Detroit — strange, but they were only feeble flickerings out of the past. Or was it strange, he reflected, that they should now seem so dim and unimportant? They had happened, that was all. A curtain had fallen over them; they were part of a bad play that had ended.

Frances ... Did the name stir anything? Yes — a little bitterness, and much compassion. He had failed her, or she had
failed him, or something else had gone wrong; anyway, it was all
mucked up and futile and nothing left to it. Not even children,
to give you the illusion, at least, that a part of you went on and
didn't die.

And if the curtain had fallen on Frances, what else was left?
Nothing. Of course, there had been the destiny awaiting him,
the destiny he had grown up with since childhood. A great
surgeon! What a destiny! A bone-hacker, a money-grubber, a
sycophant — there was your healer.

His eyes, roving about the room, fell on a mirror on his bedside table. He reached out for it and examined himself curiously.

He was unprepared for the change in his appearance. He
had watched himself losing weight steadily, but in the short time
he had been in bed his cheeks had become hollow, his hair had
turned grayer, the eyes glowed with fever.

He sank back, exhausted. "To burn with a hard gemlike
flame!" Even Pater had been an illusion....

His reverie was disturbed by footsteps. It was Frances. He
watched her as she placed his glass of milk on the table, studied
her solicitous face, let her prop up the pillows behind him, then
said in a firm voice:

"There's something we have to talk about ... I don't know
what they've told you, but I'm dying. *I'm* finished — *your* whole life
is ahead of you. I want you to divorce me and go your own way."

7

For some weeks he was treated at a local hospital, and then,
when he was strong enough to travel, he left for Calydor Sanatorium, up at Gravenhurst. He was "going home," and the irony of
his life was complete.

At the railway terminal Frances stood beside him among the
hurrying crowds, while a redcap took his luggage. He looked

about the station. Detroit, he thought — heart of a new America. Another year and another dream that the locusts had eaten.

Frances held his arm tightly. She had begged to go with him, but he had clung stubbornly to his single theme: he was dying, they would be divorced, she would find a new life for herself, and a clean break now would be the best for both. She had been stunned, then outraged, then crushed. All her feelings of loyalty, of love, cried out in protest. Whatever had happened between them, she could think of nothing but to be with him, to give him whatever frail support she could, and let the future take care of itself. But to all her pleas he had calmly replied: "It makes no sense. You have a full life ahead of you. I won't be a partner to wasting any more of it. I won't leave for the sanatorium until you agree to divorce me." That had defeated her.

As he turned to her now she tried desperately to think of what to say, how to make right and whole again everything that had slipped through their fingers.

He bent to kiss her. "Goodbye ... dear, unspeakable Scot," he said softly. "Go back to Edinburgh — you'll be happier there. Sell everything and go back ..." He turned and went down the station platform.

In Toronto, the next morning, his parents were waiting for him at the station to take him to Gravenhurst.

His father was older, a little stooped. His fingers trembled as he extended his hand. On his mother's strong, proud face there was a look of anguish. Together they boarded the train for northern Ontario, his mother sitting beside him.

As the train crossed the Don river he gazed silently at the clumps of trees, the fields turning brown, the last few houses on the fringe of the city. Once his mother turned her old eyes on him and asked, "Norman, is there much pain?" He shook his head. Not that kind of pain.

Sandy patches appeared in the fields, then came the stiff, green pines, the outcroppings of rock on the low hills, the first fingers of the Muskoka lakes, and at last Gravenhurst.

They drove through the town, past the little church where he had once listened to his father in the pulpit, and into the rock-capped hills. A few minutes out of the town they swung towards the lake and drove over a cinder road, between lines of carefully tended pines, into the sanatorium.

In the infirmary, while he lay back in the rough-textured hospital clothes, his mother bent her head beside his bed and prayed, her eyes brimming. He took her hand gently. "No, Mother," he said. "There's no need for prayer or tears. I have no regrets. I'm tired. Anything coming after this would be an anticlimax...."

8

He was finished with the world, but a letter from Trudeau Sanatorium changed the course of his treatment.

In Detroit his first impulse had been to gain admittance to Trudeau Sanatorium at Saranac Lake, New York. But there had been no bed available. Now, a month later, a letter from Saranac Lake informed him that he could gain admittance immediately.

Founded by Edward Livingston Trudeau, the great pioneer in sanatorium treatment in North America, the Saranac Lake hospital was highly regarded throughout the medical profession. Despite his mood of weary fatalism Bethune decided to make the change.

He arrived at Trudeau Sanatorium on December 16. Holly wreaths on the buildings gave the hospital a Christmas touch. Once again he went through the routine examinations and submitted quietly to all the tests. He was fascinated by his own X-rays. He read, he wrote letters, he lay thinking for hours. He showed no anxiety, no hope, no fear. He wore an air of neutral calm, yet managed to bend the infirmary's routine to his own whims despite anything the nurses could say. While he was confined to bed he wore an old straw hat he had brought with him. After he was permitted to get up he strolled about the corridors in his pajamas. When he was finally transferred to the "Lea," one of the sanatorium cottages on the slope of Mount Pisgah, the infirmary staff breathed a nervous sigh of relief.

In the cottages of the miniature city, the little world where January 1927 was a footnote on a medical chart, the patients awakened in the morning, their breaths clouding the air. The doctors passed along the assembly line of flushed faces, dispensing optimism. The founding father, Trudeau himself, stood sentinel before the . gate in solid bronze, new patients entering and old ones leaving before his sightless eyes. And up in the cottage called the Lea, four men with nothing to wait for closed the circle of their lives, growing attuned to each other's innermost thoughts and abandoning all pretense of privacy.

Four men — three of them doctors — all condemned to death by tuberculosis, all knowledgeable in the disease that had condemned them, all apprised of the symptoms appearing hourly, daily, weekly in notification of the time and form of eventual extinction. In two hundred and twenty-five square feet of space, they occupied four single cots, between walls of yellow pine, arranged to make the best of windows and doors opening on three sides and a fourth doorway into a tiny bathroom. As the wind blew louder and the snow piled higher against the cottage they grew into a macabre community in which they knew the special tonal quality of each member's cough, each one's special tastes, discomforts, habits, wakings, nightmares.

There was Dr. B.,★ a Southerner, with fair hair, blue eyes, a handsome face, a warm, pleasant smile. There was Dr. Lincoln Fisher, born in Michigan, brought up in New England, dark, young, eager, quick. There was Nan Li, a Chinese, short, correct, friendly. And there was Norman Bethune, assessing them quickly, liking them all immediately, and now joined with them in an intimacy that extended through every minute of every hour of every day.

For each of them the Trudeau staff had decreed bed, rest, quiet. They had their own ideas about how to spend their remaining days. They established an "underground" to the outside world through some of the attendants, and through this "underground" they smuggled in liquor, food, and anything that appealed to them. They disdained the natural boundaries of night and day.

★ Dr. B has requested that his name be withheld.

Often, when the lights blinked out in the other cottages, they squeezed into the bathroom to play Russian bank all night, a dressing gown draped over the single small window so that the light wouldn't give them away. They loved music and listened for hours to a gramophone that was "legal." Their favourite record was "Lonesome Road," and they played it over and over again. They kept a secret "pantry" from which they prepared snacks the administration would have frowned upon. Sometimes they invited other inmates to gay parties. If they kept late hours one night, they slept the next day. They talked endlessly of life, tuberculosis, books. With "scientific detachment" — real or pretended — and with an eye to the future, they kept a chart of the dates on which one expected to die.

The mood to which they were keyed was expressed in a series of murals Bethune sketched on the walls while the others watched with interest. He entitled the murals, "A T.B.'s Progress: A Drama in One Act and Nine Painful Scenes." The visual "drama" consisted of nine allegories showing the various stages of his life from womb to tomb. It had vivid colour, bold lines and the prophecy of an early end for the four of them. Under each allegory he wrote a satirical verse.

The first panel showed the Angel of Life holding the infant Bethune in her arms. The succeeding panels showed the infant beset by ferocious-looking animals, symbolizing childhood diseases. Then came early manhood, with a young man at the prow of a ship, lured from his course by four sirens labelled Fame, Wealth, Love and Art. They pointed to a castle, labelled Castle of Heart's Desire. The next panel showed the castle to be nothing but an illusion, a Hollywood stage set, where the young man was attacked by swarms of "T.B. bats." The next panels depicted him entering Trudeau, then leaving the sanatorium and dying on the plains of Arizona.

The final panel showed the Angel of Death holding Bethune in her arms. She looked down on him with a kindly expression. In the foreground was a small graveyard and a row of tombstones. Under the final scene was the verse:

> Sweet death, thou kindest angel of them all,
> In thy soft arms, at last, O let me fall;

> Bright stars are out, long gone the burning sun,
> My little act is over, and the tiresome play is done.

From the mural the Angel of Death looked down upon them with her benevolent face while spring came, and with it a letter from Frances. The divorce had become final; she was leaving for Edinburgh at once.

He reread the letter, tossed it away, pulled on his coat and went out. For hours he walked among the hills, filled with many conflicting thoughts, wanting to be away from everyone. The letter had awakened an unexpected nostalgia. Why should it matter? he asked himself. But now that it was settled, it did. He had demanded the divorce, but suddenly it seemed as if the last, thin strand connecting him with the outer worlds was gone. The knowledge that a part of him was still vulnerable, could still yearn for something he had put behind him, was a shattering revelation. As he sloshed through the wet snow he wrestled with a rising feeling of impotence, self-pity, rebellion.

It was dark when he returned to the Lea. Fisher, Li and B. were waiting for him. "Is there any drink left?" he asked.

Sitting on his bed he felt a deep need for companionship, an urge to talk. The others, sensing his disturbed mood, listened attentively.

It began to snow outside. The wet flakes spattered against the windows. The night seemed to grow white. Bethune lit one cigarette after another, talking compulsively and refilling his glass. As he rambled on, about himself, his past life, the wind rose up against the cottage like the prodding of a giant hand. The others understood his restlessness. Each of them, in his own way, had been squeezed in the same vise. But they were veterans now — they could be patient with the T.B. apprentice.

He grew silent and lay back on the cot. The letter, he thought to himself, had reminded him of something he had forgotten. He had come to Trudeau, accepting his fate; now he was discovering what it meant *to live it*. Now the thought that he would never see Frances again filled him with an unendurable emptiness, the bitter knowledge of what it meant to lose her, and losing her, of his final isolation here on Mount Pisgah, waiting for the end. He had known only the surface of death; now he was tasting its last, slow agonies.

He roused himself. "The hell with it," he said. In his lung the rot was spreading fast; soon it would put an end to all pangs and questionings. "Let's have another drink."

While Fisher fetched the bottle he pulled out the gramophone and put on a record. A rich baritone filled the room ... *The Lonesome Road*....

The voice died away, the room became still. In the darkness the others watched him, knowing there was nothing to be said, then fell quietly asleep. Switching on his bed lamp he began to write a letter to Frances:

> Dear Frances,
>
> So you are going back to Edinburgh. It's for the best. Your feathers have been sadly ruffled, and there is nothing I can do now.
>
> Here nothing happens — or nothing *seems* to happen. Actually, much *does* happen. Contemplation becomes one's special form of action, and no one here can escape the changes, the discoveries, the greater self-knowledge that are inevitably the product of such enforced contemplation....
>
> I once, vaguely, accepted the idea of my own special, personal predestination. It has disappeared in the ruins. Here, where we are excluded from the living world, we perhaps get a little closer to reality sometimes. Out of that closeness come glimmerings of understanding, with its inevitable cycle of despair, hope, resignation. But it comes too late — for me. What a terrible irony: the victim of circumstance becomes the master of his fate at the price of accepting his defeat....

He stopped writing with a sudden feeling of futility. A strange sensation was crawling through him. He struggled with the rush of loneliness and overwhelming dread. It bit into him too sharply to be denied: the taste and smell and substance of fear. It was a lie that he could purge himself of Frances. It was a lie that he had lived his life. It was a lie that there was nothing left for him. He had created nothing, he would leave nothing behind him, he had not yet even lived. He switched off the lamp and gave himself up completely to despair.

Above him, in the nine painful scenes of a T.B.'s Progress, the darkness seemed to twist the features of the Angel of Death into a hideous grin.

9

It was a warm evening in late summer. In the groves of cottages the windows were open to the warm breezes. In the Lea, the four inmates lay in bed reading. They had just returned from the library, each carrying a stack of novels, magazines, and medical journals.

Bethune had started on a current novel, grown bored and picked up a book by Dr. John Alexander, *The Surgery of Pulmonary Tuberculosis*. He riffled the pages idly, thumbed backwards, and said aloud, "Listen to this." He read,

> It is rather extraordinary that we should have been so seriously backward in doing pioneer work in the surgery of pulmonary tuberculosis. It will be a surprise to the majority of American physicians who read this book to realize the steady advance in thoracic surgery* and the definite hope offered the hopeless.

"Let's have a look at it when you're through," Fisher said sleepily.

Bethune adjusted his bed lamp, settled back once more and began to read. The opening sentence was a calm statement, but weighted with revolutionary overtones: "Surgery of the twentieth century can boast no more important advance than that now being made in the operative management of pulmonary tuberculosis."

---

* Chest surgery.

Surgery for pulmonary T.B. Done by whom? He could recall only inconclusive reports in American medical literature. *Operative management* ... Direct, drastic, surgical intervention? As opposed to the catch-all fetish, lingering, uncertain rest in bed? Hadn't he himself complained about the inadequacy of rest alone? He was seized by a sudden excitement:

> Only a few years ago any kind of surgery for the disease was considered ill-advised and meddlesome. Extra-pleural paravertebral thoracoplasty★ and allied procedures are now offering to a large group of persons with predominantly unilateral tuberculosis (i.e., T.B. in one lung mainly) an excellent chance to escape a certain tuberculosis death and to become permanently well.

He reread the passage carefully. This doctor was actually making the cold, casual statement that supposedly hopeless cases of T.B., centred mainly in one lung, could be completely cured by surgical methods! But that was precisely his own condition — infection crippling the left lung. Bethune read on swiftly, his excitement continuing to increase as Alexander, in measured words, declared that there was sufficient evidence to adopt surgical procedures, that an appalling ignorance lay behind the failure to utilize them in America, that thousands of men and women were dying because of this failure, that there had been widespread misrepresentation where the facts had not been wholly ignored. The words seemed to leap up at him:

> In view of the enormous amount of work that has been done since the days of Koch to find a cure for mankind's most widespread scourge, it is surprising that the medical profession as a whole knows so little of pulmonary compression (deflation of the lung). Without doubt it is the most valuable contribution to the therapy of pulmonary tuberculosis that has been made in

★ Removal of part of the ribs to collapse an infected lung.

the present century and, in fact since Detweiler advocated sanatorium treatment in the eighteen seventies ... The value of surgery for selected cases of pulmonary tuberculosis is no longer a matter left open for discussion ... It is incumbent upon physicians everywhere to acquaint themselves with the indications and contraindications for surgery so that the thousands of patients, who would otherwise certainly be lost, may be saved.

This volume, the first in the English language, presents the entire subject of pulmonary tuberculosis with the object of acquainting the medical profession with the principles and practical details that will enable it each year to save thousands of lives which certainly will be lost if surgery is not undertaken.

The others were asleep now. Only his bed lamp burned in the darkness, casting shifting shadows on the walls. Bethune looked thoughtfully at the book in his hands. Why hadn't he heard of it before? He searched among the pages to find the date of publication: 1926, the previous year.

So that thousands may be saved! — Hope for the hopeless! Could it be that a fresh approach had been found, that somewhere medical men, trying to pierce the unknown, had found a light, and needed only to be followed?

When dawn came his bed lamp was still burning. At last he let the book fall away, but it was a long time till he slept. A thought had begun to take shape in his mind, a slippery, elusive wisp of hope that he hardly dared acknowledge. Hope? No, not yet, he told himself — merely a growing resolution.

He fell asleep with daybreak in his eyes, Dr. John Alexander's book beside him, many of its passages heavily penciled, his life, for better or worse, profoundly, irrevocably, unshakably altered.

For the next few days he said little to anybody. He spent most of his time in the staff library, searching for everything published on surgery for pulmonary tuberculosis. He was astonished to find how little material there was on the subject. A few of the articles he found in medical journals he dismissed as inconsequential in the face of the material collated by Dr. Alexander. Apart from a few articles by Dr. Alexander himself he was forced to fall back on that expert's book. But what he did find was enough to set his mind teeming with new ideas.

For weeks he pumped every source he could find. In Alexander's book he read with admiration of the men who cast aside hidebound tradition and sought revolutionary procedures of restoring the tuberculous to health. De Cerenville in Switzerlan; Brauer, Wilms, Sauerbruch, Stuertz, in Germany; Gourdet, Tuffier, Bérard, in France; Jacobaeus, in Sweden; Davies, in England; Gekler and Murphy in the United States; Archibald in Canada. These were men who rejected the concept of medicine as something static. They attacked what was unknown, in order to make it known. If men died of T.B., they insisted the job of medicine was to discover how to keep them from dying. If the current techniques failed, they insisted new techniques had to be found. And a special thrill in the vast agitation with which Bethune was now filled was the discovery that a Canadian surgeon, Dr. Edward William Archibald of Montreal, stood forth among the men advancing the new creed that there was "hope for the hopeless."

All of these men, with their own hands, had shown there were countless cases where patients had been put to bed without improvement, but had recovered when the infected lung had been collapsed either permanently or temporarily, as the individual conditions required. As he reached deeper into the subject, Bethune went from impatience to exasperation.

The Lea now resounded constantly to discussions on artificial pneumothorax* and the drastic operation known as thoracoplasty.

"It's beyond belief," Bethune would say. "Many thousands are dying who are not only suitable for surgery, but urgently need it, and aren't getting it. Only 17 surgeons in this country have been using the methods developed by Sauerbruch, Brauer and others. And the total number of operations in the past seven years — in America, I mean — has been only 300. A drop in the bucket. At this very moment there are 30,000 men and women, in this

---

* Insertion of air into chest as to collapse one lung.

country alone, and I wonder how many in Canada — 30,000 who are dying, for whom there is no hope with the current methods, and who might be saved by surgery — compression of the afflicted lung by one method or another."

He paced the floor moodily. "That isn't mere ignorance. It isn't only conservatism. It's downright barbarism ... And what about us? Do you think any one of us stands a chance, lying in bed till doomsday?" He paused, confronting them. "Alexander has gathered all the evidence. Artificial pneumothorax, which even we have known about for some years, but of which we seem to be afraid, for some reason, as the devil fears holy water. Yet what could be simpler? Insert a hollow needle into the chest cavity. Pump air into the cavity so that the lung is deflated as much as you want to deflate it. Then the lung is truly rested. It *can't* move. Compared to that, staying in bed keeps the lung working like a fire engine ... And when that's done, keep pumping your air in every week, every month, every two months ... as often as necessary, for as long a period of time as necessary."

He waved the book in front of him "I'm tired of dying this way."

"What do you suggest? Can you say you've honestly given bed rest a fair trial?" Fisher asked.

"No, and I don't intend to. I want compression treatment. Alexander has convinced me. All of this is just horsing around. I'm going to demand artificial pneumothorax." That afternoon he stormed into the administration building while a staff meeting was in progress and demanded artificial pneumothorax. Trudeau's staff was well acquainted with his turbulent personality, and one doctor carefully suggested that there were risks involved in the treatment.

Bethune grinned, opened his shirt, and exclaimed, "Gentlemen, I welcome the risk!"

He was to comment later that despite his criticisms of the "conservative" therapy at Trudeau it had been fortunate for him that he had been treated there. Since the sanatorium's founding near the end of the nineteenth century it had been in the vanguard of the fight against tuberculosis on the North American continent.

Most of the leading T.B. therapists at the time either trained at Trudeau or made sure they saw some service there. This included such T.B. specialists such as Dr. John Alexander and Dr. Edward Archibald, both of whom Bethune was to meet before he left the sanatorium. However, the hospital administration of the period reflected, to a great extent, the then current attitude to T.B. surgery even though Trudeau's administrators were more advanced than their contemporaries in other parts of the country.

Thus, surgery was only recommended in advanced cases, and pneumothorax treatment, which was known to the hospital staff, was still considered to be a form of therapy in its experimental stages. Before long the entire world of T.B. medicine was arguing the pros and cons of Dr. Alexander's statements and theories. It was inevitable that Alexander's views would eventually prevail, but the role Bethune was destined to play was to hasten its acceptance at Trudeau. He was ready to act as a guinea pig himself.

If some of Trudeau's staff doctors were loath to try a therapeutic procedure which they weren't entirely sure about, then they must have welcomed the opportunity of having a patient insist on it, particularly when the patient was an experienced physician who understood all the risks involved. The effect of the pneumothorax treatment was quick and dramatic. His cough faded and the sputum disappeared within a month.* He felt a new vitality seeping through him, a transformation of mood and consciousness, a steady influx of restless energy and hope.

Following the prescribed routine now to the letter, he drafted a program for the rehabilitation of T.B. patients returning to normal life. The tuberculous, he argued, were somewhat in the same fix as the war veterans. They were torn from their normal routine, their lives interrupted, and if eventually cured, returned to their homes without a single preparation to take up their old lives or begin all over again. His plan envisaged a university right in the sanatorium. The professors were to be men suffering from T.B. themselves. The students were to be patients on the way back to health. The purpose would be to fit the patients vocationally and psychologically for a world which made no provisions for their

---

* Medical records at Trudeau Sanatorium.

return. The plan was looked upon as a Utopian dream but was destined to be realized eventually.★

But he was not satisfied merely to plan rehabilitation programs. He was anxious to plant his feet firmly on the future. He began preparing for his own return. He studied avidly, kept notes on his reactions for the pneumothorax treatment, plunged deeper into surgical therapy for T.B., wrote a steady stream of letters to old friends, and took over a course in physiology and anatomy for the student nurses at the D. Ogden Mills School of Nursing sponsored by the sanatorium.

Two months after he had received his first artificial pneumothorax he was X-rayed for the last time, tapped, investigated from stem to stern, and pronounced fit to leave Trudeau. The effect of compression therapy in his case had been nothing short of miraculous — almost complete recovery in two short months!

The cavities in the lung had healed under pneumothorax and a termporary phrenicectomy.★★ There was no sign of infection. For years to come his bad lung would remain artificially collapsed.

All evening doctors and fellow patients came to the Lea to say goodbye. Then they were alone, he and his three cottagemates.

"We'll miss you," Fisher said simply. "The Lea won't be the same any more."

"And a good thing, too," Bethune laughed.

He slapped Fisher on the back affectionately, "You idiots. I would miss you too, except for one thing. I expect to see you all ... soon ... in the thriving flesh ... hale, hearty, and pneumothoraxed."

In the morning, with a firm handshake all around, the four men said their farewells. In front of the administration building, in the December snow, with the sleigh waiting, they pommeled each other, grinning like a quartet of kittens. Then he was off, standing up in the sleigh and waving his arms till he had passed through the gate and down the slope to town.

★ Ten years later a Study Craft Guild was established at Saranac Lake. "Only a few friends of Bethune," says Mrs. F.H. Heise, wife of Trudeau's medical director, "realize this is an outcome of Bethune's dream."

★★ Or phrenicotomy. The phrenic nerve is interrupted to paralyze the diaphragm. This helps to compress the diseased lung.

At the station he scrawled a cable to Frances in Edinburgh and handed it in at the telegraph office: "Cured, left Trudeau today. Am feeling the same about you as always. Will you marry me?" He had a minute left for a last look at Saranac Lake, once more covered with snow, and then he was on the train, rattling through the white hills.

He pressed his face to the window in exultation. It was real; he was leaving; he was free; he had cheated the hangman. One year ago he had come through these same hills — for the last time, he thought then, resigned to his fate, uncaring, all his farewells made. In Detroit, he reflected, he had gone under; at Trudeau he had learned once more the desire to live.

Detroit ... It seemed far away to him now. City of assembly lines, fleshpots, rich man, poor man, the American myth. He had gone under, thinking himself a lonely rebel, yet gone under because he had clung to it, trying to scrape up for himself some of its glitter and riches, writhing in his own disillusionment. Yes, it was simple to face it now, he thought cheerfully. With all his easily mouthed ideals he had put fame and fortune on the throne where medicine should have sat alone. But no more.

Never again would any living being lie under his scalpel as a remote and separate organism posing a mere problem in mechanics. A man was flesh and dreams; his knife would save the dreams as well as the flesh.

How many Fishers, Lis were still left at Trudeau! How many tens, how many hundreds of thousands would come after them! Trudeau was behind him, he thought, but for a year his mind had filled with an overwhelming picture of the suffering, the despair, the wasted lives, the careers and talents swept away by tuberculosis — all aided and abetted by some men's refusal to move into the unknown, and some men's mere indifference. But there were others, the real men of medicine — not yea-sayers or nay-sayers, not scramblers after quick profits, but seekers. And he would be among them; he swore to it himself, with his left lung collapsed in his chest but his hopes soaring: *he would be among them.*

Greater than all music, paintings, poems was their gift, the gift he now felt slumbering once more in his hands and brain: life itself, for all men equally, life for all music, paintings, poems were made. Yes, he would be among the seekers, the disturbers, the givers of life, those who had raised up his faith again. And out of his renewed faith, as the train sped through the empty fields, there formed in his mind a rich, deep affirmation. He poured out his thoughts on a sheet of paper in a paraphrase of the Apostle's Creed:

> I believe in Trudeau, mighty father of the American sanatorium, maker of heaven on earth for the tuberculous; and in Artificial Pneumothorax; which was conceived by Carson, born of the labours of Forlanini; suffered under Pompous Pride and Prejudice; was criticized by Cranks whose patients are dead and buried; thousands now well, even in their third stage, rose again from their bed; ascending into Heaven of Medicine's Immortals, they sit on the right hand of Hippocrates our Father; from thence do they judge those phthisiotherapists* quick to collapse cavities or dead on their job. I believe in Bodington, Brehmer, Koch and Brauer, in Murphy, Friedrich, Wilms, Sauerbruch, Stuertz and Jacobaeus, in the unforgiveness of the sins of omission in the Collapse Therapy, in the resurrection of a healthy body from a diseased one, and long life for the tuberculous with care everlasting. Amen.

When he had finished he leaned back in his seat and watched the passing scenery once more. His life, he reflected, was like the train: slow in getting started, but now slipping into top speed under a full head of steam.

God, he would soon be thirty-seven. What a long, winding ruin of time and wasted opportunities lay behind him! But at least it was now *behind* him; dead and decently buried in a dozen cities, the rest sloughed off at Trudeau, along with his sputum cup, staff, tubercle bacillus, uncertainties, fears. Goodbye to the ruins. Goodbye to Trudeau. Hail to the cities awaiting his return.

---

* T.B. doctors.

PART TWO

THE ENEMY — TUBERCULOSIS

10

On a cold, clear day in January 1929 Dr. Norman Bethune
walked north along Montreal's Park Avenue, turned west on Pine
Avenue, and entered the grounds of the Royal Victoria Hospital, an immense, grey building on the southern slope of Mount
Royal that looked more like a traditional Scottish castle than a
modern hospital.

Somewhere inside the great building Dr. Edward Archibald
was waiting for him. Also waiting was his new career as a thoracic surgeon. For two years Bethune had been shaping his life
toward the goal that had brought him back to his homeland. In
Detroit, where he had returned briefly from Saranac Lake to
wind up his personal affairs, former colleagues had given him a
cordial welcome. His reputation, they assured him, though built
in such a short time, had endured. He could resume his lucrative
practice where he had left off. But he was no longer interested
in Detroit, regular practice or the making of money. He told his
friends he was finished with general surgery. His sole interest
now was pulmonary tuberculosis. "Compression, early compression, and still earlier compression," became his theme song to
every doctor he met.

At his old hospital he had performed enough surgery to pay
his expenses and provide some ready money. Then he had gone
to the New York State tuberculosis hospital at Ray Brook where
he worked for close to two years.

At Ray Brook he had applied the lessons learned at Trudeau.
He also conducted a series of bacteriological experiments on
lung collapse in albino mice in collaboration with two other
doctors.* When he was satisfied that he was ready to branch out,
he wrote Archibald, and the dean of Canadian thoracic surgery
agreed to take him on as his first assistant. He arrived in Montreal with a confidence based, not on the old mystical notion of

* Doctors David T. Smith and J.L. Wilson. The results of their work were published in 1930 under the names of Smith, Bethune and Wilson in the *Journal
of Bacteriology*.

predestination, but on accomplishment. He had worked hard for two years preparing himself for tutorship under Archibald. He knew he was ready.

The Royal Victoria Hospital is medically administered by McGill University's famous Faculty of Medicine. A few months after Bethune's arrival he was appointed to the University's teaching staff. He loved to teach, and his teaching methods were unorthodox. His lectures were remembered by his students as much for his caustic comments on cliché thinking, on smug acceptance of what was allegedly known, as they were for his brilliant demonstrations of operative techniques. He enjoyed dramatizing a surgical problem in terms of the *human being* lying on the operating table. He tried to make his students see the *person* as well as the way the scalpel incised, or the way the blood vessels had to be tied. His classroom lectures and his operating theatre demonstrations were among the most popular at the University.

While working at Dr. Archibald's thoracic surgery clinic at the Royal Vic, and teaching at McGill, he took time off for occasional trips to Trudeau Sanatorium to lecture and demonstrate thoracic operative techniques.

Yet, immersed as he became in his work and his teaching, he felt a disturbing loneliness during his leisure hours at his small flat, or as he wandered through the strange streets of this second-largest French-speaking city in the world. He knew the cause well: Frances.

Since his arrival in Montreal he had often written to her. At first he had been uncertain about her reaction, but he had given himself up to the yearning he could no longer suppress. It was his old self that had been entangled in the wreck of their marriage, but his old self, he reasoned, was now gone. Everything he had done for two years seemed to draw him back inevitably to her. It was as if his life followed two lines: she was one, the other was his work.

He poured all his loneliness into his letters, writing about everything, even the most minute details of his daily routine, as if nothing that he did or saw or thought could be fully experienced unless he shared it with her. Where his letters had once been filled with rebukes, or remorse, or unhappiness, or apologies, or desperate pleas, now he wrote more calmly, more tenderly, with a note of deep longing breaking out unexpectedly in the midst of descriptions of Montreal or accounts of his work. In a typical letter he wrote:

> I get up at nine, and have coffee, toast, and marmalade. Walk to the hospital (25 minutes along Sherbrooke Street) and do clinical work (surgery, etc.) till one. Lunch at the hospital. Research from two to three. Then home to bed till six. Up and make dinner. Then bed again at eleven or twelve after an evening of reading. Once in a while go to the pictures or a hockey match....
>
> My health is excellent. I had an X-ray today and it shows no disease or cavity present; nothing except healed scars.
>
> I've often thought I should like to surprise you one morning by waiting at the corner of the street for you as you walked down for the car. I'd just say "Hello — let's go for a walk."

In her replies Frances wondered tactfully whether they had really changed enough to overcome old difficulties. He replied for himself in a gentle note: "I am getting quieter and quieter! You wouldn't know me now, I swear."

As Frances still expressed fears about the possibility of joining him once more his loneliness began to oppress him. He wrote once:

> Last Sunday, having been in bed with a bad cold, I got very tired of the flat and took the train at 8:35 in the morning with my skis for the mountains (forty miles north of the city). Skied six miles. Lunch in the woods and then back to the station and home again at nine and so to bed.
>
> Today I feel much better. The skiing stopped my cough! It was very lovely in the Laurentians — like Switzerland. The train was just like the trains in Vienna. Do you remember when you and I used to go to the country? — The same

lovely young people eating sandwiches out of paper bags and going to sleep on each other's shoulders coming home. My skiing was bloody awful. I fell all over the place....

How often can I say it? I love you. I wait for you.

Your

BETH

Her letters became more affectionate, but still she tried to reason with him. They had failed so miserably before, how could they know it would work out now? She loved him too; she too was lonely; but she was terribly afraid.

But he could wait no longer. "Why should we be separate when we love each other? I can be happy with you ... But you not with me? I have been thinking that if you came, we can start out by meeting just as friends, living apart. Perhaps that is the only way for us."

Her next letter, by return mail, was only a few lines. Hang the doubts, the misery of waiting! She was packing for the trip to Montreal.

She arrived in the summer, and he had arranged everything. Though they had discussed living apart, in their last letters, taking their time to find out how matters stood between them, now he rushed her off to a clergyman. They were married again.

With Frances back, he felt that all was renewed. He was the full man now. Marriage, love, his work — and soon children, children to fulfill them both.

There had been a purpose in everything, he told himself then. A purpose to his mad searchings, disillusionment, collapse and rebirth. All of it had shaped and directed him. He had passed his fortieth birthday. The years to come would redeem the years gone to waste. He had little time left, but he knew now what he hadn't known when he lay dying in Detroit. Some day he would be gone, but perhaps after him no one ever again would need to die of tuberculosis.

11

The quiet of the operating theatre was suddenly shattered by a loud oath. The nurses and assistants looked up to find Bethune standing rigidly beside the operating table, one hand still holding a clamp projecting out of the patient's back, the other raised with a rib stripper. He was glaring at the stripper, his eyes dark above the mask that gave his face a ghoulish appearance.

"Blasted idiocy!" He threw the stripper savagely across the room.

After the operation was over he quietly picked up the instrument. In the privacy of his office he laid it on his desk, studied it for a long time, and then made a series of sketches. When he was satisfied he had what he wanted, he called the hospital mechanic.

"Look," he said, tossing him the instrument, "I've got some sketches here I'd like to give you. I want to make some changes in that silly thing." His finger traced the outlines of one of the drawings.

A week later the mechanic returned with the redesigned stripper. Dr. Archibald himself tested it during his next thoracoplasty, pronounced it a definite improvement, and from then on it became standard equipment in the clinic's chest surgery.

The designing of a modified rib stripper was only one of many indications, to those who worked with him, that the pupil was quickly becoming the inventor, the innovator. Working under Dr. Archibald convinced Bethune that the latter was one of the greatest thoracic surgeons on the continent. But for the obscure doctor who set himself the task of completely defeating tuberculosis, the necessity of learning everything to be learned was coupled with the necessity of resting content with nothing. Existing knowledge was the storehouse of the past; it had to be thoroughly explored — and constantly extended.

Even as he first began taking over complicated cases from Dr. Archibald he was already reaching out along new paths. His mind teemed with new techniques, new approaches, designs for new instruments, along which the rib stripper was almost incidental. No sooner did he master a surgical procedure than he was dissatisfied with it, searching for possible improvements. Archibald was frequently impressed with his assistant's unrelenting demand for the application of modern technology to the operating theatre.

Before he had performed his first operation by himself at the clinic he had already produced a new apparatus for artificial pneumothorax. Dissatisfied even with this, he added a foot pump and a mechanism for drawing off fluid from the pleural cavity, thus giving the apparatus a two-in-one purpose. The machine was constructed by the hospital mechanic and was soon used fairly extensively in other hospitals, including the Gravenhurst sanatorium where Bethune had spent a month in 1926.*

One day, after a thoracoplasty during which Archibald operated and Bethune exhausted himself holding the retractors (instruments for holding the wound open), he decided the current technique was altogether too primitive. In the next few weeks he designed two mechanical arms which could be fastened to any table in a matter of seconds, did the job more effectively than any human agency, and released an assistant for other work. He called the new device the Iron Intern.**

He had a profound admiration for the surgical instruments bequeathed by the masters of surgery, and an equally profound contempt for doctors whose minds were sealed to change and the possibilities of new techniques. "They are sinking slowly into quicksand and don't even know it," he would say. Men like Sauerbruch, Lilienthal and Stille, for example, had developed shears to cut the first rib which he considered works of art. But the all-purpose rib shears made him angry. Every time he used it he swore under his breath and retreated to his office to sketch numerous designs for a new instrument. The problem had aroused his

---

* Since there were already some 25 pneumothorax machines already in existence, produced in various parts of the world by masters of pulmonary surgery techniques, use of Bethune's machine was a rare tribute to its inventor.

** He used it effectively at a clinic which he later headed himself. It was also fully described and illustrated in the Dec. 1936 issue of the official publication of the Canadian Medical Association.

interest even back at Ray Brook Sanatorium. But each new type he made up was as clumsy or as heavy or as oversharp as the type it was designed to replace.

He found the key to the problem through the unorthodoxy that so often disturbed other doctors.

He was collecting a pair of shoes that had been resoled one day when he noticed the shoemaker using an interesting device for cutting nails out of shoes. If only resecting ribs, he reflected, were as simple as mending shoes. He turned to leave, and was struck by a sudden thought. He asked to look at the shears. The surprised shoemaker passed them over the counter.

A few minutes later Bethune burst into the apartment shouting "I've got it!" He took from his pocket the pair of shears which he had purchased from the shoemaker and laid it triumphantly on a table. "There. That's the answer. Staring the whole damn profession in the face, and nobody ever thought of it. A gift from the United Shoe Machinery Company to the operating theatre."

Frances was accustomed, as of old, to have him come home with new paintings, hats, books or art objects of all kinds. But this was no art object. "I hope you know exactly what you're being so ecstatic about, but all I see is a vicious-looking tool."

"Precisely," Bethune said happily. "A vicious tool. And in two weeks' time it will be a pair of nice, shiny rib shears that will simply sing through the ribs...."

During the next few days he spent his spare moments studying the cobbler's shears and drafting sketches. In the end, the Bethune Rib Shears, as it was to be known, appeared for its first test at the clinic. It was essentially the shoemaker's tool, but modified to suit its new purpose. The handles were made nine times longer than the jaws to give powerful cutting leverage, the points were somewhat blunted, a stiffer steel was used, and rubber grips were put on the handles. The instrument was an immediate success.

"The surgeon," Bethune often said, "who can't see the hints and answers that nature and the world thrust into his face should be digging ditches, not massacring the human body."

Before a bit of truth or unsuspected knowledge he was humble; as a partisan of the ideas and technical innovations forever tumbling from his agile mind he was aggressive; sometimes, to those about him, even disturbingly violent. In one case, when surgery was being discussed for a patient with adhesions from the lung and chest wall, which prevent the lung from collapsing when compression is desired, he proposed a new method he had developed for cutting the adhesions. The method was highly complicated, and involved the insertion into the pleural cavity of two slender tubes. Through one the operator could both illuminate and look into the pleural cavity. The other was a mechanism which, with delicate manipulation, fastened silver clips on each adhesion. The adhesions were cut through *between* the clips, the clips then acting like "tourniquets" and preventing the severed stumps from hemorrhaging. With the adhesions gone, the lung could be collapsed by artificial pneumothorax.

The technique was novel and intricate. Dr. Archibald was skeptical, but Bethune argued for it with the vehemence for which he was noted. In the end Dr. Archibald gave in, saying Bethune was as stubborn as a mule, but that if his method didn't work he would be the first to admit it.

The method worked and Bethune soon described and illustrated it for the medical journals. But he was finally convinced, after much experimentation, that it was inferior to the electrocoagulation procedure (cutting through the adhesions with an electrically heated metal implement) and presented his new views frankly in the Canadian Medical Association Journal.

The question of adhesions *in reverse* sent him off into one of his most interesting experiments. There were times when it was desirable, they found at the clinic, as others had also found, to *induce* adhesions between lung and chest wall in order to prevent sections of the lung from collapsing in certain forms of surgery. Many investigators had grappled with the problem, usually with poor results. Bethune developed a number of methods of actually causing adhesions to develop, but most brought complications that made them untenable. In the end he carried on experiments with six dogs and six cats. In these experiments he established that the introduction of ordinary talc-iodine powder on the desired lung surfaces (blown in through a hollow needle) quickly caused these surfaces to fasten themselves onto the chest walls through the quick growth of connective adhesions.★ These adhesions, in turn, prevented collapse of the lung areas involved. They developed, under Bethune's method, without infection or other complications in the pleural cavity. Dr. Archibald considered the Bethune Pleural Poudrage, as it came to be known, "a distinct advance." He also had no hesitation in declaring that the Poudrage and other innovations "make Bethune's genius in mechanical inventions an established fact." ★★

As his exploring mind sent him probing to the roots of one problem after another, a few men in the profession said that he was too avid for "spectacular" results, mechanical innovations — and too little interested in the effects on the patient. His public reactions to the whisperings was one of complete indifference; underneath his perpetual composure the insinuations made him writhe. Those close to him knew that there was nothing h e would attempt on a patient that he wouldn't attempt first on himself.

During the period in which his left lung was kept collapsed he experimented endlessly on himself with his pneumothorax apparatus, sampling every possible manner of making pneumothorax more efficient and every possible reaction on the patient. He had his own phrenic nerve tied again to revive the memory of what happened to the patient and to test the effectiveness of phrenicectomy.★★★ When the problem came up as to whether the presence of blood in the lungs would show on X-rays he decided to find out for himself. He withdrew blood from his arm, injected it into the tracheobronchial tree, and had himself X-rayed. The blood cast no shadow on the films. The test was not necessarily conclusive, but it revealed his approach to experimentation and illustrated his readiness to continue in the role of guinea pig as well as investigator.

★ Published later, Feb. 1935, *Journal of Thoracic Surgery*.

★★ Letter to authors, 1943.

★★★ The operation was done not only to observe the regenerative powers of the phrenic nerve but also because he was convinced that his own condition indicated the procedure at the time. This was a radical phrenicectomy with resection of the accessory phrenic nerve.

When one of the patients at the hospital died of obscure symptoms, Bethune was puzzled by strange foreign matter he found in the lungs during the post-mortem. He had a mould made for laboratory tests but these drew a blank. In an effort to discover whether the foreign matter was tuberculous he then injected some of the mould into a rabbit. When nothing happened to the rabbit he rubbed some of the mould onto his own ear. The astonished laboratory technicians were petrified at the thought of what he might have done to himself. A few weeks later he presented himself again. "Well," he asked genially, "what did you think it was?" Looking at him anxiously they confessed they didn't know. Had he discovered anything? "Nothing," he replied. "Not a damn thing's happened. Anyway, it wasn't tuberculosis, or I wouldn't be so cheerful about it. So we can conclude that in a negative sense, the experiment was successful."

Whatever the incidents of the experiments indicated to his colleagues, in the chronology of Bethune's rapidly developing career, they dovetailed with formal confirmation of his significance as an innovator.

In the summer of 1931, a year after he had launched himself along new paths under Dr. Archibald, he was buttonholed one day by a middle-aged American of dignified bearing at a medical convention in Montreal. The American introduced himself as George P. Pilling. He had for some time been trying to meet Bethune, he said, and had come to Montreal for two reasons: first, to attend the current medical convention, and second, to meet Bethune.

Mr. Pilling was the head of the Philadelphia firm of Pilling and Sons, internationally known manufacturers of surgical instruments. "I have seen some of your instruments, Dr. Bethune," he said approvingly, "and I would like to propose a contract under which we would have exclusive rights to the manufacture and distribution of all your medical inventions."

Next day Bethune arrived at Pilling's hotel room, marched in, seated himself at a desk, said, "Let's hear your contract terms," and started sketching on a pad. Pilling watched, fascinated at the rapidity with which Bethune sketched. Bethune looked up, "Don't mind me," he said. "I can listen to you while I work."

While Pilling outlined his firm's proposed royalty arrangements, Bethune continued his sketching. The American finished, somewhat uncertain that he had made himself understood. Without a break in his sketching, Bethune said, "It's a deal," and then launched into a long dissertation on what was wrong with modern surgical instruments.

The gist of his remarks was that surgery was partly in the van of twentieth-century technological development and partly in the Middle Ages. Surgery's best minds had successfully introduced breathtaking reforms, yet often seemed bogged down by prejudice and inertia. Surgeons too often blindfolded themselves to industrial developments which could make possible all types of new instruments for the operating room. There was a need to attack prejudice, lack of vision, indifference — a need for a fresh approach, based on the most advanced changes in technology, and even to make *demands* upon technology. "We need, in short, a spring cleaning in the operating room," he concluded.

Impressed by the lecture, Mr. Pilling suggested that Bethune write a medical paper on modern surgical instruments.

"I plan to do just that," Bethune announced and handed Pilling a sheaf of papers which bore the rough sketches of his pneumothorax apparatus and half a dozen other instruments.*

Mr. Pilling took cordial leave of his visitor and soon his firm was advertising the Bethune Pneumothorax Apparatus, the Bethune Rib Shears, and an assortment of other Bethune instruments. For Bethune it was to presage a new eminence. The pupil had already established himself as a master in his own right. Henceforth, wherever medical men warred against tuberculosis across the continent, the instruments bearing his name were among their indispensable weapons.

---

* He later described his inventions in the *Journal of the Canadian Medical Association*, Dec. 1936.

12

The course he had set himself stretched straight ahead. For the doctor and man reborn at Trudeau nothing seemed unattainable. Then suddenly everything collapsed. After one year of their second marriage, Frances asked for a divorce.

For the first few months of their second marriage, all had gone relatively well. Even as the old conflicts emerged once more in the routine of daily living, a deep bond remained between them. But with mixed feelings of fear and frustration, both sensed that the pattern their first marriage had followed was reasserting itself.

Neither one could isolate the exact cause, but Frances especially found herself growing increasingly restive and unhappy.

Were they simply unsuited for one another? Then what about the affection they shared, and which emerged with powerful force during their moments of reconciliation? Vaguely, both perceived the conflict was a combination of many things.

To begin with, there was Bethune's overwhelming sense of dedication. It overflowed into their marriage, making her feel she shared only a corner of his life, stifling her sometimes with the demands that it made upon her own life. Like his mother, like Eleanor Dell, she, too, was convinced he was destined for greatness and vaguely, broodingly, she often felt she was holding him back, that she was "not good" for him. With these feelings came another — that he was "not good" for her!

One afternoon she came home to find him sitting cross-legged on the floor, studying a miniature skeleton. She had asked him in the morning if he would mind shopping for her, and now she said "Did you remember to buy the meat for dinner?"

"Yes," he replied absently, "it's in the refrigerator."

When she opened the refrigerator door her gaze fell, not on the lamb chops but on a human intestine he had brought home from the hospital to study at his leisure. She gasped in horror, and that might have ended the incident, but it didn't. Somehow it stayed with her, bringing into focus many things she had kept even from herself. He had his work; he lived with it even when things went badly between them. She, however, had only their life together, and when that fell apart she had nothing.

Perhaps even then they might have gone on, content to be together despite all the recurring tensions. But unexpectedly Frances found herself awakening to the possibility of life with another man that could be as normal as she had once desired.

She spoke her mind frankly to Bethune. Under the circumstances she felt she could no longer live with him, and asked for a divorce. His reaction was a series of climactic gestures. First he staggered her with an outburst of scorching anger. Then he staggered her with an outburst of magnanimity. If she could be happy only with another man then she must have a divorce immediately.

Outwardly composed and the soul of affability, Bethune was now quite miserable. He divided his free time between a feverish social whirl and lonely brooding. At the hospital his colleagues noticed that he grew daily more irritable. He kept assuring Frances that her new marriage would have his hearty approval, but when a friend visited his room one day and noticed a huge doll in the corner, Bethune said bitterly, "That? That's Alice in Wonderland. Sole issue of my marriage. Frances and I have an understanding about her. She is to spend six months with me and six months with Frances...."

Out of all the years of love and longing he had been left only with a doll.

13

In the spring of 1933 an opportunity arose for Bethune to take temporary charge of the thoracic department of one of the largest hospitals in the United States, the Herman Kiefer Hospital in Detroit. The hospital's thoracic surgery chief, Dr. Edward O'Brien, had been seriously injured in an automobile accident and when the problem of a replacement arose, he suggested Bethune.

Bethune knew the position would only last until Dr. O'Brien recovered, but he took it because it gave him the opportunity of doing things his own way in as head of a department. With mixed feelings he said goodbye to Dr. Archibald, "the man who taught me more than any other doctor," and left for Detroit.

Here, for the better part of a year, he did all the thoracic surgery on Dr. O'Brien's service at the Herman Kiefer Hospital, the Maybury Sanatorium, Northville, and the American Legion Hospital, Battle Creek. The experience was invaluable.

Instead of returning to Montreal on O'Brien's return, Bethune went on a barnstorming trip across the states, demonstrating his surgical techniques and comparing notes with other surgeons.

When he returned to Montreal in the spring of 1934, he considered himself a better surgeon than he had ever been, but there were no other hospital appointments available. In the years after Trudeau he had never bothered about building up a private practice because he had concentrated himself as a surgeon. He had accomplished what he had set out to do but in the process, as he wrote one of his friends, he had gone "stone broke."

The man whose surgical instruments had won numerous testimonials, who had just demonstrated his advanced techniques to American doctors, whose medical articles were closely studied — was now looking for a job. He began a series of formal letters to hospitals, sanatoriums, and friends, announcing that his services were available. A number of hospitals replied, each promising that "when the occasion arises, in view of your excellent credentials, we will keep you in mind."

It was a time of universal retrenchment. Economic depression was stalking the continent. The incidence of sickness was rising sharply among all sections of the population, but the wealth of America was rusting, hospital staffs were being cut, and there seemed no room anywhere for a surgeon who had already made his mark.

Then, unexpectedly, he received a letter from the Sacré Coeur Hospital, in reply to his routine application, granting him an appointment as head of a new chest surgery department the hospital was setting up.

He accepted, and wrote Dr. B in a swift rise of good spirits:

> I was appointed Thoracic Surgeon and Bron-
> choscopist to the Sacré Coeur Hospital in
> Cartierville; 450 beds, 20 miles from Montreal.
> French-Canadian and Catholic. $1,200 a year,
> one day a week, so the strain is less strained. My
> title is: *Chef dans les Services de Chirurgie Pulmo-*
> *nare et de Bronchoscopie!* I am going to have a
> nice big white cap made with "Chef" marked
> in front. Really, I am delighted. No chest sur-
> gery has been done here up to date with the
> exception of phrenics as curiosities. I cauterized
> some adhesions there yesterday and the chorus
> of oh's and ah's from the nuns rose like a chant
> at the high altar.

Sacré Coeur stood behind great lawns and gardens along the
Cartierville highway. While there had been no chest or pulmonary surgery done at the hospital, now, under Bethune's direction,
the new department became one of the most important of the
hospital's services.

He was in many ways a disturbing phenomenon in the Catholic institution. Unlike the conventional doctor who, he was fond
of saying, "dresses like a cross between a mortician and a maître
d'hôtel," he often turned up in a pork-pie hat, dark shirt, silk tie,
English tweed jacket, expertly tailored, and grey flannels. At first
the nuns were scandalized; then they accepted him; then they loved
him. Soon his connection with Sacré Coeur became permanent.

Being in charge of the chest department, he was in a position
to try all his ideas and techniques without hindrance. He refined
and developed many of the innovations he had introduced at the
Royal Victoria under Dr. Archibald. He designed and introduced
numerous new operating instruments.

His clinic grew from nothing to the point where it was treating as many as 1,100 tubercular patients in a single year. Under
his supervision close to 300 major and minor chest operations
were eventually being performed annually, including as many as
73 thoracoplasties in a single twelve-month period.

The steady operating routine stimulated rather than dulled his zeal for experiment and new attacks on tuberculosis. His old energy was back, renewing his appetite for work. He could stay up most of the night with friends, operate in the morning, do experimental work in the afternoon, and make the round of his patients in between. If confronted with a case for which there was no precedent in medical literature, he improvised with breathtaking audacity.

In one case he was called in as consultant for an elderly male patient at the Royal Victoria Hospital. The patient had been operated on two years before for the draining of a large amount of pus from the right chest space. Now he had severe pain again in the same area and it was established that the infection had recurred. One of the difficulties involved was the advanced age of the patient and the fear that he might not be able to withstand extended surgery. The extent of the infection was indicated when Bethune removed 500 cubic centimeters of pus from the chest by aspiration (literally, sucked out through a hollow needle). Laboratory tests showed the presence of streptococci and other bacilli, but no tubercle bacilli. Studying the case, and taking into account the patient's age and absence of tuberculosis, Bethune decided on a novel treatment. He cut through to the pocket of infection and kept the wound open to drain for nine days. On the tenth day he introduced a test-tubeful of live maggots directly into the open wound, covered it securely with a wire screen, and suspended an electric light near the screen to drive the maggots into the depths of the wound.

He was basing this treatment on something known but mostly ignored since the days of Ambroïse Paré (1509–1590): Neglected wounds infested by maggots tend to heal rather than become worse. Controlled experiments had on several occasions established that maggots seemed to "eat" infection. Now Bethune, with nothing but maggots in the patient's wound, waited for results.

The day after being screened in the maggots showed themselves very lively. Two days later they were still lively, but less so, and were also larger. The discharge from the wound now was markedly less and thinner. The next day the maggots were dead and the discharge even more improved, with many less streptococci showing up in laboratory tests and the exposed lung surface taking on a healthy appearance. The dead maggots were washed out with saline solution and two days later new living maggots were introduced once more. Six days later, when these maggots were in turn washed out, the cavity originally established by the infection had been reduced five times. Six days later the patient was out of bed, and two weeks later, with the cavity fully closed, he was discharged from the hospital with no further recurrence of his troublesome infection. It was the first time maggots had been so used.*

Bethune experimented further along the same lines. He published his findings in the March 1935 *Canadian Medical Association Journal* and the *Journal of Thoracic Surgery*.

There were the years now of work, growth, achievement and recognition. He was his own master. He could follow his own leads and set up his own goals. His temper came into conflict with no superior authority. He was free to put his views into practice and could argue them against all comers on equal terms.

He became a frequent contributor to the medical journals, sometimes departing from the conventional patterns of medical writing to raise controversial issues. He was a well-known figure at continental gatherings of chest surgeons, and came to be numbered among the top few. Only four years after he had begun to work under Dr. Archibald he was elected to the Council of the American Association for Thoracic Surgery. He sat on the council alongside Dr. John Alexander, whose book had so profoundly influenced his outlook while he was still at Trudeau Sanatorium. As his reputation grew he was appointed consultant to the sanatorium at St. Agathe des Monts, and to the health departments of the Federal and Provincial governments. And as Sacré Coeur expanded its role in the surgical treatment of tuberculosis in French Canada, he himself began to branch out from the techniques of surgical treatment to a theoretical evaluation of the disease.

---

* It should be recalled that this was before the development of sulfa or the various antibiotics.

Just as he had become dissatisfied with the fears about radical treatment when he himself was dying, he now became dissatisfied with what he considered a piecemeal approach to the disease. He declared in all his writings that it was necessary to abandon the idea that T.B. was merely a disease of the lungs. It was in reality a disease of the body. The bacillus's attack on the lungs was the end product of the environment's attack on the whole organism. "Any scheme to cure this disease," he often said, "which does not consider man as a whole, as the resultant of environmental strain and stress, is bound to fail."

In the middle of 1932 he had first published his *Plea for Early Compression in Pulmonary Tuberculosis*. Restating the thesis that the final cure might come through a direct attack on the tubercle bacillus, he held that T.B. could be wiped out before that time. He continued to argue that early, rather than late, compression of the affected lung should be attempted in order to permit the body to throw off the disease. "Pulmonary tuberculosis," he said, "shows an inherent tendency, a willingness for recovery, which when considered beside chronic heart, kidney or liver diseases which show little or no tendency to cure, makes it unique among the diseases of long duration affecting man.... We, as a people, can get rid of tuberculosis, when we make up our minds it is worthwhile to spend enough money to do so. Better education of doctors, public education ... enforced periodic physical and X-ray examinations, early diagnosis, early bed-rest, early compression, isolation and protection of the young are our remedies."

His attitude towards conservatism and inertia in the profession grew more and more critical. The refusal to move forward, he declared, was taking its toll in lost lives and in the end forcing expenditure of state money on illnesses and hospitalization that could have been avoided. Those who opposed "active treatment" for early precavernous and frankly cavernous tuberculosis were merely echoing "objections raised at the beginning of the century against operations for appendicitis." Precautionary measures, early diagnosis, early treatment and full utilization of surgical procedures — these were his constant cry.

At Sacré Coeur his ideas brought encouraging results. Cases which ten, perhaps even five years earlier might have been considered hopeless were either cured by surgical techniques or substantially improved. But as he studied the figures on incoming patients and the percentage of those released as cured, a strange contradiction, at first vague but then unmistakable, began to vex him. "There's something wrong," he would say. "The more advanced our curative surgery, the more cases of T.B. we get. Precisely at the moment when scientific knowledge on how to attack the disease has reached its highest point, the incidence of the disease has equally reached its highest point." In the province of Quebec there was a higher percentage of T.B. cases than in any other Canadian province. There were more victims than the hospitals and sanatoriums could accommodate. The province with the lowest standard of living had the highest T.B. rate. And throughout the country, in the city slums and bankrupt farm hinterlands, there were many thousands of people slowly succumbing before the disease without even knowing they had it.

Why? The question made him uneasy even as he continued to expound his theory of early lung compression. His search for the answers led him to another disease that was engulfing the world — a disease more deadly than tubercle bacillus and swifter than medieval cholera.

Like any other serious medical practitioner he had always known that T.B. fed on poverty. But now poverty, for some reason, seemed to be spreading everywhere, spewing forth ten new cases of T.B. infection for every single case he and other doctors cured. Now when he asked himself why, the answer beckoned him along many strange, new and disturbing paths.

The papers were full of crisis, depression, bankruptcy, unemployment, relief, controversy. In October 1929 there had been a tremor on the New York stock market, and then much more than a tremor. There had been no need, of course, for undue alarm — so everybody had assured everybody else — but without undue alarm banks, factories and mines had fallen into bankruptcy like a house of cards, and the prophets of "cautious optimism" had followed one another out of the high windows of their Wall Street offices.

Bethune had, of course, been aware of some economic malaise that was causing a lot of discussion, but it was one of those cyclical things, the economists said, and would soon straighten itself out. Now, however, five years had passed; nothing was straightening itself out. The man who had set out to cure T.B. became obsessed by the fear that all his nice theories, so practical in the operating theatre, were being undermined outside the operating theatre.

One million people, a tenth of the entire Canadian population,* were dependent on government relief. When Bethune read of the living standards of the unemployed his indignation rose at the revelation that the families of the unemployed lived on a government stipend of $1.20 a week per adult and 80 cents a week per child. That was obviously ridiculous and would have to be changed. But when he said so, his colleagues looked at him as if he were a little touched in the head. Didn't he know that it was the same everywhere? And indeed he found that it was. While presidents and ministers talked of "prosperity around the corner," unemployment, bankruptcy and fear gripped every continent. Dislocation and collapse stretched from Spain, where Primo de Rivera ruled through military dictatorship; to Germany, where a strange creature and a strange movement, Hitler and National Socialism, had seized power; to China, where Chiang Kai-shek was busily reducing the population by massacres of opposition elements; to Japan, where a militarist clique dreamed of ruling all Asia.

To Bethune it began to appear as if some mass mania had laid hold of the world. Night seemed to be day and day never seemed to come. "Pull in your belts," cabinet spokesmen of ample girth advised, and stopped counting when the number of unemployed around the globe hit 40,000,000. It was a simple matter of overproduction, they said, but everywhere the people had nothing.

In the world at large he noted a disturbing contradiction. Millions were without clothes, and the United States ploughed under its own cotton fields. Tens of millions were hungry, but Canada burned its wheat. On street corners men begged a nickel for a cup of coffee, but Brazil dumped its coffee into the ocean. In Montreal's working-class districts the children were bowlegged with rickets, but oranges from the South were destroyed by the carload. And from the head of the Canadian Medical Association came a warning that disaster lay ahead for the profession and the

---

* By 1952 Canada's population exceeded 14,000,000.

people of Canada unless emergency measures were taken to provide medical services for the majority of citizens who couldn't afford to pay, and for the doctors who couldn't afford to treat their patients without payment.

One night Bethune stood before the easel he had set up in the living room of his apartment, daubing away idly, trying to catch the night scene through his large windows overlooking Beaver Hall Square. He had had the windows put in himself, replacing smaller ones which had not let in enough light. At night he could look out and see the lower city, at the foot of Beaver Hall Hill, the lights of the harbor, and the massive skyscrapers which were centred just south and west of the apartment. From his window the sound of tugboats on the St. Lawrence were distinct and mournful. Northwards ran St. Catherine Street, the busiest street in the city around him, and now he tried to catch the feeling of it on canvas.

He daubed away but was dissatisfied with what he had painted and replaced the canvas with a clean one. Then he sat down at his typewriter. He had for some time been turning over in his mind a statement of the doubts and fears gnawing at him. He thought of the hundreds of people coming into his ward, and wondered whether their charts should be labelled "pulmonary tuberculosis" or "economic poverty." At Trudeau it had seemed clear to him that surgery would be the answer to T.B. Now nothing seemed clear, except ... Yes, one thing, at least, seemed clear.

Tuberculosis, he wrote, was the specific response of the human organism to a specific environment. Well, that was hardly new; it had to be stated more precisely. Trudeau had written: "There is a rich man's tuberculosis and a poor man's tuberculosis." That, he reflected, was what now needed to be said again, and would have to be shouted from the rooftops. "There is a rich man's tuberculosis and a poor man's tuberculosis. The rich man recovers and the poor man dies. This succinctly expresses the close embrace of economics and pathology." The conditions breeding T.B. in man were spreading. "Let him persist in continuing in such an environment and he will die!"

Men, women, and children were dying every year of T.B. He had no way of helping them. As a surgeon he never even saw them, and even if it were physically possible to get enough doctors to handle them, others would follow from the same homes, the same streets, the same cities. It was necessary to sound a warning!

"The incurable tuberculous who will fill our sanatoriums for the next five years are now waling the streets, working at desks with early curable tuberculosis ... Lack of time and money kills more cases of pulmonary disease than lack of resistance to that disease. The poor man dies because he cannot afford to live. Here the economist and sociologist meet the compressionist on common ground."

He reread what he had written with a sense of frustration. What did he know of economics or surgery? He had spent most of his life becoming a surgeon; as a surgeon he could heal the human body, not the whole damn stupid mess called society. "We, as physicians," he continued, "can do but little to change the external environmental forces which predispose to infection and re-infection. Poverty, poor food, unsanitary surroundings, contact with infectious foci, overwork and mental strain are beyond our control. Essential and radical adjustments of these are problems for the economists and sociologists."*

He reread the article many times. Did it say anything new and worthwhile? Did it make sense? Or was he moving into still another blind alley?

He felt satisfied with what he had written, with himself, with everything. Perhaps he was simply *thinking* too much about things he didn't understand. He went back to his easel.

He painted long into the night, at breakneck speed, his depression gradually slipping away. When he was finished he felt tired but relaxed. He stood away from the easel and studied his work with satisfaction.

Dominating the centre of the canvas was an impressionistic Godhead, a powerful embodiment of justice and impartiality. Before him, humbly, fearfully, stood a surgeon, awaiting the final verdict. Surrounding the surgeon were the spirits of men and

---

* Published later in *Canadian Medical Association Journal*.

women he had treated on earth, pointing at him, crying out to God in their agony and wrath.

Across the back of the canvas he penciled the title: "The Surgeon at the Day of Judgment."

14

He had become a successful surgeon, a social lion, an available bachelor, a prize catch for a never-ending cycle of endless soirees. Snobs, cynics, and socialites pursued him, yet felt out of their depths when they captured him.

Among some of his colleagues, for whom the pillars of life were a comfortable home, payment of the mortgage, insurance and a growing bank account, his improvidence was staggering. He earned a lot of money — and spent it all. Even Frances, after all these years, could still gasp at some of his gifts. He bought everything that pleased him, no matter what the cost. He was especially a boon to struggling young Montreal artists, whose work he bought on sight if it pleased him. To those who found his freehanded dispensing of money disturbing he had a ready reply: "Money? Only the medium of exchange."

When he met a colleague given to pontificating about his profession he liked to say that the surgeon was no different from a plumber, except that he wasn't always as skilled. If he was with a group of people who bored him he left without ceremony or excuses. "He's a terribly exhausting man to know," one of his friends said resignedly after one of his typically swift arrivals and departures.

His apartment on Beaver Hall Hill was furnished with sybaritic touches — an echo to his early hedonistic days in London. The furniture was of his own design. The paintings included his own and those of many young Canadian artists. Books overflowed every room. The *objets d'art*, the rugs, the drapes had been selected with an eye for colour, design and quality. But just as his turtle-neck sweaters satirized the dinner jackets of stuffy acquaintances, so the sensuous appearance of his home was lightened by a satiric quality all his own. His diplomas, often the carefully displayed self-advertisement of the doctor, were consigned to his bathroom walls.

Nothing that pleased him was too expensive for his purse. Yet all his friends knew that there was nothing that pleased him that he didn't delight in sharing. Every book in his astonishing library carried a simply designed bookplate with the legend, "This book belongs to Norman Bethune and his friends." As with his books, so with his home. Artists who laboured in obscure poverty, actors who in the existing state of Canadian arts dreamed only of raising enough money to go to New York or London, bright young people who had yet to taste economic security — all were welcome, and all discerned a genuine affection beneath the airy affability with which he received them. Sometimes they would congregate while he was dressing in his bedroom. They would read his books, play his records, and he would come out, and say cheerfully: "I'm off to attend a patient. There's food in the refrigerator and liquor in the bathroom. Have fun while I'm away."

He startled even his closest friends with Shavian sallies against the smugness of ownership. One evening a young lady brought to his apartment by a mutual acquaintance was struck by a pair of vivid drapes over the window. They were long, full, and made of blood-red velveteen.

"You like them?" he asked.

"They're wonderful!"

He picked up a pair of scissors, cut away half of one of the hangings, and tossed it across the room to her. "My own selection," he said.

"What have you done!" she cried.

He looked at her sideways, veiling his amusement. "I've given you something you like. What else?"

Among the gossips — and those who knew him only from a distance — there was a good deal of eyebrow-raising about his "antics" with women. His attitude was frank and often disconcerting to the strait-laced. He looked appreciatively at every neat ankle that passed his way. His comments were uniformly uninhibited in the street, the living room and at the dinner table. "What a magnificent pair of hips...." "What a pelvis for childbearing...." "What a beautiful back for a thoracoplasty...."

He loved beauty as the artist, the doctor, the man. But more than beauty, the *minds* of women intrigued him. "Did you ever get so bored with a woman," he once asked a startled colleague, "that you had to make love to her?"

Renée Adorée, a beautiful Hollywood film star of the period, for whom he devised a special phrenicectomy necklace when she was suffering from T.B.,* credited him with transforming her whole life in their conversations before and after the operation. In a felicitous poem she wrote to him after her recovery she said that everything meaningful in her life she now owed to him.

Theories about the "special mind" of women angered him. "Women have been slaves too long," he often said, "I am tired of the idiots who try to keep 'explaining' the female mind. The female mind is a human mind. Under inhuman conditions it will suffer. The myths created about the so-called female mind are kept alive by men who would like to keep women in bondage."

Hypocrisy between the sexes irritated him as much as pompousness in the medical profession. He could shatter airs and "respectability" with deadly sarcasm, yet astonished those who showed him the least affection with a paternal tenderness.

Most people who attempted to define him floundered among all the catchwords. He was mad, some said; vain, charming, irresponsible, sensitive, arrogant, a loyal friend, a great surgeon, a showman, a genius, a demanding child — in short, a zigzagging comet of a man flashing in and out of the lives of many people, leaving some enchanted, some disturbed, some grateful, some saddened, some angered, and some exultant, but none untouched.

There were a few who truly knew him — a few who had come close to the son of evangelists, the one-time patient meditating on death and man's fate at Trudeau Sanatorium, the one-time disciple of Pater and Giotto.

There was Frances, whom he still called "my wife." Sometimes it would seem to her that she had deserted him, that all would have gone well had she only given him more love. But whatever her tortured thoughts, lying awake at night, or

---

* He performed the operation on Miss Adorée in Tucson, Arizona.

meeting the procession of people he brought for her approval, she knew … knew what so many others, who thought him either interesting, or different, or talented, didn't know.

Frances knew … His quips and his moods and his angers could be real and frightening; but the sometimes impossibly irascible man was also the reverently softened doctor. He sneered at medical men's pretensions with harsh words. But to Frances he would say moodily, "We should be like monks, yes, going about in sandals and bare garments. Our purpose is to guard and resurrect the human body. It should be a holy purpose, and our dedication should be as holy as our purpose."

In the world at large he was the *bon vivant*, quick to defend his pride and vanities. In the hospital ward he was the father, ageless, transformed, sensing in himself all the suffering and yearnings of his patients. In the world at large no two people thought of him in any one pattern; in the ward his patients all loved him devotedly, just as the nuns loved him, and all who knew the doctor as well as the man.

That Christmas, of the year 1934, those who received his Christmas card were intrigued by it. On one side of the card was his Compressionist's Creed On the other was a sketch of a pneumothorax apparatus under which was the legend, "Wishing you a happy pneumothorax." At the bottom of the card he had printed the words of Whitman:

"I do not pity the wounded; I become the wounded."

He could administer a terrible tongue-lashing to a nun for some little inefficiency, but at the next moment, when the young woman patient she was attending, dying from virulent and hopeless tuberculosis, whispered, "Will you kiss me?" he looked down at her with the memory of how he had once lain like this himself, how he had once himself grasped at the few remaining things in life like the flower leaning towards the sun. He hesitated only for a moment, then bent and kissed her, while the very nurse he had just spoken to so harshly pulled his arm in warning. For days afterwards he gave himself prophylaxis, but when a staff member asked him how he could take such changes with a virulent case, he shrugged and said shortly, "The doctor works with more than medicine."

He cherished life. He cherished his mind and his hands and his heart and everything that gave him the power to give it and redeem it. And in a world where his private dream was assessed as a piece of softheaded sentimentality, where he saw life equated to cash dollars, he kept his dream well hidden from prying eyes.

He felt himself *bonded* to life. Frances knew him as the guardian and father to all who came to him broken and diseased. The man snarled; the doctor smiled. The man's lips derided the ways of the world; the doctor's lips kissed the young woman aching for a little human affection before her end. The man's face took on many aspects; the doctor's face was always tender.

All this, and where it came from, Frances knew — not all at once but in bits and pieces. From the way he had come home sometimes, silently, everything shut out but his particularly difficult cases of the moment, his thoughts moving restlessly from symptom, to ailment, to cure, to prevention, his moods sensitized to his patients' every shade of feeling.

She remembered it all again when he telephoned her one day and said quickly, "I must see you right away. Can you come up to the apartment?" His voice was agitated.

She found him pacing back and forth in his living room, mute thanks in his eyes as she entered, his face grey, his hands seizing hers tightly.

"I just lost a patient and I had to see you. He was a young monk. Far gone, and full of complications. Only surgery could help.... I thought — perhaps I could save him.... He was quite young ... a monk ... all those years away from life ... now finished altogether.... He died on the table while I was operating...."

Whatever she could never understand about him, this she understood. Not death itself plagued him, but the loss of a life he wanted to save; a life that would rise up to haunt him like the spirits in his painting of "The Surgeon at the Day of Judgment."

"It's hard to explain," he went on restlessly. "I ask myself: am I at fault? Should I know more, am I not good enough? Are we all at fault? I can't explain it; but when they die like that a part of me dies with them."

She tried to soothe him. He had done everything possible, she reasoned, everything known, and it was futile to blame himself for what was inevitable. But she knew he was baring a part of himself where she feared almost to look.

"When they die, a part of me dies with them...." So many of them would die, and he would suffer every last agony; tortured, twisting in the grip of his own impotence.

15

MARCH 1935

Hitler roared in the Berlin Sports Palast. Prime Minster Baldwin talked of collective security at Downing Street, while Neville Chamberlain awaited the summons to destroy it. The peasants, workers and middle classes of Spain stirred restlessly. Mussolini cast covetous looks across the Mediterranean from Rome. In Moscow the newspapers were filled with studies of progress in the current Five Year Plan. In China the civil war pursued its zigzag course. In Montreal the warm weather brought slush, unemployed demonstrations and the forty-fifth birthday of Dr. Norman Bethune.

In the dismal thirty-fifth year of the twentieth century spring came to Montreal as usual. In the centre of the city it unwrapped warm brown patches of Mount Royal. In the suburbs it thawed the sod of last year's lawns. In the East End it left a dark sooty cake of ice that would remain long after the rest of the city lay bared to the warm sun. Spring wore a different face in every section of Montreal.

Things were going well at the hospital; Bethune's ideas and techniques were making headway — but new misgivings began to stir in his mind.

To his assistant and loyal friend, Dr. Georges Deshaies, he confided some of the things disturbing him. Tuberculosis could be wiped out, he would complain, but was actually increasing. On the operating table the surgeon treated only the violent effects of the disease in the individual, not its general origins.

And how many thousands of people were going about with T.B. who never came to the clinics — because they hadn't the money, or the knowledge of what was wrong with them? Sometimes he felt he might just as well throw the knife away and stand on street corners, shouting a warning to the people passing by. Maybe that would do more good than surgery alone.

To Frances, whom he saw infrequently now, he raged and stormed, while she sat quietly, listening, her bright eyes patient and sympathetic. "Medicine!" he would cry. "You don't know how much of it ends up in a blind alley. Some day the textbooks will describe us as the men of the *pre*medical era." Long ago, in Detroit, he had complained that too many doctors were concerned only with "surface" medicine. Now his mind was filled with ideas that sounded strange, yet fascinating to Frances.

"The doctor," he would say, "is supposed to be dedicated to the maintenance of the people's health. How many doctors practice according to that concept? And is it always their fault? No, it's all wrong. We casually accept the idea that every street in every city has its water mains, sewage pipes, sanitation, electricity and other services. But do we include genuine medical services among these? No. And why not? Because there's no such thing as the right to a healthy life. It still has to be purchased, like a can of beans at the corner grocery. You've got to pay for it in dollars and cents. We set ourselves up in practice, all smug and satisfied — like tailor shops. We patch an arm, a leg, the way a tailor patches an old coat. We're not practising medicine, really — we're carrying on a cash-and-carry trade. I'll tell you what's needed: a new medical concept, a new concept of universal health protection, a new concept of the functions of the doctor."

One day he visited Frances unexpectedly. He seemed filled with tense elation. "My work is completely out of whack," he said.

"Now really, Beth," Frances said. "What is it that's got you now?"

For a moment he was irritated, then ignored the question. He had once thought that by perfecting himself as doctor and surgeon he would be able to do something to wipe out T.B. But it didn't work that way. They had to take medicine right down to the people. And how were they going to do that? "We go to the people! *We go to the people!* No more private practice; we change the whole system of medical service. Look out the window — a whole street of houses. That's where the doctor must go. Into every house, into every city, into every village. From door to door. We take medicine right down to the last individual. We don't wait until the invalid drags himself down to our offices at so much per consultation; we go to *him* before he is ill and show him how to remain healthy. And if he is ill already, we arrest it by prompt action. From house to house, street to street, city to city...."

"And who," Frances inquired, "do you mean by 'we'?"

"Me," he said, "and others who will go with me. Others who will believe as I do that the doctor's duty is to act, to go to the source of the disease." His excitement rose. He was anxious to convince her.

"And where will you find such men?"

"Where did the church find its priests?" he retorted. "If there were men who responded to the appeal of the church sufficiently to abandon all their worldly possessions and take up the frugal life of a monastery, then there will be doctors ready to set aside private gain in order to become priests in the service of the people's health. Doctors will band together in a community of medical practitioners. We'll go into the slums, into the districts where the need is greatest." Did Frances know that in the rural areas of Quebec there was more disease than any other part of the country? Did she know that 20 miles from Montreal, in Lachine, one third of all the babies died at birth? Did she know that more children died at birth in Montreal and Quebec City than almost anywhere in the world except backward cities like Bombay and Madras?[*]

"But where," she interrupted, "will the money come from to pay for it all? Suppose you persuade others to join you — what will you live on?"

"Ah, well — money...." He waved it aside impatiently. "For ourselves we will need nothing. We'll live on what we can get ...

---

[*] Bethune's statements were based on Provincial Government statistics. These were the years of severe economic depression. Infant mortality rates have improved since then in Quebec.

nickels, dimes, dollars. It will be enough. Whatever people can afford will keep us. Medicines, supplies, equipment — all these are technical details. If necessary we'll shame the government into giving them to us."

He paced about, talking quickly and eloquently of his plans, then stopped in front of her, seizing her hands. "What do you think?"

"I don't know," she said slowly. "The way you talk makes it sound like the most wonderful thing I've ever heard of — or the most impractical."

16

A few days later he began the outline for a booklet exposing the health conditions in the province of Quebec. "Bring it out into the light of day," he told his friends, "and then stir up enough feeling to get something done. Put it in terms that the people can understand, and maybe some of the babies now dying in this benighted land will have a chance to be saved. The facts will be more eloquent than all the pious platitudes in the world."

The problem seemed to be more than poverty in the midst of plenty. The whole country, the whole world was seething. Everywhere there were challenges, denunciations, high-blown speeches, diplomatic threats — all recorded in a jargon that was not only new to him but bewildering. What the devil did Hitler want? How did a civilized nation permit such a madman to rule in their name? Why did the Western diplomats treat him with such strange delicacy? And that other mountebank, Mussolini, ranting from the Piazza Venezia — how come he, Bethune, had hardly been aware of the peacock's existence back in Italy? And why didn't someone stand up and tell him to pipe down in good, round, four letter words? And what about this hubbub at home? What were all these groups demanding, attacking, organizing, counterorganizing?

"If the daily newspapers confuse *me*," he said, "they must be confusing a lot of other people." He decided to draft a little booklet to provide simple explanations for terms applied daily to current events. On the first page he wrote: "A Newspaper Reader's Dictionary — or 100 Definitions as a Guide to the Daily Press." He never got beyond the first few pages, but before forgetting about the project he did 53 terms for definition, most of them indicating the direction in which his mind was searching. The list included: dictatorship, democracy, unemployment, employer, employee, wages, trade unions, capitalism, socialism, communism, strike, the working class, the *bourgeoisie*, the Soviet, patriotism, nationalism....

Landing squarely in the developing controversies between labour and industry, communism, socialism and capitalism, he set to work to find out the characteristic features of each. With typical thoroughness he covered sheets of paper with ruled columns, headed one column "capitalism," one "fascism," and one "communism." Underneath he wrote: "the definition ..." Further down he wrote: "the facts ..." He filled the columns with all the data he could find, changing his mind often about "the definition" and "the facts" as he went along.

Some of his friends now began looking at him askance. When they saw radical pamphlets on his table they began to ask: "Are you becoming a communist?" "I wouldn't know," he would say blandly, "for the simple reason I'm not sure just what a communist is yet. What I do know is that according to the communist, it isn't what the anticommunist says it is, and vice versa. And what I'm equally sure of is that it's damned easy to get yourself tagged as a communist. If you're going to yell 'communist' at every nonconformist, then by God you'll have to count me the reddest of the red."

He read everything he could lay his hands on, his ideas on politics, economics, philosophy developing in neat progression on the endless sheets of paper with their precise captions and columns of data. But he was soon to find that the answers he was seeking overran the simple summaries of his notes and pamphlets.

One afternoon he was driving some colleagues to his apartment when he suddenly found himself wedged into a traffic jam, with masses of people appearing as if from nowhere and running frantically along the sidewalks.

As he opened his door to look out, several police patrol cars came twisting through the stalled cars, sirens screaming. "Must be a bad accident," he thought and got out of his car.

What he saw when he wriggled through the line of honking cars into a clear area up ahead was no accident. Two lines of mounted city police were coming down the slight incline of St. Lawrence Boulevard from Craig Street, in close formation stretching clear across the street from sidewalk to sidewalk. They moved forward slowly, flank to flank, driving before them a crowd of several thousand men and women. The police rode their horses as if on display, their faces impassive, almost bored.

The crowd was wedged together compactly and the men and women fell back in unison, step by step, silently, their faces turned towards the line of horsemen advancing behind them. Above their heads, suspended between two slender poles held by unseen hands, a white banner flapped in the wind: "Milk for our Children! Bread for our Wives! Jobs, not Breadlines!"

Then, as if by prearranged signal, the double line of horsemen broke their mounts into a trot.

An angry roar rose from the crowd. The demonstrators drew together, joining hands. For a moment they held their ground. The police came on at a canter, their splendid horses making an awesome sight.

"*A bas la police!*" a voice cried. "Down with the police!"

The police came on, the boredom gone from their faces, their lips drawn, their arms rising in unison with truncheons strapped around their wrists. A ripple of indecision ran through the crowd. A deep sigh echoed through the street for the moment, a gasp of protest and disbelief — followed by a sudden hush. Then the horsemen were plunging deep into the crowd, flailing about them with their truncheons, their horses rearing wildly, men and women falling to the ground, clutching each other, screaming in fear and pain.

Bethune was caught up in the first ranks of the fleeing demonstrators and pressed back against the stalled automobiles. He was wedged against the side of a car, catching a glimpse of the driver's panic-stricken face, then the press of bodies carried him to the sidewalk where he stumbled into a doorway.

He saw a man with his hands covering his face, cringing, his shirt ripped at the shoulder, coming towards him, tossed like a cork on water, blood streaming through his fingers. Bethune tried to get to him, but a motorcycle sidecar, pushing ahead in a straight line, caught the man beneath the groin, lifted him on its streamlined point and tossed him aside.

"Murderer!" someone shouted. A young woman with a thin face hung onto the motorcycle, trying to upset it, screaming, "*Maudit cochon!* — Damned pig!" The policeman in the sidecar calmly flung a beefy hand into her face and sent her sprawling.

Bethune finally managed to force his way into the street, stumbling over a woman with a child in her arms crouching beside an automobile. Some of the demonstrators were trying to escape among the stalled cars. He now had only one thought: to get back to his own car for his bag. When he reached his open convertible, one of his colleagues was waiting for him tensely. "What's happening?" he asked.

"Murder," Bethune rasped. "Cold-blooded, brutal assault and murder!"

A young man came up, leaned over the hood and retched violently. One side of his face was raw and swollen, his shabby clothes were spattered. "Here, come around this way. I'm a doctor." He turned to his colleague. "Hand me my bag and give me a hand."

He helped the young man into the back seat, laid him out gently and reached into his bag, listening to the roar of the trapped demonstrators, the sound of the galloping hoofs, the screaming sirens, the sounds of pain and terror and hate.

The next day leaders of the Montreal Unemployed Association were meeting in their dingy office when the door flew open and an expensively tailored individual walked in. He extended a card to them and said: "I'm Dr. Norman Bethune. Any man, woman or child you send to me will receive medical treatment free of charge. By next week I hope to have another ten doctors doing the same…."

To his fame as an innovator in chest surgery he now added laurels that went unrecorded in the medical journals. His name became known on the breadlines. He began to mingle with the men who had forgotten the sensation of a decent meal. He went to their homes, stood among them as "block committees" prevented their evictions for nonpayment of rent, accompanied them to meetings where orators spoke movingly of the plight of the jobless, met their leaders, made friends with people who called themselves communists, CCFers,* socialists, liberals.

He found it a strange, new, stimulating environment, where men and women spoke with passion of the future as well as the present, discussed philosophy and organized trade unions, and accepted him with a warm camaraderie which he relished.

His notes and occasional diary records now took on a new flavour:

> My "bad side" is back to normal. I had forgotten all about it, but it's reassuring news all the same, for there's no time now to get dragged back into the mire again. Am I on the right track? The answer seems to be dictated by necessity rather than theory. The problem is to *participate*, not merely to assemble academic facts. The rich can take care of themselves; who will look after the poor? They live without even the knowledge, so many of them, of their natural right to healthy bodies. My new friends and "nonpaying" patients, however, aren't backward about asserting their natural rights. One can't help admiring the spirit of some of these people. They have nothing, yet in their murky meeting halls, under the police clubs, they weave a rich and optimistic dream. It is hard to follow them sometimes, even harder sometimes to agree with their knotty theorizing, but easy to share the excitement and enthusiasm minted of their wants, deprivations and single-mindedness. They have handed me a new honorary degree: I

---

* The Co-operative Commonwealth Federation — the Canadian Social-Democratic party.

115

am now a Doctor of Medicine, a Fellow of the Royal College of Surgeons, and "*Comrade Beth.*" It is an honourable title. I feel I have set my feet on a new road. Where will it lead ...?

17

It led him first to the Soviet Union, whose attempts to create a socialist society had increasingly roused his interest. The self-appointed physician to Montreal's needy left Montreal in the summer of 1935 to attend an International Physiological Congress being held in Leningrad, after arranging with his first assistant, Dr. Georges Deshaies, to take charge of the work at the hospital during his absence.

Among other Canadian representatives were Sir Frederick Banting, Dr. John S.L. Browne and Dr. Hans Selye. Banting was world-famous as the co-discoverer, with Charles H. Best, of insulin. Dr. Selye had not yet published his famous paper on the "adaptation syndrome" nor had he yet outlined his theory of the diseases of adaptation. For Selye the trip to Leingrad meant meeting the great Pavlov, whose work had foreshadowed his own experiments. For Dr. Browne, the Physiological Congress meant comparing notes, corroborating his own findings in biochemistry, part of the preparation which was to see him become one of Canada's outstanding professors of medicine and head of an internationally famous clinic at the Royal Victoria Hospital. For Bethune, the Physiological Congress was frankly an opportunity to see how "socialized medicine" functioned in practice.

He decided he could study all the papers read at the Congress by reading them; in Leningrad he attended the first session of the Congress and then went his own way. He arranged a private interview with Pavlov, and then spent the rest of his time "looking at people" and investigating tuberculosis therapy.

His reaction to Pavlov was summed up in a letter to a medical colleague in Montreal:*

> I attended the session of the Congress where I had a chance to see and hear Pavlov. He reminded everybody of George Bernard Shaw — his looks, that is. I think we're now beginning to appreciate what Pavlov has done for the science of human behaviour. He's given us a new approach to the basic problems of disease, or rather he's given us new evidence to prove that disease must be seen in its proper context — we react to our conditioning. Not only our reflexes, mind you, but even our tissues, even our blood cells....

Through the Russian Commissariat of Public Health he received permission to visit hospitals and sanatoriums, and to study Soviet methods of dealing with tuberculosis. Here he launched into an inquiry which became the climax of his stay in the U.S.S.R. and left him at a high-peak of excitement.

Bearing out his own belief that tuberculosis could be fought to a standstill, he found that in 18 years, almost half of which were spent in rebuilding the country's ruined economy, the Soviet Union had cut the incidence of tuberculosis by more than fifty percent.

His excitement grew as he pursued his inquiry further. The rest homes, convalescent homes and outright sanatoriums were the most lavish he had ever seen, with industrial workers receiving priority in the institutional treatment, the exact reverse of the situation back home. In the dispensaries and sanatoriums all treatment was free, not as a matter of charity but as a constitutional right of the invalid. Included in the officially prescribed preventive measures were tuberculin tests for children from an early age, something he had long championed at home.

A decade earlier, at Trudeau Sanatorium, he had talked of the need for special rehabilitation measures for patients leaving T.B. institutions. Now, in Russia, he found a large-scale rehabilitation

---

* Letter to Dr. H.S. Sept. 9, 1935.

system that he immediately declared to be the finest in the world. Under this system Russia had a series of day and night sanatoriums exclusively for overnight or daytime patients. The latter were men and women who were back at work after having been released from regular sanatoriums, or a few with early chest conditions not sufficiently menacing to warrant full hospitalization.

Although he had no time to visit the many sanatoriums in other parts of the country, he had now seen enough to be convinced and elated. He wanted to stay on, to spend more time studying the medical services, to travel through other parts of the country, but he had already overstayed his leave. Two months after his arrival, he left for home, armed with books, pamphlets, medical articles and the feeling that something new was being tested in ancient Russia that would profoundly affect the pattern of men's lives throughout the world.

At the time, Canada and the Soviet Union had no diplomatic relations of any kind and curiosity about the "Soviet experiment" was spreading. As a consequence, Bethune was flooded with invitations to speak in public about his trip.

He accepted as many invitations as he could, speaking to students, medical bodies and organizations of diverse interest. His platform manner was completely unorthodox. Not matter how large the audience, he chatted as casually as if he were talking to a few friends in his own living room. Sometimes he sat on the chairman's table; sometimes he hauled his chair along to the front of the platform, put one knee over it and carried on, disregarding the textbook rules on public speaking.

In all his talks he followed a simple strategy: to present the facts and *to shatter smugness* while doing so. He hated cliché thinking, in left-wing circles as well as right-wing, and he enjoyed nothing better than to challenge peoples' accepted views and to make them think. In Toronto, Banting was to create an even greater stir with glowing reports on the Soviet Union. His Soviet tour, Banting declared, had been the most stimulating experience of his life. In articles and speeches he lauded the U.S.S.R. for "building a gigantic structure on the solid rock of science and research.... No people in the world so fully realize that the research of today is the science of tomorrow." As one of Canada's national heroes, Banting's statements created greater receptivity for the things Bethune was saying, although both drew sharp criticism from some conservative quarters.

The summing up, the implications of the facts he had gathered, Bethune left for his report to the members of the medical profession at a meeting sponsored by the Medico-Chirurgical Society of Montreal.

The meeting was held on September 20, 1935. The hall was filled by doctors, their families and some laymen who had managed to secure coveted invitations. Dr. Selye spoke first, dealing only with the scientific reports and discussions at the Congress. Dr. Browne was next and, in a facetious mood, he discussed not only the Congress but also related his personal experiences with sinks that had no plugs, with Intourist Guides who didn't understand English but tried to make out they did, with red tape, with difficulties in getting railway tickets. He presented his personal adventures in a highly amusing manner and sat down amid warm applause. Bethune had known beforehand that Selye would speak primarily of the Congress, and that Browne would also speak of his personal misadventures with plugless sinks and beautifully tiled bathrooms without toilet paper.

As he stepped to the speaker's stand there was polite applause. He acknowledged the chairman's laudatory remarks on his position in the world of thoracic surgery, and lit a cigarette.

"My position as the last speaker of the evening," he opened conversationally, "was of my own choosing. I had decided to take up a position opposite to that of my fellow Lenin graduates." He paused as a titter ran through the audience. "I felt fairly sure they would be unanimous. And I had decided that if they deprecated Russia, I would praise her; if they praised her, I would diminish her. This would not be done in a spirit of pure perversity — but rather from a concern for truth which appears to me to consist, not infrequently, in the conjunction of apparently irreconcilable aspects of reality."

He drew on his cigarette and savored his listeners' curious looks as they pondered this unexpected opening. Then he continued from his prepared text:

All accounts of returned travellers from strange lands and foreign shores are essentially self-disclosatory and unwittingly autobiographical in character. Criticism [he sharpened the words ever so slightly] ... becomes the critique of the critic. This is traditionally true of all the returned travellers, from those Biblical gentlemen who reported Palestine to be a land flowing with milk and honey — when it was nothing of the sort — to Marco Polo, Christopher Columbus and Baron Munchausen.

At this point he smiled, while audience and speakers alike seemed to stir, to sit forward in anticipation of what was to come.

Now, I did not go to Russia, frankly, like the others, to attend a Physiological Congress. I went to Russia for more important reasons than that. *I went primarily to look at the Russians.* And secondarily, I went to see what they were doing about eradicating one of the most easily eradicable of all contagious diseases, namely, tuberculosis. I happen to possess some very definite ideas on how this might be done, given the necessary courage and currency. I shall not say anything about the Congress, since I only attended one session — the opening one — being much too busy swimming in the Neva, walking about unhindered in the streets, looking into windows and making the rounds of the picture galleries — a combination Peeping Tom and an Innocent Abroad.

He paused for another puff from his cigarette and slipped into a more jocular tone again.

Perhaps the title of my address should really be: Reflections Through a Looking Glass. This might lead one to suppose I was about to draw a comparison between Looking-Glass Land and

Russia. It would be easy enough to parody that fairy-tale or write, with tongue in cheek, an article entitled, *Malice in Blunderland*. But derision and denial are interesting psychological phenomena which are essentially protective in nature. It is easier to deride than to praise …

It should be remembered that in calling Russia a land of topsy-turvy, as it has been called, a reasonable doubt may arise as to whether the things one sees there are really upside-down. For this disturbing optical illusion may also be obtained by an observer standing on his head! Certainly, over the portals of Russia should be inscribed, "Abandon Old Conceptions All Ye Who Enter Here."

He snuffed out his cigarette, dropped the stub into a side pocket, and proceeded to draw on his beloved "Alice" books for further parallels with what he had seen in the Soviet Union. He found counterparts in the Soviet scene to the White Knight, the White Queen, the Red King, Humpty Dumpty, the Mad Hatter, Tweedledum and Tweedledee:

Stalin might be given the role of the Walrus, Lenin that of the Carpenter, and the NEP men that of the Oysters who were taken for such a disastrous walk down the Beach in 1921.

To take without benefit of context some of the sayings of the characters in *Through a Looking Glass* as applicable to Russia today would be interesting; such as, Russia might be compared to the Looking Glass room which Alice found looking so like her own drawing room — only the things went the other way, and the books were like her books, except that the words also went the wrong way….That it's "jam tomorrow, and jam yesterday — but never jam *today*" might be taken as the complaint of those who are impatient of what they think is the slow progress of improvement in living conditions. The White Queen's remembrance of things which happened the week after next might be taken as an example of the unlimited optimism and the faith the Russians have in their own future. And it would also be true of Russia to use the White Queen's reply to the protest of Alice, who said "Oh, I can't believe that."

"Can't you?" said the Queen. "Try again; draw a long breath and shut your eyes."

Alice laughed, "One can't believe such impossible things."

The Queen: "I dare say you haven't had much practice. Why I sometimes believe as many as six impossible things before breakfast."

Like the Queen, the Russians find it quite a simple matter to believe many impossible things — at least things that *others* consider impossible.

Then there would be as much truth in Alice's delighted exclamation when she found that the fire in the fireplace was real. "So I shall be as warm here in the old room, warmer in fact because there will be no one here to scold me away from the fire." And then she looked down from a little hill and saw the whole country as a huge chessboard and life itself a game of chess, which was being played all over the world, and said: "I should like to be Queen best." To this the Queen replied: "That is easily managed. You be the White Queen's pawn if you like and you are in the second square to begin with, and then when you get to the eighth square you will be a Queen and we shall be Queen together, and it will be all feasting and fun." And that statement would be the faith and hope of Communism in a nutshell.

While the audience was enjoying these sallies his voice and manner suddenly changed. Casting aside his jocular manner, he concluded with these words:

Isadora Duncan, in the story of her life, describes her confinement ... "There I lay," she wrote, a fountain of spouting blood, milk and tears." What would a person think, watching for the first time a woman in labor and not knowing what was happening to her? Would he not be appalled at the blood, the agony, the apparent cruelty of the attendants, the whole revolting technique of delivery? He would cry: "Stop this! Do something! Please! Police! Murder!"

Then tell him he was seeing a new life brought into the world and that the pains would pass, that the agony and ugliness were necessary and always would be necessary to birth. Knowing this, then, what could he say truthfully about this woman as she lies there? Is she not ugly? Yes. Is she not beautiful? Yes. Is she not pitiful, ludicrous, grotesque and absurd? Yes! Is she not magnificent and sublime? Yes! And all these things would be true.

Now, Russia is going through her delivery, and the midwives and obstetricians have been so busy keeping the baby alive that they haven't got around as yet to cleaning up the mess, and it is this mess, this ugly and uncomfortable mess, which affronts the eyes and elevates the noses of those timid male and female virgins suffering from sterility of the soul, who lack the imagination to see behind the blood the significance of birth.

Creation is not and never has been a genteel gesture. It is rude, violent and revolutionary. But to those courageous hearts who believe in the unlimited future of man, in the divine destiny which lies in his own hand to make of what he will — to these Russia presents today the most exciting spectacle of the evolutionary, emergent and heroic spirit of man which has appeared on earth since the Reformation. To deny this is to deny our faith in men — and that is the unforgiveable sin, the final apostasy.

A few days after the public announcement of his new political faith, Bethune took the next logical step. He joined the Communist Party. His formal membership in the party was kept secret in order to protect him professionally. But in a country wracked by division, crisis and unprecedented human suffering, he made no attempt to hide the fact that he was now no longer merely a reformer, but a revolutionary, consciously fighting to change the world.

18

It was a few weeks later that he came across the name of Fritz Brandtner at the Montreal Art Gallery, when a painting by Brandtner attracted his attention. As he often did in such cases, he bought the painting and made inquiries about Brandtner. Learning that the painter had recently left Germany rather than live under the Hitler regime, Bethune wrote to tell him how much he liked his work. They soon became good friends, and out of this friendship came a unique project.

Describing his work in Europe one day, Brandtner mentioned that for some time he had studied in Vienna under Dr. Cizek, the originator of a progressive theory of art education for children. Bethune listened, questioned him closely, and the next day was back to see Brandtner with a plan for a creation of a Children's Art School. The painter had supplied an answer to a question that had been plaguing him: what could he do — he, a doctor and a reformer — for the children growing up in the dark corners of the city? It was a very small answer, he knew, but it was a beginning from which bigger things could grow.

His plan was simple: under his sponsorship and Brandtner's guidance to set up an art school for children using Dr. Cizek's methods. There would be no fees, no costs of any kind. His home might house the school. Every child would be welcome. As the school developed it might eventually be able to finance itself through the subscriptions of interested individuals. Until then, Bethune would meet all expenses.

So began the Children's Art School of Montreal, the first such project in Canada, dedicated to the job of bringing the joy and creativity of the arts to the children of the slums.

To help supervise the school Bethune called on another artist, Marian Scott, whom he had met on his trip overseas and with whom he had become close friends.

Three afternoons a week Mrs. Scott and Brandtner received the children, welcoming them into Bethune's large living room, where they spread out on the floor, painting the colours and images that intrigued their budding senses.

Though hard pressed by work at the hospital and his outside activities Bethune tried to get home as frequently as possible when classes were being held. He would come into the studio, a look of pleasure on his face, asking, "And how are my children today?"

Every Saturday morning he took them to the art galleries, explaining the paintings to them, describing what the artist tried to accomplish, acting as guide among the masterpieces of the past and the modern painters of Canada. These Saturday mornings were among his happiest hours in Montreal.

It was during this period that he put away Alice, the make-believe Alice, the ghostly reminder of his marriage. He had found his children in a real world, at last.*

It was in painting too that he found immeasurable happiness; it provided him not only with a source of relaxation but a new form of creativity. His paintings were bold and imaginative. His sculpture pieces showed the same characteristics. The art critics of Montreal were unanimous in their praise of the paintings he exhibited in the autumn of 1935 at one of the local art shows.

---

* Two of the children won the first and third prizes in an International Art Festival sponsored by the French Government.

He considered himself as much an artist as he did a surgeon and often said that the two were inseparable. He once wrote:

> Bound by the rigid and inexorable laws of his medium, the human body, the surgeon is permitted but few of the liberties his fellow craftsmen may take who work with stone, wood or metal.
>
> He is not allowed the exhibition of playful fancies, wit or humour, which other craftsmen enjoy in their productions. But, for all that, our craftsman often has the soul of a creative artist, although the nature of his plastic medium restricts the free play of his artistic nature. Like most other men, his creative force is confined to one channel and allowed but one escape. The modern introduction of anaesthesia has liberated the craft from the hurried expediency of the past to the more leisurely procedures of today. Modern surgical craftsmanship with its new leisure and, as an immediate consequence, its new precision, permits and encourages the artistic sensibilities of the operator. These artistic desires and their approximate satisfaction are contained, to a large extent, in what is known as "surgical technique."*

19

With the Children's Art School launched and operating, Bethune took up the larger issue toward which, it seemed to him, he had been groping all these years. He set himself the task of canvassing the whole history of medical care, examining the systems of medical services throughout the world, and drafting a public

---

* *American Review of Tuberculosis*, Sept. 1932.

health care program that would be practical, simple enough to be easily implemented, and comprehensive enough to assure adequate protection to the mass of the people. The project was big enough to stagger his most sympathetic colleagues. When he discussed it with a prominent American public health authority, I. S. Falk, the latter was helpful but full of warnings about the monumental research work involved.

"The problem is not only one of bookish investigations," Bethune answered. "It's the problem of finding a solution to the mass illness brought by seven years of crisis and depression, by greed and stupidity."

One of his colleagues had once complained that Bethune's zest for action overshadowed his appetite for study. Whatever the merit of the criticism, now his zest for action led him to plough through every tract on medical organization he could lay his hands on. He read all the available documents of the medical associations of Canada and the United States, received long briefs on Britain's experiences in public health from colleagues working in London, corresponded with interested government departments at Ottawa, and exchanged views by letter with any and every expert he could track down on the continent. He prepared bibliographies listing hundreds of books and pamphlets on the subject. He immersed himself in the statistical handbooks of the International Labour Office and the relevant branches of the League of Nations. He combined his studies of the public health system in each country with research into its economic and political background, average wages, governmental structure, the social awareness of its political parties and population. And when he felt sufficiently sure of his ground he called a group of doctors and community workers to his apartment and put his ideas before them.

Out of this gathering grew something new in Canadian medical history: The Montreal Group for the Security of the People's Health. The name of the group was unwieldy and went through a number of modifications, but its purposes were simple enough. Just as the Children's Art School was dedicated to the advancement of deprived children, so the new organization as dedicated to the bringing of proper medical care to the people who needed it most.

One hundred doctors, dentists, nurses and social workers joined the group, making Bethune their secretary. By July 1936 they were ready to fire their first public broadside. After preliminary conversations between Bethune and government officials, the Group issued a declaration over Bethune's signature drawing attention to the terrible plight of hundreds of thousands of people in the province of Quebec, emphasizing that the health of the people could be guarded only if accepted as a government responsibility. It put forward a number of practical suggestions to bring immediate improvements in the public health situation.

Among steps recommended for trial were: a program of compulsory healthy insurance, covering all wage-earners; teams of doctors, nurses and dentists to work out of special hospitals in the municipalities; a scheme under which all the unemployed would be assigned to local donors in groups of 500, with treatment to be paid out of government funds.

In the profession itself some fears were expressed about where all this talk about state responsibility for public health would lead. In a report sent to members of the Group Bethune wrote, "Up to the present the reaction to the tentative draft sent to members of the Montreal Medico-Chirurgical Society has been very reserved."

Though the program he was proposing was not socialized medicine, he was not hesitant in declaring that socialized medicine was the ultimate form in which medicine would achieve its liberation and its greatest opportunity to perform its proper functions. If anybody wanted to raise the cry of socialized medicine to frighten people away, then he was prepared to come to its defence.

In the discussion that followed the declaration of principles of the People's Health Group, various views developed in the ranks of Montreal's medical society. The controversy eventually reached the floor of the organized medical groups, when the Montreal Chirurgical society organized a panel discussion on economic problems of medicine. This was the opportunity for which Bethune had been waiting.

20

Three leading Montreal doctors were to participate in the panel discussion. Drs. A.H. Gordon, B. Cuddihy, and Bethune.

Dr. Gordon presented the viewpoint that stated any attempts to make the government responsible for private health threatened the foundations of the medical profession.

Dr. Cuddihy took the middle-of-the-road position, conceding that the economic crisis demanded new measures, that doctors everywhere faced big problems, and advocated health insurance schemes, without government interference.

Dr. Bethune took the radical position. He advocated social medicine outright. Both the previous speakers had argued against socialized medicine with various degrees of vehemence. Bethune opened his remarks with some sharp words:

"Tonight there has been brought before you the most interesting 'case' ever presented to this Society. It is — the Case of the People versus the Doctors. In the problem now under discussion it is necessary to emphasize that medical men themselves are being weighed in the balance. Yet we are acting both as defendant and judge. That behooves us to apply our minds with the utmost objectivity to this question."

Dr. Gordon had dwelt on the question of what might happen to the individual medical practitioner under a system of socialized medicine.

That [Bethune argued] makes it necessary to bring the problem back to its proper setting.★ For the health of the nation involves more than the personal fate of the private doctor. What we have here is an ethical and moral problem in the field of social and political economics, and not medical economics alone. Medicine must be seen as part of the social structure. It is the *product* of any given social environment. Every social structure has an economic base, and in Canada this economic base is called capitalism, avowedly founded on individualism, competition and private profit. But this system of capitalism is undergoing an economic crisis — a deadly disease requiring systemic treatment.

★ Material from here to the end of the chapter is quoted from Bethune's speech.

And here a problem presents itself with special urgency. There are those who are trying to treat the systemic disease as if it is only a temporary illness. They are doomed to failure.

The palliative measures suggested by most of our political quacks are like aspirin tablets given for a syphilitic headache. They may relieve; they never will cure.

Medicine [he continued calmly, relying more on understatement than on oratorical effect] is a typical, loosely organized, basically individualistic industry in this "catch as catch can" capitalistic system operating as a monopoly on a private profit basis. Now, it is inevitable that medicine should undergo much the same crisis as the rest of the capitalistic world and should present much the same interesting and uncomfortable phenomena. This may be epitomized as "poverty of health in the midst of scientific abundance in a country of disease." Just as thousands of people are hungry in a country which produces more food than the people can consume (we even burn coffee, kill hogs, and pay farmers not to plant wheat and cotton), just as thousands are wretchedly clothed though the manufacturers can make more clothing than they can sell, so millions are sick, hundreds of thousands suffer pain, and tens of thousands die prematurely through lack of adequate medical care, which is available but for which they cannot pay. Inability to purchase is combined with poor distribution. The problem of medical economics is a part of the problem of world economics and is inseparable and indivisible from it. Medicine, as we are practising it, is a luxury trade. *We are selling bread at the price of jewels.* The poor, who comprise fifty percent of our population, cannot pay, and starve; we, the doctors, cannot sell, and suffer. The people have no health protection and we have no economic security. This brings us to the point of the two aspects of this problem.

There are in this country three great economic groups: first, the comfortable; second, the uncomfortable; third, the miserable. In the upper bracket are those who are moderately uncomfortable and insecure; and in the lower, those vast masses, not in brackets but in chains, who are living on the edge of the subsistence level. These people in the lower income class are receiving only one-third of the home, office and clinic services from physicians that a fundamental standard of health requires. Only fifty-five percent of as many cases are being hospitalized as an adequate standard would prescribe, and only fifty-four percent of as many days are being spent in hospitals as are desirable.

In short, one has to suffer a major surgical catastrophe to have even approximate adequate care. The report of the Committee on the Cost of Medical Care (American Medical Association) showed that 46.6% of people whose income is less than $1,200 a year received no medical, dental or eye care whatsoever in a year. If this is combined with those whose income is $10,000 or more (13.8% of such persons received no similar care) we are faced with the appalling fact that 30.2% of all people, irrespective of income, received no medical, dental, or eye care whatsoever. What is the cause of this alarming state of affairs? First, financial inability to pay is the major cause; second, ignorance; third, apathy; fourth, lack of medical service.

Enormous accumulation of scientific knowledge has made it practically impossible for any one man to have an entire grasp of even the facts — much less their application — of the sum total of medical knowledge. This has brought specialization in concentrated centers of population. The general practitioner, unsupported by specialists, knows that he cannot give the people their money's worth, yet the financial cost of specialization bars many from proceeding to such fields. The necessity to make money after a difficult financial struggle to pay for medical education drives the young doctor too often into any remunerative work, however uncongenial it may be. There he is, caught up in the coils of economics, from which not one in a thousand can ever escape. The fee-for-service is very disturbing morally to practitioners. The patient is frequently unable to appraise morally the value of the doctor's service or disservice. Perrot and Collins in 1933, in an investigation of 9,130 families in America, found the depression poor had a larger incidence of illness than any other group. Also that 61% of all physicians' calls to such a class were free, that 33% of calls to the moderately comfortable were free, and that 26% of calls to even those comfortably well off were not paid for.

Permit me a few categorical statements, for dogmatism has a certain role in the realm of vacillation:

The best form of providing health protection would be to change the economic system which produces ill health, and to liquidate ignorance, poverty, and unemployment. The practice of each individual purchasing his own medical care does not work. It is unjust, inefficient, wasteful and completely outmoded. Doctors, private charity and philanthropic institutions have kept it alive for as long as possible. It should have died a natural death a hundred years ago, with the coming of the industrial revolution in the opening years of the 19th century. In our highly geared, modern industrial society there is no such thing as private health — all health is public. The illness and maladjustments of one unit of the mass effects all other members. The protection of the people's health should be recognized by the Government as its primary obligation and duty to its citizens.

Socialized medicine and the abolition or restriction of private practice would appear to be the realistic solution of the problem. Let us take the profit, the private economic profit, out of medicine, and purify our profession of rapacious individualism. Let us make it disgraceful to enrich ourselves at the expense of the miseries of our fellow men. Let us organize ourselves so that we can no longer be exploited as we are being exploited by our politicians.

Let us redefine medical ethics — not as a code of professional etiquette between doctors, but as a code of fundamental morality and justice between medicine and the people.

In our medical societies, let us discuss more often the great problems of our age and not merely interesting cases; the relationship of medicine to the State; the duties of the profession to the people; the matrix of economics and sociology in which we exist. Let us recognize that our most important contemporaneous problems are economic and social and not merely technical and scientific in the narrow sense that we employ the words.

Medicine, like any other organization today, whether it be the Church or the Bar, is judging its leaders by their attitude to the fundamental social and economic issues of the day. We need fewer leading physicians and famous surgeons in modern medicine and more farsighted, socially-imaginative statesmen.

The medical profession must — as the traditional, historical and altruistic guardians of the people's health — present to the Government a complete, comprehensive program of planned medical service for all the people. Then, in whatever position the profession finds itself after such a plan has been evolved, that position it must accept. This apparent immolation as a burnt offering on the altar of ideal public health will result in the profession rising like a glorious Phoenix from the dead ashes of its former self.

Medicine must be entirely reorganized and unified, welded into a great army of doctors, dentists, nurses, technicians and social service workers, to make a collectivized attack on disease and utilizing all the present scientific knowledge of its members to that end. Let us say to the people — not "How much have you got?" — but, "How best can we serve you?"

Socialized medicine means:

First, that health protection becomes public property, like the post office, the army, the navy, the judiciary and the school.

Second, that it is supported by public funds.

Third, that service is available to all, not according to income but according to need. Charity must be abolished and justice substituted. Charity debases the donor and debauches the recipient.

Fourth, its workers are to be paid by the State, with assured salaries and pensions.

Fifth, there should be democratic self-government by the health workers themselves.

Twenty-five years ago it was thought contemptible to be called a socialist. Today it is ridiculous not to be one.

Medical reforms, such as limited health insurance schemes, are not socialized medicine. They are bastard forms of socialism produced by belated humanitarianism out of necessity.

The three major objections which the opponents of socialized medicine emphasize are:

First: Loss of Initiative. Although it is alleged the human donkey probably needs, in this state of modern barbarism, some sort of vegetable dangled in front of his nose, these need not be golden carrots; a posy of prestige will do it as well.

Second: Bureaucracy. This can be checked by democratic control of organization from bottom to top.

Third: The Importance of the Patient's Own Selection of a Doctor. This is a myth; its only proponents are the doctors themselves — not the patients. Give a limited choice — say two or three doctors, then if the patient is not satisfied, send him to a psychiatrist! Sauce for the goose is sauce for the gander — the doctor must be given some measure of selection of patients! Ninety-nine percent of patients want results, not personalities.

Our profession must arouse itself from its scientific and intensely personal preoccupation and become socially-minded, realizing the inseparability of health from economic security.

Let us abandon our isolation and grasp the realities of the present economic crisis. The world is changing beneath our very eyes and already the barque of Aesculapius is beginning to feel beneath its keel the great surge and movement of the rising world tide which is sweeping on, obliterating old landscapes and old scenes. We must go with the tide or be wrecked.

The people are ready for socialized medicine. The obstructionists to the people's health security lie within the profession itself as well as outside it. Recognize this fact. It is the all-important fact of the situation. These men with the mocking face of the reactionary or the listnesses of the futilitarian proclaim their principles under the guise of "maintenance of the sacred relationship between doctor and patient," "inefficiency of other non-profit nationalized enterprises," "the danger of Socialism," the freedom of individualism." These are the enemies of the people, and make no mistake — they are the enemies of medicine too.

The situation which is confronting medicine today is a contest of two forces in medicine itself. One holds that the important thing is the maintenance of our vested historical interest, our private property, our monopoly of health distribution. The other contends that the function of medicine is greater than the maintenance of the doctor's position, that the security of the people's health is our primary duty, that we are above professional privileges. So the old challenge of Shakespeare's character in Henry IV still rings out across the centuries: "Under which King, Bezonian, stand or die!"

21

A few days later Bethune scrawled some memos on his desk pad:

1: Get all background material on war in Spain.…
2: Have the Case for Socialized Medicine retyped
for circulation and comment. 3: Prepare select
list of people to be sent plans for model city
for tuberculous rehabilitation after release from
sanatoria. 4: Look up medical literature for any
previous experience with condition similar to
that of the child.…."

War, the imbroglio of politics, projects for the rehabilitation
of broken lives, the fate of nations, the plight of a single child.

To someone looking over his shoulder his jottings might
have seemed curiously disjointed. At one time he would have
tabulated them as separate areas of concern. Now he found them
all interwoven, all demanding consideration and action as related
whorls of the same intricate pattern.

While he had been launching the Group for the Security of
the People's Health he had spent many an evening designing an
entire city. He had shown sketches to his friend, fellow artist and
now co-worker at the Children's Art School, Marian Scott. "My
purpose," he had explained, "may seem novel, yet I'm satisfied
it's also practical." In Russia they had the special day and night
sanatoria for sanatorium "graduates" — patients who were sufficiently recovered to return to work, but still needed surveillance,
attention, and lighter work. In Canada there were no provisions
for that type of care. But, he asked, why should it be impossible
to build completely new towns, with suitable housing, parks and
light industries, all catering to the needs of those who had suffered from T.B.? The purpose, of course, was to provide them
with an environment offering them the maximum health, the
opportunity to live normally and to earn a livelihood at trades
making no excessive demands on them.

The plans he showed Marian had a special appeal to her
artist's eye. They included designs for homes, parks, children's
playgrounds, dispensaries, hospitals and industrial buildings. The
actual cost if state-sponsored, he stressed, would come to less
money Canada eventually had to spend on repairing the damage
wrought by disease. That was the final place. He was not content merely to champion the principle of the citizen's right to

health and security. With the graphic approach of the artist and the technical approach of the doctor he felt impelled to show on paper that it was possible — and cheaper, in the long run — for people to live in pleasant surroundings, with the sun playing through the window and a garden behind the back porch.

But his dream, circulating soon among government officials and community leaders, came up against the chain effect of cause and effect that had so often swept him away from his moorings in a vicious cycle. When someone inquired one day what happened to his plan, he unfurled the daily paper and pointed to the headline: INSURGENT PLANES BOMB MADRID.

"That's what's happening to it," he said. "The cities of the future lie buried under the rubble of the cities that never had a chance. I have a child at the hospital who is dying because the human lung was not created to breathe slum air. But if I take my plea to Ottawa on her behalf, if I say to the men in office: Here are plans for a city in which my child can live and grow without fear, whom will I be addressing? The very men who sit down to their comfortable dinners with a comfortable conscience and don't give a damn for the cities now not only diseased but dying under the bombs."

So it was all one: the child at the hospital, the dream of the doctor and artist, the falling bombs, the indifferent politicians, the cities of Spain now crying out to the world for aid.

He was haunted by the headlines and the face of a child.

The fascists were moving towards Madrid, and in a bed at Sacré Coeur a child lay near death. He felt as frustrated when he looked at her as when he read the communiqués from Spain.

One of his colleagues, noticing his depression, asked what was wrong. He replied absently: "My child is very bad. There's little chance I can save her."

"Oh, sorry.... Didn't know you had any children."

"No, no. I don't mean my own. I mean a little girl at the hospital. Very sick...."

Her name was Yvette P.... She was French-Canadian. She was ten years old. She was dying.

Her father, a poor storekeeper in the French East End, had come to the hospital with his wife. In the strange atmosphere of the hospital, conscious of their threadbare appearance, they struggled to keep their composure, but as they talked to Bethune they broke down. For a year now, they said, they had watched Yvette waste away slowly. They had no money, they could afford no expensive consultations, they had been forced to go to the public clinics. They had dragged her from one clinic to another, but still she wasted away. Now they had come to him. They had heard of the famous doctor who went to the homes of the poor, who asked no money of those who had none, who said everywhere in public that health belonged to the poor as much as to the rich.

The father said fiercely: "Believe me, we do not ask for charity. We will sell everything — whatever we have. You can have it all. *Only cure her.*"

The mother, sitting in her plain dress, her roughened hands in her lap, said: "It is our only child, *Monsieur le Docteur....*"

While he examined the child the parents sat in the waiting room.

At the clinics where they had waited in the long lines of unemployed for a chance to see the weary doctors, many diagnoses had been made. One said the trouble lay in the stomach. "It will work itself out." Another had said it was a respiratory ailment. "Bronchitis, nothing very serious." Another had said: "Manifestly a persistent cough. I will give you a cough medicine." Still another had looked at the thin arms and chest and complained: "What do you expect? Malnutrition."

As Bethune examined her he soon suspected the truth. When he finished he gave instructions for her chest to be X-rayed and put her to bed.

"But she will be better — with these X-rays?" the father asked.

Bethune led them out of the ward. With a confidence he didn't feel, he explained that the X-rays would show them what was wrong. Nothing could be done till he examined them.

A nun led them away....

Bethune drove home thoughtfully that evening. The memory of Yvette's sunken black eyes filled him with depression. Would the X-rays confirm his fears? He hoped, prayerfully, that they would not. Even a virulent, full-blown case of tuberculosis would be better.

He parked his car, went up to his apartment, and walked into the living room. The room was a shambles. The children's paintings had been fiendishly, methodically torn into strips and strewn about the floor. The sculptured heads he had done were smashed as if with a baseball bat. Dripping black swastikas covered the walls. His finest pieces of furniture were broken.

He called the police and several detectives arrived to ask if he had any enemies. He pointed to the swastikas on the wall. "Does that look like the job of a personal enemy?" Yes, yes, they understood; they would investigate, Meanwhile it would be best if he stayed with some friends — just to be on the safe side. "If you look among those idiot Storm Troopers in the local fascist organization," he shot after them as they left, "you might find something." He suspected the incident was closed and he would hear nothing further.

At the hospital the next morning his worst fears were confirmed. The X-rays showed the entire right lung in a state of abscess. He studied them carefully and called in Dr. Deshaies for the latter's opinion. Dr. Deshaies looked at the films and shook his head dubiously.

Bethune looked inquiringly at his assistant. He could do nothing for the lung. She couldn't live with it. "To remain alive she must have it removed."

"And you will try to remove it?"

Bethune shifted in his chair. "I don't know ... I haven't been able to decide yet." After a while he burst out angrily: "What a rotten, damnable piece of business!"

He got to his feet and paced about the office. One year ago the child might have been cured easily. Now it was a toss of the coin. If he operated and she died, somebody would say he killed her. But who would have killed her really? That wasn't for the doctor to answer, was it? Well, for him it was. "I'll tell you who's been killing her. You, me, everybody who goes his own way while the whole damn world goes to hell!"

It was plain she was dying, and because things were so arranged that nobody seemed to give a damn about what happened to children, he was handed the alternative of letting her die or perhaps killing her on the operating table.

He walked about moodily. After a while he said more calmly, "Well, set up the operating theatre for tomorrow ... Just in case."

All evening he paced the floor of his living room. Should he operate? *Could* he operate? The principle of collapsing a lung was simple and universally accepted. But *removing* the lung completely from the chest was another matter. Nissen had done it in Berlin a few years back, and several others had followed in his footsteps. It had been done perhaps in a score of cases. But never in a ten-year-old child. Could her system survive the shock? Did he have the right to put her to the test?

Again the century-old question rose up to torment him: operate and perhaps save her, or do nothing and let her die?

Suddenly he cursed himself for a fool. That was strange reasoning! Hadn't he been confronted with exactly the same cautious nonsense when he had demanded artificial pneumothorax for himself? Was he *afraid*, perhaps?

At four o'clock in the morning he made up his mind. He wanted Yvette to live. That meant he would have to dare all consequences. Otherwise everything he had ever said, written, or practised was a monstrous fraud.

He went to bed and fell into a deep sleep, every detail of the operation firmly anticipated, ribs, pleural bag, lung mass, bronchial tubes, arteries fixed in his mind like a painting. He awoke at eight o'clock with the "tight" feeling he knew would keep him razor-sharp till the middle of the day.

He drove to one of the large department stores and bought the biggest doll he could find. At the hospital he laid it beside Yvette, then issued final instructions for the operation.

When he walked into the operating room in gown and mask, Yvette, clutching her doll, was already drifting under anesthesia. She lay on her stomach between the supporting chest rest, head tilted to one side, a corner of her mouth pulled open. The word had spread quickly, and the theatre was crowded with doctors. Only a few years ago there had been practically no thoracic surgery done at Sacré Coeur; now the *chef* was going to do something nobody in the whole country had ever attempted before. Assistants, doctors and observers were taught with suspense. "*Le chef*," the young interns whispered to one another, "is going to perform an autopsy this morning.

139

The anesthetist made a last-minute check, the first sister drew back the sheet, and Bethune looked down at the narrow back, the pathetic little shoulderblades. He felt the scalpel in his hand, and paused a moment. There, a little below the right shoulder blade, and to the side, his scalpel would enter. He forgot about the crowded theatre. In the darkness through which she was now floating, his thoughts pursued her.

The darkness clings to you now, Yvette, he thought, but I should lead you back into the spring sun.

See how many have come to watch? They look at my hands, and sometimes I find it difficult to explain that it is not with my hands alone that I press the searching knife, but something else — something powerful, assertive, born with me in the womb, sneered at and attacked everywhere, but carried deep inside me nevertheless. Remember it when the pain comes, and your mind finds it hard to understand why your *docteur* should have done this to you. I do it out of love — the secret, passionate word they have expurgated as cruelly as they have tried to expurgate *you*.

Now the retractors, the mimic, metallic hands that pull open the costal sheath with brutal necessity. Mop up the dark, mysterious flow, like wine from desert vineyards. Here are the ribs, miraculously curving, but how tragically brittle.

Now the rib shears, long and powerful, biting clean.... Then the pleura, and it is all revealed like the canvas, the painting I have carried in my head since early morning.

Careful now. The rest was mere preparation, entrance. Now we look upon the naked lung, the festering, soft mass, where life has already been extinguished by the seeping abscess. Here there is no hope. The decision is inexorable. It must come out.

Careful! The lung no longer breathes, but it is still vindictive. The abscess borders living tissue. Thus it runs throughout the world, the dirt infiltrating everything that yearns to live. It is vengeful; it is capable of ugly reprisals.

Careful! This is the real contest. Cut through the adhesions. Now the blood flows like no wine on earth. Oh, to have only two hands when death leers at me from the severed flesh. What? Of course the pulse is down. Prepare to transfuse. Oxygen. The first lung lies only half-severed in its cavity and already the heart weakens. But we will speed up nature's efficiency. More oxygen — hurry!

What time is it? Too much time has gone.

More oxygen!

Now you must steel yourself.

Now the mask gently breathes into your single lung; one lung alone, from this moment on, will know the heady quality of oxygen. Now you must want to live. Now or later, there is no life without desire.

Desire now to live and we will spit at the marauders who come pushing into my house, the house of my children! They smear the twisted cross over my children's heads. They shout in their devils' voices you have no special right to live. They drop bombs from their bats' wings and worship the ruins like a flower. But here we answer them, soon there will be no children left, no laughter, only the dreary hell-flowers of their slums and bomb pits....

There, it is done.

You are free. The gentlemen who have come to watch the carpentry are pleased. But I watch only your life flickering steadily on the nonchalant dial faces. It lifts the mercury in the tube, heavier at this point than all the burdens in the world. Now the pleura gapes with unaccustomed emptiness. The other lung, the heart and viscera will yearn to close the vacuum later. Now to bring order out of this clearing in the wilderness. Life is indivisible: the brambles of veins, arteries, stumps each reek an individual villainy. The least must be soothed with the greatest. Now the yeaning, sorrowful gulf is stitched together. Now the retractors release the wounded tissue and the slender needle tenderly reunites the delicate flesh....

A few hours after the operation Yvette asked for water. Bethune, standing by, touched her lips with a wet cloth.

In the hallway the parents waited with hope and dread. "She will recover," Bethune said. The father stood mutely for a moment, then threw his arms around the doctor while the mother clasped her hands and sobbed.

That night, tired, exultant, he wrote about the operation and sent a note to Marian Scott:

My child is well.

It was a beautiful operation. I felt very happy doing it ... except for a few bad moments. The entire right lung was removed — the first time this has been done in a child of ten in Canada.... Isn't it nice?

Yes, I will sleep deeply tonight. Last night was a *"nuit blanche"* — not whether I could do it but whether I should. But my child is well and I shall sleep deeply now.... Goodnight.

BETH

22

A week after the operation on Yvette he received an unexpected visitor — a spokesman from the Committee to Aid Spanish Democracy. Headquarters had been set up in Toronto under the chairmanship of the Reverend Ben Spence, with the support of a number of clergymen, labour leaders and public figures. As its first act of assistance to the Spanish Republic it had decided to send a medical unit to Madrid, financed by a direct appeal to the Canadian people. The Committee agreed that the one man in Canada to head the unit was Dr. Norman Bethune, if he would accept.

After his visitor had gone he sat alone for a long time, lost in thought. The he went absent-mindedly through the pile of papers on his desk, writing in occasional notes:

Go to Spain? Last week I had to decide whether to operate on my child. Now I have to decide whether I go to Spain. I am surprised, honoured — and perplexed. Am I the right person? Am I ready? Yesterday's answers seem to prepare new questions for today. And tomorrow — what? The times impose cruel and irreversible decisions on us!

The committee to aid Spain accepted the fact he needed time to make up his mind; the war in Spain did not. Every day brought more news of the blockading of the Loyalists and the fascist advance towards Madrid.

What should he do? It was a grim question. For nine years he had grappled with a problem that baffled medicine for centuries: the wiping out of tuberculosis. He thought he had found a way at last, but it would need work, persuasion, an unceasing crusade, the unorthodox methods of popular agitation. Could he now throw it all up?

And then, he asked himself, what about his personal position? Suppose he did go to Spain? Where would he be afterwards? He was now 46 years old, with not too many years ahead of him as a surgeon. He had only *begun* thoracic surgery at the age of 39, when the average doctor was already well launched in his career.

He was now Chief of Thoracic Surgery at the Sacré Coeur Hospital; Consulting Surgeon to the Dominion Department of Pensions and National Health; Consulting Surgeon to the Mount Sinai Sanatorium at St. Agathe, Quebec, and the Grace Dart Home Hospital in Montreal. He was one of the highest paid men in his profession. Medical pilgrims came to Sacré Coeur from all over the world to study his work. Many of the doctors now practising thoracic surgery in Canada and the United States had studied under him, observing his techniques and the use of his own instruments. He was a member of the top, select Council of the American Association for Thoracic Surgery, looked up to now by his former heroes.

All of this, perhaps his whole career as a thoracic surgeon, would have to be thrown into the discard. At what point, he asked himself, did the personal element fall away before the larger considerations?

The larger considerations left him no opportunity to think in terms of the personal element. The news from Spain became more urgent, and at home, native fascist groups, encouraged by the success of their cohorts abroad, began running amok in the streets. Franco's drive towards Madrid was accompanied by attacks on Jewish citizens in Montreal, depredations against Jewish shopkeepers, racist propaganda imported from Berlin. "The insanity is spreading too quickly," he would suddenly burst out ro friends. "They've begun in Germany, in Japan, now in Spain, and they're coming out into the open everywhere. If we don't stop them in Spain while we still can, they'll turn the world into a slaughterhouse."

One night, alone in his apartment, he stood at the window for a long time, gazing down at the square. Then he sat at his desk, went through his papers, wrote letters of resignation to his superiors, and drew up his will. Until it could sustain itself from public contributions, the Children's Art School would draw money from his bank account. Frances was to have power-of-attorney to handle all his financial affairs. In the event of his death all of his worldly possessions would go to her.

When he went to bed that night a typed draft of a poem lay across his desk:

> And this same pallid moon tonight,
> Which rides so quiet — clear and high —
> The mirror on our pale and troubled gaze,
> Raised to a cool, Canadian sky,
> Above the shattered Spanish mountain tops
> Last night rose low and wild and red,
> Reflecting back from her illumined shield
> The blood-bespattered faces of the dead.
> To that pale moon I raise my angry fist,
> And to all those nameless dead my vows renew:
> Comrades who fall in angry loneliness,
> Who die for us — I will remember you.

Three weeks later he left for Spain.

PART THREE

THE ENEMY — FASCISM

23

A station wagon manoeuvres along the blacked-out Gran Via, skirting the ripped pavements and shell holes. It moves without lights, slowly, cautiously. At the end of the thoroughfare it turns right and crawls through the shattered streets leading to Casa del Campo. This is no longer the city under siege — it is the battle zone itself.

The night is suddenly convulsed. Great sheets of light flash through the sky. The silence is shredded by a deafening cannonade that sickens the ear. The pavement trembles like a living being seized by fear.

In the orange-red glare of an exploding shell the station wagon lurches to the side of the street, then speeds forward as if there is no longer need for caution. Soon it is roaring into Casa del Campo, the Royal Park, heading straight for the trenches, which are pinpointed in the darkness by a blaze of guns and sounds of battle.

This is Madrid on the night of December 23, 1936.

The Christmas season has come, but Madrid lies in darkness, under curfew, stabbed by the enemy's steel-sheathed forces. Soon, perhaps, if the moon cuts through the clouds, the bombers will come, filling the sky with their angry snarl.

Today the enemy's shelling began promptly at four in the afternoon; the shells droned methodically into the streets, searching out the most densely populated districts. At dinnertime it began again, continued for an hour, precisely at the moment men and women filled the streets on their way home from work. "We are saving Spain from Bolshevism," say the communiqués issued at Burgos and written in Berlin; to "save" Spain the traitor generals are destroying Madrid.

During the noon hour a crowd of workers on the Gran Via listened to one of their leaders report on the war. From the meeting the volunteers marched directly to the trenches in Casa del Campo. Their guns were old, but their songs were new and their faces shining. This afternoon the women in the working-class district of Cuatro Caminos bore the brunt of the shelling, some losing a home, some a roof, some a bed, some a child; but tonight the women of the working class labour behind the men from their own streets, digging defences in the frozen earth and carrying the banner of their new emancipation: WE WOULD RATHER BE WIDOWS OF HEROES THAN WIVES OF SLAVES!

Madrid! Gored, bloodied, shaken, betrayed ... but defended. For thirty-seven days the city has been fighting for its life. Now, on the thirty-seventh day, the idea of defence is as natural and automatic in the lives of the people as eating and sleeping. "We must decide whether we will be hammer or anvil," a speaker cried the other day at one of the great political rallies held despite the bombers. The audience understood, and cheered wildly. It understood; for as long ago as the February days of the Frente Popular electoral victory the Madrileño cast himself in the role of hammer, with history as his anvil and Spain to be forged anew. Now the hammer is on the anvil, and at Burgos the generals are trying to discover where their easy victory went astray.

In the rape of a city the voices of its people have joined in the vast harmonies of unity. For thirty-seven days and thirty-seven nights — each day and each night with its compressed quota of anguish — the city has heard its women weeping, its men cursing, its evacuee children saying goodbye. But now, too, the traitors are being run to the ground, and the lowliest citizen has turned parliamentarian, critic, soldier, organizer. La Pasionaria, daughter of the dark Austrian mines, has gone on foot through the streets, into the seamiest corners of the city, into the bars of the shiftless and the homes of the thoughtless — lifting her voice with the unspoken hopes of all the inarticulate, speaking to the heart of each ardent citizen and the collective will of the nation, putting into simple words the meaning of all the terror, agony, and resistance: *Better to die on our feet than live on our knees!* The response rolls across the city of bloodstained streets, a chorus in which optimism rises above the bitter chords, and notes of gaiety already challenge the minor key.

The Republic has inherited a score of factions, a hundred conflicting viewpoints, a thousand stupidities. But from the mass of Madrileños, uprooted from old ways and old allegiances, the demand rises irresistibly for only one purpose: solidarity of all, resistance to the end, death to the enemy, and long live the Republic!

Madrid knows its desperate plight and its collective power. The city that is now at the heart of the world's crossroad earned its eminence by becoming the heart of the Popular Front. It is here that the demand first rose for action against the traitor generals left by the old regime, here that unarmed men and women, while the government fumbled, forced the gates of the Montana barracks in the centre of the city, made prisoners of the rebel troops barricaded inside, and seized the arms with which to defend the February vote and the revived Republic.

It is the knowledge of this collective power, tested in battle, that lightens Madrid's every painful hour with vitality and confidence. On the Gran Via, the Telefónica building, Madrid's lonely skyscraper, rears audaciously towards the skies in which the bombers flaunt their German origin. The upper floors have been hit again and again, but government offices continue to function on the lower ones. No matter where a city is hit, it too continues to function.

At first there was fear under enemy bombardment. Now the people have learned to live with the fear. Pedestrians on the Gran Via know that the enemy's shells land on only one side of the street; so they walk calmly on the other side. And the local army command, knowing that the enemy never shells the residential districts of the wealthy, has discreetly hidden its guns in the untouched parks gracing the lavish mansions of the pro-Franco upper class.

Since November 6 the sense of impotence has gone out of the citizen's fear. That was the day on which the sirens sounded as usual, the bombers appeared, the people rushed to subways and flimsy shelters. But as they fled they heard a new sound in the skies. They stopped in their tracks, looking upward. "*Nuestros!*" they shouted. Men and women sobbed with joy, they pounded each other, they threw their berets in the air, they hugged and danced and sang and cried defiance. "Ours! Our planes! *Nuestros!*"

High above the city a squadron of tiny pursuit planes bore the markings of the Republic. They flew with dazzling speed into the surprised attackers, their guns ripping the enemy. They were the government's first real combat planes, and for the first time since the July days they dispersed the enemy, bomb load and all.

"*Chatos*," the Madrileños nicknamed them delightedly — "the pugnoses." They had arrived at Cartagena from Russia in crates only four days before. They have taken the sport out of the enemy's bombing.

On November 6 the *chatos* flashed their wings over the city and on November 8 the first of the International Brigades were hastily assembled at Albacete, outfitted with trousers, jackets, indifferent weapons and moved into the lines. The approach to their battle stations lay through the streets of Madrid. Fresh from the villages and cities of the world, Mussolini's prisons, Hitler's concentration camps and the "neutrality" blockade of the Western powers, they marched through the wild acclaim of delirious Madrileños. Most of them are dead or wounded, but others have followed across the forbidden frontiers, and after six months of invasion from abroad, treason from within and betrayal by the Western governments, Madrid fights to the exultant cry: "We are not alone!"

The people of Madrid know that their cause lacks no followers — only arms; they know that the enemy lacks no arms, — only followers. They know who is sending men to the enemy and who is depriving Republican Spain of arms. They know that if Franco wins they will live under the double dictatorship of the old regime and its foreign manipulators. They know the generals and the grandees have fitted their treason into the Axis blueprint for world conquest. They know that the future of London, Warsaw, Paris, Shanghai, is being shaped in the streets where they were born. And what they think, what they feel and understand, surges trough the city from the moment, at dawn, when the first street cleaner sets up the hose, Spanish style, and washes the blood from the pavement, till the moment when the last militiamen speaks of the curfew challenge.

Isolated by fascist guns, lonely but not alone, Madrid reveals its soul in its curfew passwords. Last night those permitted on the streets during curfew heard the challenge on the darkened street corners, "Where is the army of the Republic tonight?" and replied, "Advancing." Tonight, while it waits for the bombers, while it sends its men to the trenches, while it sleeps in cold rooms with pangs of hunger — tonight, Madrid under curfew has chosen the password, "What will be free?" And the answer, "*El mundo todo!*" The whole world will be free!

The station wagon that has sped from the Gran Via into Casa del Campo comes to a jarring stop under a clump of trees, close to the trenches.

Two men jump out. Here, under the trees, is their rendez-vous: a casualty station.

They pause a moment to take stock of the figures hurrying between them in the dark. There are muffled curses from the trenches, the angry chatter of machine guns, the frightening detonations of trench mortars and the anguished cries of the wounded. They can make out the bent forms of light and quick darkness of a night battle.

The wounded are lying on the ground all around them. The moon emerges suddenly from the clouds. Near the clump of trees the light is welcome. For the wounded it reveals the world again, the familiar surroundings that tell them they are still alive. For the two men it makes easier the task of unloading the strange paraphernalia from their station wagon.

They exchange documents with a harassed medical officer in charge of the casualty station. They are an unexpected pair: two strangers, foreigners, speaking little Spanish, suddenly material-izing out of the night at the precise sector where the government troops have launched a local attack. The Spanish doctor, beset by more casualties than he can properly handle, is confused by their arrival. Where do they come from? Who are they? What do they want? They introduce themselves from their store of half-a-dozen words and sign language. One of them is tall, lean, long-faced. He is young but moves with care and deliberations of an older man. The other, the one in command, is not easily classified. He gives an impression of slender height, yet is not tall. His face is strong, showing no definite age, yet his finely shaped head is fringed by thick grey-white hair that gives him a sculptured appearance. He is dressed in a blue, zippered uniform designed for rough-and-ready use: a military tunic with patch pockets, trousers tucked into heavy boots, the insignia of a colonel of the Republican Army on his chest, a Maple Leaf on both shoulders.

The Spanish doctor glances at the uniform. His manner shows it puzzles him as much as the instructions he has just received from its wearer. He hands back the documents, salutes, says, "*Si, comandante*," and extends his arm in a gesture signifying they can begin.

Under the trees swaying in the wind, with stretcher bearers bringing up more casualties, with bullets singing over their heads, with the wounded moaning at their feet, they begin....

The comandante kneels beside the first soldier in the line of casualties. He looks into the soldier's face. The features are twisted by pain but the very pain signifies the strength with which life holds fast in the wounded body. The comandante pats the soldier's arm and moves on.

The next man is no longer wounded; he is dead. His face shows the bitter loneliness in which he died. The comandante has seen the faces of many dead, but none so reproachful as this. He unbuttons the soldier's shirt, loosens the trousers. "Not much of a wound, but much blood lost," he whispers.

He rises again and continues along the line, making his examinations and decisions swiftly. To some of the men he speaks words of encouragement; they don't understand the meaning of the words but they understand the intent, and smile with the easy grace of children. Beside others he nods his head and says to his tall, silent companion, "This one ..."

When he has made the rounds of all the wounded he walks back unerringly to a still form covered by a coat. He drops down on one knee and gently raises the man's head — but when he looks at the face it is not the face of a man; it is the face of a boy, perhaps sixteen or seventeen, pale even in the moonlight under the black crop of disordered hair. The comandante reads the face easily: the lips slack, the cheeks sunken, the skin clammy, the eyes half closed in utter weariness. The features show no recognition, no fear, no hope. "Bad shock," the comandante murmurs. "We'll begin with him...."

The waspish sounds of the bullets is suddenly lost in a deeper tone: the whine of a shell. The men laid out on the ground listen; the medical orderlies throw themselves down, covering their ears.

The whine lengthens. There is the unnatural noise like ripping canvas, then the explosion, the blinding glare, the earth heaving, the trees shivering. The boy in the comandante's arms groans, clutching his abdomen feebly. The thunder in his stomach is as staggering as the noise in his ears. Pain brings him back briefly from the dark tide on which he is slipping away. He looks up at the stranger with the grey hair, seeing nothing, perhaps, but the night and the blackness pressing against his eyeballs, straining for a glimpse nevertheless of what his mind dimly remembers.

The comandante rests the lolling head gently on the ground. While the medical orderlies hurry by, and the echoes of the blast die away, he sets to work with efficient hands. He rips the sleeve of the lad's jacket with one motion, rolls back the shirt, and swiftly explores the exposed forearm. "Ready, now." He speaks without looking up, but his tall companion is at his side to hand him the slender rubber tube with the glinting needle at the end. In the slack flesh the comandante's fingers find the vein and follow it to the end of the elbow. The moon is no substitute for the arc lights of the operating theatre, but the comandante's fingers know the routes of the soldier's dwindling life stream and the jab of the needle can bring only a merciful pain.

There is the whine of another shell, closer and more intimate this time, followed by still another before the first explodes. The enemy is searching for the target, bending the barrage closer to the Republic's lines. But there is now no time to gauge the danger. In the orange-red brilliance that now spreads in a chain of flaming geysers across the Royal Park the comandante tapes the needle onto the arm with adhesive, rises, and runs his hand along the tubing to the squat bottle his companion is holding. "Right, I'll take it," he says. "You can get more bottles out of the car."

He stands erect now, his head bare, his face thoughtful, ignoring the bullets that ping into the trees, the flares, the confusion, the shouts, the warnings of the medical officer hurrying by, the shells that ravish the night, the rumblings that penetrate to his very bones. He holds the bottle above the young soldier, moving to the soldier's head so as to put his own body between the bottle and the front room from which the bullets come.

It is an ordinary bottle but it stores a precious fluid. Blood! Dark, mysterious, inconstant. Blood — universal in type, thick and cohesive still from the veins of the living donor, live-giving with the accumulated experiences, sacrifices, yearnings of men questing for knowledge over a score of centuries. Here, on the thundering battlefield, all the textbooks, searchings, errors, corrections, scientific certainties since the mythical days of Medea and her sorcery — all are stored in a squat glass bottle.

From the grooved bellies of German guns a new salvo bursts across the casualty station. And from the ardent veins of an anonymous Madrileño the comandante sends the first warm drops of blood into the depleted veins of the dying soldier at his feet.

He releases the clamp on the tubing slowly, carefully. The lad is far gone. In the hours since he was wounded and dragged from no man's land the twilight between life and death has seeped into his organs. He shivers, his teeth chatter.

The comandante opens the clamp fully. Now the blood flows in a steady stream, and the miracle is near. The comandante has seen it many times before, but it is always new: like a wasted flower suddenly blooming again with rich-hued petals.

The boy stirs. His teeth no longer chatter. He begins to move his head. He opens his eyes, blankly at first, then with a painful effort to remember. But it is only the beginning. Casting aside the now empty bottle the comandante prepares the second. Soon, after the second bottle, the miracle is complete. The lad smiles: the comandante knows, without being able to see, that the colour has returned to his face, that after a few minutes of chill his skin will grow warm again, that after his wounds are tended he will live.

"*Bueno, bueno*," the comandante says cheerfully. He lights a cigarette and puts it to the soldier's lips. The soldier takes a deep puff. He suddenly realizes he is alive. "*Gracias*," he murmurs joyfully, but the comandante has already vanished.

For thirty minutes the comandante moves back and forth among the wounded, instructing the station doctor, refusing to accept the textbook signs of death, repeating the transfusions on the worst cases, holding his bottles aloft, screening them from the enemy with his broad shoulders, opening veins to the salty river that washes life back into the bodies of the near- dead with its strange chemistry. At last the containers in the station wagon are empty. There is no more blood to be transfused, but of the men who stormed out of the trenches to seize a strong point from the Moors and Germans one hour ago, twelve who would have died are still alive; twelve soldiers of the Republic who will be smiling when they reach the hospital, who will remember this night under the trees, and the thoughtful face of the man with the grey-white hair and his magic bottles of blood.

"*No más?*" the Spanish doctor has followed the comandante to the station wagon. "*No más?*" he asks. "No more?"

The comandante, fastening the back doors of his car, shakes his head. He makes signs that he has to return to the city for a fresh supply of blood. As he talks and waves his hands he is surrounded by a group of orderlies and soldiers with minor wounds.

The Spanish doctor raises his fist in the Republican salute. Solemnly, speaking the Spanish words with special care, as if to bridge the barrier of language by his very intensity, he says: "Dr. Alvarez Ruiz.* *Muchas Gracias.*"

The Canadian doctor stands erect, his fist raised too. "I am Dr. Norman Bethune. My friend, Hazen Sise. It is we who thank you."

In sudden silence the Canadians and Spaniards look at each other in a burst of feeling neither knows how to express, here, on this flaring sector of the war that has tossed them together in the jumble of pain and death. Then one of the soldiers points to the lettering on the station wagon that is visible in the light of the nearby flames, "Instituto Hispano-Canadense de Transfusión de Sangre."

He cries out, "*Viva la transfusión de sangre!*"

The response sweeps along the line of wounded: "*Viva!*"

"*Viva el Canada!*"

"*Viva!*"

A small voice cuts thinly through the bass chorus. "*Viva yo!*" Everybody turns. It is the voice of the boy who received the first transfusion. He has risen on his elbow, his other hand stretched out before him, his eyes burning on his young face. "*Viva yo!*" he cries. "Long live *me!*"

There is laughter; they all understand.

"*Viva!*" they cry. For themselves, for these strangers from abroad, for Spain, for the world.

---

* This is a pseudonym.

The word spreads, this morning of December 23 1936, through the lines in Casa del Campo. From somewhere beyond the seas a friend has come with a miracle for the soldiers of the Republic.

Tomorrow it will be broadcast all over Madrid, reaching out to Teruel, Guadalajara, Valencia, all the fronts, to the women who wait in dread for sons and husbands, finally, beyond the borders of Spain, to all the world.

For the first time since humans learned to kill their brothers, a man had appeared on the battlefield to reverse history — *to give blood, not to shed it.*

24

He had arrived in Madrid on November 3, a cold rainy morning, and registered at the Hotel Gran Via, just opposite the Telefónica building. In the lobby he was met by a pleasant-looking, fair-haired man who introduced himself as Henning Sorensen, in Madrid as correspondent for the *New Commonwealth* and *Canadian Forum*.*

Outside the hotel soldiers patrolled the streets in twos and threes. All the streets leading to the city boasted barricades. Bethune asked Sorensen if the situation was as bad as they had told him it was in Valencia.

"As bad or as good," Sorensen replied. "Madrid is Madrid, Valencia is, after all, only Valencia. The fascist have entered University City. Madrid women are busy filling bottles of gasoline. The people have barricaded all the streets. The fascists will have to take the city house by house."

The press offices were on the third floor of the Telefónica. Bethune and Sorensen called there that afternoon to get the

---

* A newspaper and a magazine both reflecting the viewpoint of the Co-operative Commonwealth Federation.

latest news. Suddenly, the building shook, hit by a shell; everyone looked up, waited, and then resumed work.

Bethune could look down from the windows and see the streetcar attendant on the corner switching the rails of a tram to make a turn. On the same corner the subway kiosk was plastered with posters urging the Madrileños to join the Fifth Regiment, to evacuate their children, to help the peasants gather in the wheat.

Sorensen chuckled, "You could take a tram or subway and get within a hundred yards of the trenches. You see, Madrid goes about its business as usual. It's true that the situation is serious ... but I doubt if Madrid will fall."

As Bethune walked the streets that day he could see that the rest of Madrid shared Sorensen's optimism.

With Sorensen as guide and interpreter he set out to find the best method of organizing Canadian medical aid for the Loyalist troops.

He made a swift tour of the city's military hospitals where the tensions and uncertainties were such that he could get few definite answers to the questions he asked about the medical situation at the front. To get the answers he went into the trenches of University City itself, visiting the fronts outside Madrid. He inspected casualty stations behind the lines and worked with army surgeons at several base hospitals. Here he studied the types of wounds the soldiers suffered and kept notes on the percentage of fatalities and the recoveries after surgery.

In a cellar headquarters of University City he met General Kleber, who had once lived in Canada and was now in command of the International Brigades helping to defend Madrid. Kleber gave him a résumé of the military situation, declared Madrid would hold out, and referred him to one of the chief medical officers of the International Brigades, a Czech doctor by the name of Erwin Kisch.

Dr. Kisch welcomed him enthusiastically in broken English, overjoyed to hear that a thoracic surgeon of Bethune's standing was available for service "We must put you to work at once!" he cried.

For Kisch, who had been in Spain two months, operating constantly, it seemed clear where Bethune was needed. For Bethune himself it had not yet become clear. He asked for a few more days to make up his mind and the interview ended coolly.

On November 6, he went to the headquarters of the Fifth Regiment to confer with Carlos Contreras, its political commander.*

The Loyalist military forces still consisted of the various militia groups spontaneously organized by the trade unions, and with varying political affiliations. There was, as yet, no unified command. All units fought bravely, but not as part of a disciplined military establishment. The Fifth Regiment had been set up shortly after the outbreak of the war by the Spanish Communist Party which had from the beginning, along with the Negrin-Del Vayo** Socialists and some sections of the liberal Republicans, demanded a unified command. The Fifth Regiment was designed to set an example of a disciplined fighting force. By now it had become a legend throughout Loyalist Spain and was acknowledged to be the heart of Madrid's resistance. From British and American correspondents Bethune had heard that Political Commander Contreras was the man "who gets things done."

His interview with Carlos Contreras*** took place in a car on the way to Albacete, the only time, Contreras explained, that he could spare. It was a bizarre interview, followed by bizarre events:

> Before leaving Madrid in Contreras's car [Bethune reported later], we stopped for a few minutes at the Montana Barracks, where young volunteers were getting their first military instructions. We heard the rifles had arrived from Mexico and some tanks from Russia. There was noticeable optimism. We got to Albacete around 3:30 in the morning. Here we heard that the government headed by Largo Caballero had

---

* Enrique Lister was Military Commander.

** Alvarez del Vayo was Spain's Foreign Minister; Juan Negrin later became Premier.

*** Contreras spoke fluent English.

moved to Valencia, leaving a Military Junta in charge of Madrid.

On the way Carlos gave us his views of the political and military situation. He obviously didn't think very much of old Caballero who, he said, couldn't forget that it wasn't a trade union he was now leading but an armed struggle. He was afraid that Caballero was not up to the situation, and implied that the UGT leader was resisting demands for a unified command. Army units in various parts of the country (particularly the Aragon) were operating on their own. Certain anarchist battalions went into action only under orders from their own-appointed commanders. Without a central, unified command, Contreras held, the Republic could never hope to defeat the mechanized units of Germany and Italy.*

I could not help but remark on the difference between the spirit of Madrid and that of Valencia or Barcelona. In reply, Carlos made the point that the spirit was best where the fighting was most bitter. The Communist Party was stronger in Madrid than anywhere else in Spain, and the bulk of the Socialist Youth Organization, also was in Madrid.** The lessons of the war were moving the Socialist rank-and-file to the left, while Caballero seemed to be moving toward a closer alliance with the Anarchists and certain right-wing Republican elements. Carlos saw Caballero's moves as an attempt to offset the growing influence of the left-wing Socialists, Communists and the liberal Republican groups who demanded a dynamic program to

---

* A unified command came into existence in May 1937, when Caballero resigned and was replaced as Premier by Juan Negrin.

** The 100,000 members of the Socialist Youth had enrolled *en bloc* in the Spanish Communist Party a few months before.

transform the unorganized mass of militia into an efficient, unified fighting organization.

Carlos didn't think the Popular Front was threatened but seemed to indicate that a new alignment within the Popular Front was necessary if Spain's resources were to be properly organized to fight a prolonged war. It was evident that the traitorous army generals had been defeated; it was also evident that Germany and Italy were determined to prolong the war as long as they could, not only to guarantee their Mediterranean flank, but to use Spain as a testing ground for their equipment and their strategy.

When we came to the question of what I could do for Spain, Contreras said there was a number of alternatives. I could function as a surgeon in one of the hospitals, or for the International Brigades, or I could establish a Canadian Medical Unit to work in the cities or the Front. He assured me that anything I decided to do would be helpful, told me to see him if I needed any help in anything I decided to do, and then left to attend to his urgent business. He returned to Madrid next morning but Sorensen and I went to see the chief of the Sanidad Extranjera (Foreign Health Service, attached to the International brigade), a little Frenchman who suggested I work with him. It was something to consider, and we left Albacete with him the following day (November 8) to "inspect the front lines." We never got anywhere near a front line and we lost our way four times. That was enough for me. We wasted two days with him for nothing. I told him politely as I could that I had other plans, and we returned to Madrid, luckily getting transportation on a truck.

Henning and I arrived in Madrid on the 11th and I made another tour of the casualty stations. By now I had a feeling about what had to be done.

When he became certain of what was missing in the army's medical services, he went back to Dr. Kisch to outline the novel project that had taken shape in his mind. In all modern wars, he pointed out, even the most highly organized medical services suffered from a serious defect. Never had provisions been made for those would who bled to death on the battlefield, or between the trip from the front to the base hospital, or who were so weakened by loss of blood or shock they were unable to survive surgery once they arrived at a base hospital. In Barcelona, Dr. Duran Jorda had done great work in storing blood and organizing blood banks. But the main problem had not yet been tackled decisively. *The problem was to provide transfusion directly at the front, as close to the battlefield as possible.* Bethune was convinced that it was feasible, and would result in a sharp decrease in death among the wounded. He was therefore proposing the organization of a *mobile* blood transfusion unit that would gather blood from volunteers in the cities, store it, make it available to casualty stations and field hospitals, and above all, provide transfusions at the front while fighting was in progress.

For a long time Kisch sat back in his chair, staring at Bethune. "If you can do it," he said at last, a new note of respect in his voice, "you will be making medical history."

At the Socorro Rojo* Headquarters in Valencia, Bethune outlined his plans to the top officials who had to approve them on behalf of the government. They listened to him carefully, among them two Spanish doctors, then looked at one another and finally gave their opinion.

"Impractical."

They studied his figures again, wrestled with the uncomfortable statistics of men who might have been saved but had died from loss of blood or shock.

One of the older Spanish doctors looked about his colleagues, then at Bethune. "But as you say, 'perhaps impossible,

---

* Socorro Rojo was a Spanish trade union which functioned as the only effective medical service in Loyalist Spain until the newly organized Sanidad Militar took over its functions in the spring of 1937.

but necessary.' And if necessary, then not impossible. And if not impossible, then it is made so because it required somebody to say so."

They decided without having to make a decision. "How soon," the old doctor asked, "can you get your plans into operation?"

"As fast as it takes to get to Paris and London, and back again with the necessary equipment. And as soon, after that, as you can give me a place to work along with technicians, doctors, nurses."

An hour later Bethune sent a long cable to the Spanish Aid Committee in Toronto. He outlined the situation at the front, his plans, the government's approval, the methods he proposed to use, the technical innovations he intended to introduce. He ended the cable with an appeal for immediate action:

> Need a lot of apparatus, sterilizers, instruments in sets, microscopes, et cetera. Have many new ideas for improved apparatus. Am leaving with Sorensen for Paris and London to buy necessary equipment. Cable as much money as possible to committee representative in Paris.

The next morning he set out for Paris with Sorensen without waiting for a reply. When he arrived he found ten thousand dollars had been cabled from the Canadian Committee with a message expressing approval of the project and promising him full financial support.

He made a quick tour of medical suppliers in Paris, established contacts for future supplies and moved on to London.

After the battlefields of Spain, England was quiet, grim and grey. To newspapermen who flocked to interview him, he described the project he was preparing, declared his conviction that Spain would hold out, and labelled as "damnable," English, French, and American refusal to sell arms to Republican Spain.

When he had completed his purchases he armed himself with all the available literature, from every part of the world, on latest techniques of transfusion, locked himself in his hotel room and plunged into the story of blood, a story that had dazzled and tantalized men for more than two thousand years.

25

The story was everywhere: in the British Museum, in the musty reference books, in a million hospital wards around the world, in the hazards hovering over every city street and modern machine, in the ills of civilization, in men's despairing resistance to the seeming cruelty of death which equated them in the end to the lowest weeds of the sea.

Bethune too had been caught up in it. He too had helped shape it — casually, in the days of his apprenticeship in the operating theatre; consciously, now he had apprenticed himself to the battlefield.

From the days of antiquity men had written their history in blood before they recorded it in tablets. They looked upon its mysteries with awe and fear. They endowed it with the same magic attributed to the elements that lashed and warmed them. Moving forward to the higher levels of civilization they gazed backward upon the lower animals with superstitious envy, dreaming sometimes that perhaps they might revitalize their failing organs with the blood of four-legged creatures.

For thousands of years they knew nothing of the fluid that washed back and forth through their bodies, nothing of the channels it followed, of the life-giving substances it deposited in vital organs, like silt left on barren fields by the rivers of the earth. They knew only that in every breast there beat a rhythm, and in every wrist a pulse, and when the thickening fluid burst from its unknown labyrinth, the body returned to silence and decay.

Through Stone Age, Bronze Age, the migrations of vast primitive hordes, the first civilizations of Asia, the first stirrings in Europe, the gestating centuries of the Dark Ages — through it all the ever more certain knowledge that to bleed meant death carried no novelty and little stimulus. Without reverence for life, few arms reached out to build barriers against death. Even the handful of Greek patricians, full of philosophy and love of the body's external shapes, assigned to man the anatomy of the dog. In medieval Europe, when the sportive spirit and searchings of the Greeks became overlaid by dust, life was riotous for the few and a mere burden for the many. The people were serfs, chattels, tied to the land others owned; ignored, not even despised, by the rare minds stirring occasionally into thought.

Men looked neither to the stars nor to the light once glowing in the past, nor to the future. The spur of necessity had first to drive them forth beyond their own shores, to distant, forgotten places; to open the rest of the world; to seek the riches of the East; to navigate the seas; to find the earth round and not flat; to spread trade; to map shorter routes to the Orient; to discover America.

While Columbus, in 1492, sought out the secrets hidden by an ocean, a doctor in Rome sought the secrets hidden in the life stream. While Columbus's sailors were sighting land, the doctor was transfusing blood from the veins of three young boys into the veins of old Pope Innocent VIII. History as recorded that Columbus fared the better of the two. Though he missed the Orient he discovered America, whereas the doctor killed both boys and pope. But from the discovery of America and the first attempted blood transfusion known, there would come together many streams of human effort that would some day be the heritage of Dr. Norman Bethune on the battlefields of Spain.

To establish that heritage other seekers first had to brave prejudice, fear, punishment. Dissection of the body was forbidden; those who came to understand that the body had to be dissected if it was to be known, worked in secret, sometimes suffering imprisonment and exile. In 1613 William Harvey changed the course of medicine with his discovery of the circulation of the blood. Only now could the dream of the anonymous Roman doctor become a reality. To make it a reality many men worked and searched and experimented — and added to their reverence of life the possibility of preserving it.

In England, half a century after Harvey's discovery, Richard Lower transfused blood between two dogs by running quills from the cervical artery of one to the jugular vein of the other. In Paris, at the same time, Jean Baptiste Denis transfused the blood of a lamb into the veins of a fifteen-year-old boy suffering from anemia and some unknown fever. When his patient recovered, French medical men were highly impressed and Denis continued to transfuse for many ailments. His very success, however, proved his undoing in the end. Noting that some patients fell into a state of shock after receiving blood he decided to attempt the cure of a mental patient by transfusion. While the shock brought about by incompatible blood is different from that produced by insulin injections or electric charges, Denis was anticipating a therapeutic approach for certain forms of mental illness by 250 years. But he was working in the dark, though working better than he knew. When some of his patients died, prejudice, fear and conservatism rose up in righteous anger; all blood transfusions were banned in France and the ban spread to most of Europe.

For almost 200 years medicine then turned away from the mystery it didn't understand. Transfusions became the black market calling of quacks. Human blood was tampered with for every purpose, except the simple one of maintaining the body's normal supply or overcoming the effects of hemorrhage, shock, burns. Respectable doctors bled their patients for everything from pimples to plague. Unprincipled frauds secretly prescribed transfusions for exactly the same ailments. The orgy of black magic reached its solemn, stupid climax with the announcement of a German doctor that he had discovered the secret of domestic bliss in the blood. Where there were difficulties between husband and wife, he declared, transfusion of the wife's blood into the husband, and vice versa, would immediately end all discord. In the existing state of medical knowledge, it would have ended husband and wife as well.

The disrepute which held up further investigation was merely a reflection of the disrepute in which life itself was held. The French Revolution had to put a new emphasis on the dignity of life before the men of science could counterattack the obscurantists. On the barricades of 1792 the proclamation of Liberty, Equality, Fraternity changed the course of history. Henceforth the dead rot of feudalism was challenged. From America, the Continent had heard Thomas Paine's bold talk of the rights of man. Modern industrial society, slowly germinating in the shadow of medievalism, burst the bonds of feudalism. As the new era emerged, unevenly, in turmoil and bloodshed, but with the promise of a limitless future, it freed the scientist to cut a path before the world-conquering capitalist. The serfs turned men were herded into new factories, the miseries of industrial exploitation tarnished the bright slogan of Liberty, Equality, Fraternity, but science was let loose to probe all mysteries and a new generation of thinkers arose to denounce all exploitations.

And so, three decades after the French Revolution had lit up the way for the nineteenth century, an English doctor, James Blundell, returned to the field which had remained untouched for so long. He was guided by compassion and the new spirit that rejected the unknowable. For years he watched women die in childbirth from hemorrhage. He rebelled at the fate which destroyed so many mothers in the very act of giving life. If it was from blood loss that they died, he reasoned, why not defeat the hemorrhage by mechanical means? Why not give back to the arterial system Harvey had already discovered an amount of blood equal to the amount lost during confinement? He pondered the problem and finally created a syringe with which he transferred blood from a healthy individual to a hemorrhaging mother. Like other medical men, he knew nothing about blood itself, but his syringe worked. Some of the mothers died for reasons he couldn't fathom, but some of them were saved. And those who were saved brought blood transfusions back into the field of serious medicine.

Other doctors took up where Blundell left off, often for reasons they couldn't understand, but saving lives nevertheless that would otherwise have been lost. And now there came onto the scene men who looked for answers in blood itself. Why did transfusion save some and kill others? How could blood be prevented from coagulating while being transfused? The Frenchman Landois studied and experimented and finally came up with the startling discovery: something in one blood stream could agglutinate and dissolve the cells of another bloodstream. But what? Though he was on the right track he missed the full truth.

Then came another Englishman, Dr. Braxton Hicks, working to defeat coagulation and finally coming close by adding sodium phosphate to blood to preserve it. It was close, but not close enough.

Then came the "black period." While medical men were still ignorant of the blood's strange secrets, transfusions became a craze. They were given for boils and tuberculosis and everything in between, with the cure usually more devastating than the original disease. In despair, doctors sought a substitute for the life-giving discovery which led them on and in the end always baffled them:

for blood they substituted salt solutions, which mimicked the blood until the body produced its own. Now there were no complications. Hemorrhages were relieved and post-operative shock was lightened. For fifty years blood transfusions were used only rarely, replaced almost entirely by transfusions of salt solutions.

That might have been the end, but science and technique and the widening concern for human life refused to be stilled. Again there were men who rejected the unknowable, who kept studying, searching, experimenting, until at last the secrets were secrets no longer.

In 1902 the Viennese bacteriologist, Dr. Karl Landsteiner, emerged from his laboratory with the first answer. He had peered into the depths of human blood. He had found that like the oceans it also had its "flora and fauna." It was, in fact as if the timeless river running through the veins of men had three tributaries, all flowing from the mother river but each with its special flora and fauna. In his test tubes Landsteiner separated them, and then brought them together. And when he brought them together he saw with startled eyes how one seemed to turn upon the other, to stir up a strange tempest, as if all the living being of the ocean were suddenly engaged in fearful combat.

His discovery put the crown of success on Landois's failure. There were certain protein substances, he showed, which typed blood in three categories, depending on the manner in which they were present. He called the proteins isoagglutinins, and announced there were two such separate, distinct and hostile isoagglutinins. Individuals with one of the proteins in their blood were type A. Those with the second type were type B. Those with a combination of both types were type AB. The cells of one type destroyed the cells of the other two; to mix them was to invite disaster and death. Only when a patient was transfused with blood from an individual with his own blood grouping could the transfusion be successful. Now the failures of three centuries were explained! The basis was laid for the saving of untold lives.

When Descastello and Sturli in Italy, following in Landsteiner's footsteps, announced the discovery of a *fourth* tributary, a blood type with *none* of Landsteiner's proteins in it, the incompatibilities of the blood were finally defeated. The fourth type, O, or universal type, could be transfused safely to individuals of all types.

Henceforth no one would need to die because of transfused blood of a different type. And yet victory was still incomplete. The mother river remained perverse. It could flow from human veins from generation to generation, from Neanderthal man to the pilot hurtling through the skies, renewing itself, mortal in the body of individual man, immortal in the bodies of the race. But exposed to air and light it was no longer a flowing river. It became like a stream cut off from its source. It thickened. It grew sluggish like mud and water. It coagulated.

Now the risks of transfusing were almost gone, yet the act of transfusion itself remained a problem. In the very act of transfusion, blood often coagulated, the flow stopped, the patient died. And again the experiments started, the work in the laboratories went on unheralded, till at last still another answer was found, this time in America.

In 1915 the mother river was kept flowing for the first time outside the body's arterial system. Dr. Richard Lewisohn in New York and Professor L. Agote in Buenos Aires, working separately, added sodium citrate to some test tubes of blood and reported that the sodium kept it fluid longer than it had ever remained by itself.

From Lewisohn and Agote the surgeons took over, perfecting the tools of transfusion and devising simpler methods. A decade later the Russians, with their own special approach to tradition and pioneering, took over in turn, showing eventually that citrated blood could be stored in refrigerators for six weeks and still be used successfully.

By 1936 the Russians had established the world's most advanced system of blood banks. And by 1936 the first shots of the second world war had already been fired in Manchuria, Ethiopia had been swallowed up by fascism, and Spain was bleeding under the invader's bombs.

The testing time had come — for those who had followed the mother river to its source, for those who had harnessed it to feed life, for those who would shortly cry themselves under bombs like those wracking Spain.

What now for the long, twisting agonized story build on the ruins and hopes of so many men, over so many centuries, in so many lands? Now, for those still filled with the reverence for life, the story moved to Spain, to Dr. Duran Jorda of Barcelona, and to Dr. Norman Bethune of Gravenhurst, London, Vienna, Berlin, Detroit, Saranac Lake, Montreal, and Madrid.

In Barcelona, Dr. Jorda* had set up a blood bank using the latest findings of the Russians and some of his own. He had developed a highly technical system of pooling, bottling, and transfusing blood. Dr. Jorda's blood-bank clinic was to achieve glory during the days when Catalonia itself became a fighting front, but at the time, in Madrid, where the fighting was fierce and decisive, there were no mobile blood banks.

This was where Bethune stepped in. Perhaps the situation called for a man who was poet as well as a doctor, soldier as well as student, painter as well as healer of the body, dreamer as well as scientist — a man, above all, filled with a vast affection for the people, a vast hate for the disturbers of life and a vast belief in the future he and others could fashion. Here, it would some day be recorded, Norman Bethune took up where the explorers of the mother river had left off.

What would they have said of him — the Roman doctor, Landois, Denis, Blundell, Landsteiner?

In his London hotel room, tracing the story to which they had given their minds and lives, he gave it no thought. He was too busy with such practical matters as containers, refrigerators, needles, syringes, antiseptics, station wagons, personnel.

Others would come after him. The mother river itself would soon be broken down into serum and plasma, and yield still further secrets. But in the story without end he would be counted as among the first to offer his life for every life he salvaged from the terror engulfing Spain and the world.

26

On December 6, at six o'clock in the morning, Bethune returned to Madrid with a station wagon loaded with medical

---

* Dr. Jorda later became chief of the Blood Transfusion Service of the Spanish Republican Army.

instruments and supplies. With him were Sorensen and his latest recruit, Hazen Sise, a young Canadian who had run into Bethune in London and volunteered to serve with the unit.

In Madrid there was open jubilation. The fascists had thrown the most powerful attacks of the war against it from the south, but had been stopped. The city flexed its muscles like a young giant who has suddenly been faced with a staggering test of strength and emerged a little dazzled by his unsuspected stamina. Now the military command could pass from exhortation to a calm appraisal of the city's clear ability to hold out. It would be a long time till Franco's officers lunched in Madrid.

The Socorro Rojo had not been idle. In preparation for one of the most novel medical projects in military history the Spanish authorities had selected special quarters for the blood transfusion unit. Within a few days Bethune, Sorensen and Sise moved into a palatial eleven-room apartment formerly occupied by the German Embassy's legal counsel. It was situated on Principe de Vergara, a wide boulevard lined with trees in one of Madrid's wealthiest residential sections. "Here," a Socorro official said wryly, "you will not be disturbed by the bombs. Franco is careful with the property of the rich."

Three of the rooms were to be used by the Canadians as living quarters. The rest were to be used as laboratories, refrigerator rooms for storaging of blood, and transfusion rooms. Two young Spanish doctors were assigned to Bethune as assistants, along with two laboratory technicians, three nurses, a cook and housekeeper, a clerk and a doorman.

In a state of mounting excitement the laboratory was set up, two refrigeration units assembled, and the transfusion equipment moved in. The unit was to function along a 400-mile front. Bethune and the two Spanish doctors were each to be in charge of a separate sector of the front. As comandante of the unit, with the rank of colonel of the Republican Army, Bethune was directly responsible to the Army for the entire project. Sorensen was named liaison officer, and Sise was to be in charge of transportation. From the moment the service began it would never stop — part of the unit would be on duty every moment of the day or night, ready to rush blood to any section of the front the moment a signal was received from military headquarters that fighting was in progress.

Once everything had been installed on Principe de Vergara, small refrigeration units were distributed to the hospitals and field stations on the three sectors for the storing of blood in between emergencies.

Now everything was ready. Returning from a last check-up of arrangements at the front, Bethune called the members of the unit and Socorro Rojo officials into session.

"Our glorified milk delivery system," he reported, "has been set up — to the last detail. We're ready to start 'delivering.' There's only one thing we need. The 'milk.' Without that we might all just as well go home." He turned inquiringly to a Socorro representative.

The Spaniard nodded confidently. "We shall see to it that you have all the blood donors you need."

"The need for donors will continue as long as the unit is operated. To have a sufficient store of blood on hand to meet all emergencies, donors will have to come forward every day."

The Spaniard looked baffled as if he failed to understand why the matter had to be discussed. "You shall have the donors," he said simply.

For three days an appeal went out to the people of Madrid through press and radio. Blood was needed for the men at the front!

On the third night Bethune sat listening to the radio announcement, then wandered through the laboratory with its gleaming equipment, the refrigeration room with the waiting bottles, the transfusion room with its three beds for donors. Everything was in order, but he felt a sudden stab of uncertainty. Suppose the morning came and only a few stragglers showed up? It was easy to buy equipment, to make grandiose plans, to assume titles — it would all be worthless without blood, and that was something you couldn't buy in Paris or London. Was there a home in Madrid without hunger, without its casualties, without its men at the front? With their own bodies the men and women of Madrid had fashioned an impenetrable shield about their city. What more could one ask of them? The women who built fortifications and lived on beans; the men who worked all day and slept "with one eye open" at night — had they not been bled and starved themselves? It occurred to him that he might have overlooked the chief element in the project: the *human element*, the imponderables that rose up to confront every surgeon as the body lay revealed under the knife. And how many imponderables were here, he reflected, looking out the window at the darkened street. One air raid tonight, and in the morning all Madrid would be haggard and sleepless. Keep a man sleepless long enough, ad his brain would become as soppy as a sponge.

He awakened Sise in a fit of restlessness. "I was just wondering about tomorrow," he said. "Do you think they'll show up? It's all fine on paper, but without enough donors —"

Sise yawned sleepily in the dark. "That Socorro chap seemed to think there'd be no problem."

"Yes…. Still…." Bethune prowled about the room. "Yes … he should know. Well, good night, we'll need plenty of sleep by morning. We'll know soon enough."

It seemed to him he had hardly gone to bed before someone was calling him.

"Dr. Bethune … comandante …" Dr. Lopez,* one of the Spanish doctors, beckoned him to a terrace off the study, pointing silently at the spectacle below.

Over two thousand people filled the street, with more arriving every minute. They stood close together, from sidewalk to sidewalk, eyes fixed on the Institute. There were men and women, young and old, gaunt and portly, civilians and soldiers, poorly clad workers and well-dressed housewives. They were waiting patiently, silently, without laughter.

As the two doctors stood on the balcony the people on the street nudged one another expectantly. Bethune gazed at the upturned faces for a moment, then went inside. His face betrayed nothing of the turmoil he felt, he issued quick orders, the doors were opened, and the first donors filed in.

All morning and far into the afternoon they worked, registering, taking malaria and syphilis tests, checking the blood counts, filling the liter bottles — and still the donors came. A militia detachment had to be called out to keep traffic moving outside. From the Socorro Rojo extra clerks were sent to help. And finally there were no more bottles and even the kitchen refrigerator had been emptied for makeshift storage space.

From the balcony Dr. Lopez announced that no more donors

---

* This is a pseudonym.

could be taken till the next day. But the men and women who had waited for hours cried out in disappointment.

"*Mañana?*"

"*Hombre! Porque?*"

Shouting above the din, Lopez tried to explain that there were no more containers for the blood, and no more space to store it. But the protests continued.

"*Hombre ... camarada ... por favor.... ahora!* You must take the blood now! Our men need it now!"

With a harassed look Lopez turned to Bethune. "What shall we do? They will not leave!"

Bethune leaned over to the balcony railing to look at the shouting crowd below. Turning back to the Spaniard, his face lit up with pride, he said: "If they won't leave, then we'll stay open. We'll admit them all. Let the clerks register them, take their names and addresses. We'll make as many blood tests as we can today, and explain to all of them that we will be calling them back within a few days...."

Ten days later, on December 23, the first transfusions from stored blood delivered by the mobile Spanish-Canadian blood unit were given in University City.

The following day Bethune sent a cable to the Spanish Aid Committee in Toronto:

> Institute launched. Magnificent response from the people of Madrid. First test transfusions at front carried out last night with complete success. Greetings from all.

27

The war was like a flood: blocked at one point, it broke out at another.

In November it had swirled round Madrid; now, in the new year, it threatened to engulf the south.

Franco had thrown everything into the assault against Madrid — and failed. A stalemate now would have gained the Loyalists time to strengthen their defences — and the fascists, a moral defeat. To surround Loyalist Spain, to cut it off from the rest of the world, to reassure Rome and Berlin — that was now viewed at Burgos as a prime necessity. By the end of January massed German, Italian, and Moorish troops, deployed in the south after the stalemate at Madrid, began heavy attacks northward. Their strategic aim was occupation of the coast and a flanking movement against the Loyalists. Standing in their way were Málaga, Motril, Almería, a string of sun-baked towns, and the poorly equipped troops of the Republic. If successful, the drive could sweep along the coast to Cartagena, Murcia, Valencia, and perhaps, eventually, into Catalonia. For Franco it would be a resounding victory; for the Republic, disaster.

At the Blood Institute on Principe de Vergara Bethune tapped veins, kept up his relays to the front, followed the government communiqués, and studied the map of Spain. It was clear that a new phase of the war was opening, and therefore a new phase in the work of the Institute. In November and December, Franco had made Madrid the hub of the war, and the Republic's defensive effort had pushed out of the city like the spokes of a wheel. One of these spokes had been the Institute. Now, with the blood transfusion system working efficiently on fronts covering 1,000 kilometres, and with the new fascist attack gaining momentum in the South, Bethune drafted plans to extend the work of the Institute. It was a war of blood and iron, and the blood had to follow the fighting.

He laid his plans before the Socorro Rojo and his colleagues at the end of January. The decisive thing now, he contended, was to extend operations to the areas and fronts directly in the path of the latest fascist attack. His proposals received immediate endorsement. On February 4, accompanied by Sise, he left the Institute in charge of Dr. Lopez and Sorensen and set out for Málaga. They travelled in a new truck fitted out with special refrigerators, stored blood, and transfusion equipment. Their last news on the situation came from an English correspondent who had just arrived from Málaga. "You're going to have your work cut out for you," he said. "It was the hottest spot in all Spain when I got out a few days ago, and I don't mean the weather."

As they drove along the highway to the coast Bethune made notes on the work ahead of them. "On the way down from Valencia we'll make preliminary inquiries at the hospitals. We'll find out their blood needs, plan deliveries and establish the number of casualty stations they can service. That means we'll have to get more drivers, more doctors, more technicians and blood donors in each area." It would also mean that the Institute, from the great arc around Madrid, would be servicing the fronts all the way south to within a few miles of Gibraltar. When they arrived at Valencia on February 6, the news at Socorro Rojo headquarters was somber. The situation in the south, an official said, was "fluid." It was suggested that the trip down the coast now would be too risky. There was no telling how the fighting might go, and it might be more prudent to establish the subsidiary blood bank in Valencia itself. Bethune agreed that it might be more "prudent," but they left the next morning nevertheless, joined by a young Englishman, Thomas Worsley, who was to be a relief driver.

For three days, in an atmosphere of increasing uncertainty, they followed the coastline, feeling the tension growing in every town along their route. On February 10 the reached Almería and heard the worst: Málaga had fallen. "You can go no further," a spokesman at the Governor's office said. "There is nowhere for you to go. We don't know where our troops are. There will be nothing ..."

"But wounded," Bethune said. "There will be plenty of wounded."

"Chaos! Where will you find the wounded? The fascists are in Málaga and advancing north — that's all we know. Perhaps you can do something here?"

"Our instructions are to take blood and transfusion equipment to the furthest point in the south," Bethune replied tersely.

They drove through the town silently, viewing the small port below. An old destroyer ready for scrapping lay in port. From a villa overlooking the sea there fluttered a Union Jack.

Under the palm trees gracing the port Sise stopped the lorry. "Well," he inquired, "what do we do now?"

"Exactly what we set out to do." Bethune pointed to a marker at the side of the road: 169 kilometres. The markers ran northward from Málaga. That meant they were one hundred and sixty-nine kilometres from the fascists — from the front.

28

Bethune himself recorded the events that took place after they left Almería:

> We spent one hour in Almería: long enough to look for a meal that was unobtainable. The little seaport had been bombed from the air and blockaded from the sea. One could sense the hunger in the streets. A street-urchin led us to a little bar, but it was completely filled with militiamen, all of them eating the same steaming, soupy mixture. Ragged youngsters roved among the tables, pouncing on the leavings. At a hotel in the centre of the town the proprietor apologetically served the one-course, standard fare: beans. When we started out again the streets were filling with people. The news about Málaga was spreading.
>
> Men stood about in groups, debating: was it wise to stay? Was it possible the fascists had come this far?
>
> Sise drove by the port and into the hills. From here to Málaga there was only one road. From Almería it followed the jagged line of the coast. It circled round steep curves, banked on the right by grey cliffs, overlooking the sea on the left. Behind us Almería was cut off from view; below us the Mediterranean tossed its breakers against the rocks.

Ten miles out of Almería my reveries were
interrupted by a strange procession. I peered
through the windshield accordingly. Peasants?
Yes, plodding along with the ever-present donkey. Yet as they drew closer they were no longer
merely peasants.

Coming towards us we saw a man leading
a donkey by a string, dragging his feet, his head
hanging, a child tied onto his back with a shawl.
The donkey was heaped high with a mattress,
pots and pans, a pair of books, blankets, a water
jug. A boy hung onto the donkey's tail. Behind
him came a woman with an infant in her arms,
and behind her an old man hobbling with a
stick, dragging another child by the hand.

The refugees passed the car without seeming to notice it. They plodded along wearily,
their feet scuffing the hard road, their shoulders
drooping as if to pull them forward, their mouths
hanging open, their eyes rolling upwards in the
unconscious symptom of complete exhaustion.

Further down the road another group was
filing round the bend. They were like mourn-
ers following a hearse. The men staggered under
their wide hats, the women trailed haltingly in
their traditional dark cotton cloaks, the children
wore only short pants or shifts, their half-naked
bodies hot in the sun.

The second group stumbled by us and I felt
a jab of pity, anger, impatience. We drove on, and
around every bend there were more refugees.
At first they came on in scattered groups, then
at more frequent intervals — a hundred yards
apart, fifty yards, then following on each others'
heels: a thin line flowing without break along
the side of the road, with the hot sun above and
the sea below.

There were families walking together, carrying a few trivial possessions; men and women

who seemed to be alone, moving without choice at the pace set by others; children with tired, bewildered faces, passing from hand to hand. They seemed to have sprung from the ground; they were like shadows moving from nowhere to nowhere. Between the noise of the sea and the echoing cliffs the only sound they made was the scuffling of sandals on stone, the hiss of labored breathing, the moaning that burst from cracked lips and travelled along the wavering line till it expired in the distance.

They were of all ages, but their faces were drawn with the same weariness. They flowed past our truck without expression: a young girl, hardly sixteen, straddling a donkey, her head drooping over an infant at her breast; a grandmother, her old face half-hidden in her dark shawl, dragging along between two men; a patriarch, shrivelled down to skin and bones, his bare feet dripping blood on the road; a young man with a pile of bedding strapped to his shoulders, the leather thongs cutting into his flesh with every step; a woman holding her stomach, her eyes wide and fearful — a silent, haggard, tortured flood of men and animals, the animals bellowing in complaint like humans, the humans as uncomplaining as animals.

Sise stopped the car. I got out and stood in the centre of the road. Where were they from? Where were they going? What had happened? They looked at me slowly, sideways. They had no strength to go on, but feared to linger. The fascists were behind them, they said. Málaga? Yes, they were from Málaga, and Málaga had fallen. Málaga! *Nada más!* Where were they going? Wherever the road led. There was no other road. The fascists had come to Málaga, the guns had roared, the houses had crumbled, the city had been gored and everyone able to walk

had taken to the roads. Turn about, they advised;
there was nothing left ... nothing behind them
but more people on the road, and behind them
again, the fascists.

I came back to the truck. Hazen had his
camera ready. I watched grimly while he took
pictures from the roadside and the top of the
truck. I thought of Málaga; a stunning defeat!
How had it happened? But it was no use thinking about that now. What mattered was that
somewhere this side of the captured city Loyalist lines, surely, would be reforming. Somewhere
down there would be new defences, more bitterly contested now. Somewhere down the road
there would be fighting, rear-guard actions at
the very least, wounded, dying, needing the
blood we had brought from Madrid.

We drove more quickly now and as the road
banked steeply the line of refugees grew wider.
Then there was a sharp turn away from the sea,
a slow climb, and suddenly we breasted a hill
falling away to a long, level plain. Sise rammed
his foot on the brake with a surprised grunt. The
truck jolted to a stop against a shuddering wall of
refugees and animals. They filled the entire road.
Women screamed, donkeys reared, faces pressed
in upon us, and as quickly as we had reached the
hilltop, the wall of refugees reformed to move
around the truck.

But it was the scene below that held us
speechless.

The plain stretched into the distance as far as
the eye could see, and across the plain, where the
road should have been, there wriggled twenty
miles of human beings, like a giant caterpillar,
its many limbs raising a cloud of dust, moving
slowly, ponderously, stretching from beyond the
horizon, across the arid, flat country and up into
the foothills.

I hoisted myself onto the running board, shielding my eyes to look down onto the plain. Nowhere was the road visible. It was blotted out by the refugees, thousands upon thousands of them, pressed together, falling against each other, like bees swarming in a hive, and like bees filling the plain with the hum of voices, cries, wailings, the grotesque noises of the animals.

We began to descend slowly, Sise sounding his horn without stop. On the running board I tried to wave the refugees aside. They paid no attention to my shouts or the sound of the horn; they merely flowed around the car with down-cast eyes, bumping against its sides and then spreading across the road behind it again.

If they were from Málaga they had been walking at least five days and five nights. Was it possible? That old woman with the open ulcers on her legs — could she have survived five days and five nights on the open road? Yet there she was, her cloak trailing in the dust, swallowed up now behind the truck. And the children ... of all ages, most of them barefoot — could they too have survived? Too many children! One quick glance along the road immediately ahead gave a sickening wrench. Five squirming miles of people, and among them thousands of children!

We drove past stragglers, families resting by the roadside, men and women huddled together, sleeping on the bare earth; through wretched villages emptied by the general retreat; along-side bomb-pits and burnt-out peasants' hovels. Then the plodding mass changed imperceptibly, like a spring suddenly filled with mud. I swore under my breath: militiamen! At first there were only a few, lost among the refugees, but a mile further they came on in hundreds, then in thousands. Their uniforms were torn, their weapons gone, their faces covered with stubble,

their eyes hollow with defeat. What were they
doing among the refugees? Political irrespon-
sibles? Deserters? I had no time to wonder, for
behind the militiamen came lines of cavalry.
Horses and riders were spent. Some of the cav-
alrymen slouched along with their boots slung
about their necks, leading their mounts, women
or children clinging to the saddle. They were no
longer cavalry; they were refugees like the rest,
silent, grim, in flight.

... The Spanish sun was as merciless as the
fascists that day. The heat became a tangible,
hated enemy. The road swerved back to the
sea, and we heard the sound of the surf on the
rocky coast again, rumbling like a distant drum
beneath the sounds of the exodus.

Now there were more signs of panic, hurry,
disorder. We had to manoeuvre around broken-
down carts and abandoned trucks. Dying burros
had been pushed onto the beaches below, where
people lay stretched in exhaustion, their swollen
tongues hanging from puckered mouths. More
children, more militiamen, more deserted villages. Stopped momentarily by an obstruction
on the road, we were engulfed by shouted pleas,
hands reaching out towards us, people begging for water, for transport to Almería. I threw
my water canisters out of the window and we
pushed ahead.

We passed an empty bus with a militiaman
at the wheel. As we passed, the militiaman stuck
his head out of the bus, waving his hands and
shouting, "Petrol...." Sise shook his head and
cried back "*Al frente!*" Behind the bus a little
girl crouched beside the road, all alone, howling
with her thumb in her mouth. Out of the line of
refugees I saw a militiaman's hand reach out and

hoist her on his back. Beside the militiaman a peasant was carrying a woman over his shoulder, like a sack of potatoes.

The coast fell away again and we drove between fields of sugar cane. The heads of the sugar cane swayed gently in the breeze. Green leaves drifted across the road and under the bare feet. Beside another stalled bus a group of militiamen waved at us to turn back. Through the window we shouted the refrain, *"Al frente!"*

We came out on the coastline again just as the sun mercifully began to set. The sky glowed, long tongues of flame trembled in the Mediterranean, then it was suddenly dark. We sensed the quickened pace of the refugees about us. Sise switched on the headlights. Immediately we heard angry cries: *"Luz* — lights!" In the besieged cities children were growing up, unaware that man had long ago conquered the darkness, and here too, on the pleasant coast that had once drawn ecstatic tourists, lights were a menace and only the black night held safety.

Without headlights it was almost impossible to drive. We sounded the horn, we shouted, but it was no good. In an hour we moved a short distance, then we moved no further. We sat in the lorry cabin, thinking, then a group of militiamen came up, harassed, but with some semblance of discipline. They asked for our documents, examined them carefully, saluted, and reported the situation behind them. The fascists were coming eastwards swiftly, they said. The next town was Motril, and it was already in enemy hands or would be soon. There was no front; no stand was being made anywhere this side of Almería. It was more than a rout — it was a collapse, with the southern coastal region falling like a ripe plum into the hands of Franco's foreign troops.

The door of the lorry flew open. In the darkness a man held it with his shoulder, his wide eyes fixed on me, a five-year-old child in his arms. He held out the child, emaciated, shivering with fever, and began to talk quickly, the words spilling from his mouth, hoarsely at first, then his voice rising till it was like the wail of a desolate flamenco. I needed no translation; the words were universal; they would have been understood in any language: "*Mi chico — muy malo*.... My child is very ill.... He will die before I carry him to Almería.... I will stay behind.... I ask only for him.... Take him — leave him wherever there is a hospital.... Tell them that I will follow.... Tell them this one is Juan Blas and that I will come soon to find him."

I took the child and laid him gently on the seat. The Spaniard seized my hand convulsively and made the sign of the cross over me. I needed more than Spanish to speak my heart to this stranger, to the faces coming out of the tumult and the night, the faces gathering aout me, twitching with fear, to the arms reaching out like a wavering, stricken forest, to the voices beseeching me.

"*Camarada ... por favor ...* save us," they cried, and I understood their pleas without understanding the words.

"Take our women and children ... the fascists will be upon us soon...."

"Have pity, *camarada*, save us, for the love of God...."

"Let us go with you in your vehicle, we can walk no further...."

"*Camarada, los niños* — the children...."

I hoisted myself onto the running board. They surrounded me, plucking at my clothes. The bitter thought burned into my mind: Where were they tonight, the appointed ministers to the Christian God, bearers on earth of His love and salvation — where are they, that they hear nothing of those who cry out to the Lord? Into what dark cave has the love of *man* been hounded? Where the mercy and conscience of a world going its sickly way?

Words — bah! Everywhere a deluge of fat words, and under the deluge, here on the Málaga road, the lost and the damned. If only I had a thousand pairs of hands, and in each hand a thousand deadly guns, and for each gun a thousand bullets, and each bullet marked for an assigned child-killer — then I would know how to speak! From every gun in every hand I would speak death for the corrupted breed, and with a voice like Gabriel's trumpet I would roar at the ears of the slumbering world, drowning the fools and liars still spreading their clamorous deceit abroad. With a voice like Gabriel's trumpet I would awaken the indifferent millions beyond Spain's invaded borders: "Your hands are polluted with innocent blood, all you who sleep peacefully tonight! Your cities are Sodom and Gomorrah if you care nothing for the shame on Málaga road tonight! Your children will wander in their own wilderness of death and terror, all you who hear the anguish of Spain and stay silent tonight!"

I bent down to peer at Sise across the shivering body of the child. "They're right," I said. "It's senseless now to go further. There's only one thing we can do — get as many of these people to Almería as we can manage. We'll unload everything in the back to make room, and send the stuff along with the first ambulance that comes by. We'll take children only...."

We turned the truck about on the narrow road, unloaded the equipment and stores of blood, and when we were finished I opened the back doors of the van. A thrill of excitement ran through the refugees, all of them waiting but none daring to hope. I inspected the van, calculated the number of people it would accommodate, and jumped to the ground. *"Solamente niños!"* I announced, but the words were lost in the hubbub and I was thrown back by the sudden surge of bodies. The doors to safety had opened, and to every refugee it seemed rescue was a matter of now or never. As I fell back under their frantic charge, I flung my arms across the open doors. "Children only!" I shouted furiously, holding them off. *"Niños!* Children only!" Sise came plunging to my side to help.

"How will we manage it?" Sise panted, pushing against the milling crowd. "They'll go mad — those left behind!"

"No adults," I felt my voice harsh against the pleading and weeping. "There's nothing we can do except fill up with children. I'll pass them to you — let nobody else in even if you have to do it by force."

Slowly, methodically, I fought my way into the hysterical ranks of the refugees, shouting, *"Niños! — Solamente niños!"* It seemed gruesome now to decide who would go and who would stay, more terrible even than to be a helpless onlooker. "You," I called, pointing over the heads at a woman holding her baby about her neck. "We'll take your child!" Willing hands pushed her towards me. Soon I reached her, standing close in the press of bodies. "We'll take the child," I repeated, but the mother merely looked at me with great, dark, sunken eyes and held the child tighter. Perhaps she didn't understand? I put out my arms, but still she made no move, looking up at me without expression, and I saw that the child was too young to be separated from the mother. I felt a stab of uncertainty. It was easy to say, "Children only," but this woman's dark, sunken eyes replied: "Take my child alone, and you kill us both." I put my arms about her, opened a way for her into to the truck, and into Hazen's waiting arms. "Both of them," I said, and pushed into the crowd again.

Back and forth I went, ordering, trying to soothe the women, selecting the youngest, grimly turning adults away, carrying the children in my arms. And as I filled the truck the anguished voices pursued me. I heard men and women calling for families lost somewhere in the night. Mothers whose children were in the truck stood nearby and whispered encouragement. Men who watched silently, their hopes sinking as the truck filled up, went off into the fields to throw themselves on the ground. "Who am I to decide their fate?" I asked myself.

"How many more?" I called to Sise.

"Two more — with a tight squeeze."

I felt a touch on my arm. I looked over my shoulder and saw an old face, a stooped back, tears, and the unspoken inquiry glimmering through the tears. I looked at the old man, waiting for my wind to come back, then slowly shook my head. "Your face will haunt my dreams, friend," I thought, but I put aside the hand at my sleeve — an old man's hand at my sleeve like that of a child.

Two more to go — and there was a sudden silence as the truth dawned on the waiting refugees with a blinding vision: this was the silence that filled the prison courtyard as the hangman fitted the noose about his victim's neck and the spectators braced themselves for the last

unbelievable act. But here there were no spectators. Here all were victims, all felt the noose
tightening about their own necks.

I passed a woman of fifty, old before her
time, but still too young for death. She could
hardly stand erect. Her legs were gigantic, the
varicose veins visible in the darkness, knotted
like swollen throngs of torture, blood seeping
into the cuffs of her linen sandals. I came back to
her. What if this were my own mother — how
would I decide? I stood before her, touching her
bony shoulder. My own mother? But if not my
own, then someone else's — a mother of Spain,
and therefore my own. I steadied her swaying
shoulders, but she looked calmly away, as if she
had nothing to ask.

I took the last child for the last precious
space — plucking it from the arms of a woman
who held it, screaming, then screaming gave
it up as if it was issuing once more, in blood
and pain, from her very womb. I carried the
child, a little girl, through the silent crowd to
the truck. Suddenly a woman pushed in front
of me, seized the door-jambs and clambered on
the truck. I caught her ankle in mid-air and
swore, but she shook free and turned about
in the confined space to face me. "Get out!" I
ordered, holding the child towards her. "It's you
or the child! Do you understand? Will you take
the place of the child?

The woman was young. Her long black
hair fell about her pale face. She looked at me
with hunted eyes, then flung open her cloak and
raised her cotton shift high. She was distended
with child.

For a moment we looked at each other, I
with the child in my arms, she with the child
in her womb. She pressed herself down on the
tiny space of flooring on her feet, her great

stomach between her knees, smiled at me and held out her arms. With her eyes and arms and her smile she seemed to be saying "See, I will take the child, and it will be as if I am not here, as if I am taking nobody's place." She placed the girl on her knees, pillowing the little head on her shoulders.

Now it was done. Forty children and two women were jammed together in the truck and the front cab. Half of them sat on the floor, for the remainder there was only space to stand. For better or worse, it was done.

I banged the doors shut and ordered Sise to take them directly to the hospital in Almería and to stop for nothing and nobody. If he could pick up a few armed militia men to ride the running boards and keep the others off, all the better. He was to make sure they got food and medical attention, then report to the governor's office, inform the governor of the situation, and tell him he must send transport at once or there would be more dead from hunger and exhaustion than from enemy action. Then he was to get the tank filled with gas and come back for another load. He turned, walked back to the cab without looking back, climbed in, and started the motor....*

The truck was gone, the women wept for their departed children, for the children let behind, the men hoisted the packs to their backs, they moved forward again, the thought of the enemy like a hot wind on their necks.

At the side of the road, I found the old woman with the bleeding legs. She was sitting on the ground, her head on her knees. She

---

* The Englishman, Worsley, remained with Bethune on the first night. Later he drove the truck alone, or helped Sise. Other references to Worsley appear in sections of the journal which we have omitted for lack of space.

looked up, the same calm resignation on her gaunt face. I took a tube and bandage from my kit and bandaged her feet. "Come," I said, "it's a long way to Almería. We'll walk a while, till it's safe for you to rest." She understood nothing of what I said, but she gave me her hands. I raised her gently, talking to her in the strange language she had never heard before.

Together we joined the other refugees on the road, her head resting on my shoulder. Together, with the others falling in behind, we began the trek to Almería....

... Carried along by the stream of refugees I peered at the illuminated dial of my wristwatch. Was it only midnight? Had I been walking only four hours? Four hours that seemed like an eternity, yet the others had been walking at least four days!

I had left the old woman two hours ago when she could go no further, after making a bed of earth for her in an open field, among the many others who owned nothing now but a bed of earth. Perhaps, I thought, a stray ambulance would pick her up; perhaps, on the other hand, the fascists would reach her first.

I had used up my last bandage, administered my last pill, given away my last chocolate bar, smoked my last cigarette, and thrown away my empty kit. I had only my bare hands now, and my impatience for Hazen's return. And then — what? Then it would be like trying to drain the ocean with a thimble.

... There was a commotion on the road. I made out our truck, crawling along with dimmed headlights. Sise jumped out, haggard but elated.

Back and forth we shuttled, for four days and four nights working furiously to evacuate the remnants of a whole city. For 48 hours Sise stayed behind the wheel while I stayed on the road, assembling the next group to be transported. We grew white-faced with lack of sleep. We lost track of time. We lived with the heartbreak of those left behind, and the weary joy of those brought to safety. We worked with the knowledge that every trip might be the last, with the fear that the evacuees furthest from the city would be swept up by the fascists.

On every trip to Almería, Sise stopped at the governor's office to clamor for trucks, carts, for anything moveable to speed the evacuation. But there was nothing left on wheels in the city.

On the second day I decided it was no longer possible to take children only: the sight of parents separated from their children became too ghastly to bear. We began to move whole families, giving preference to those with children. On the second day we tasted too what the others had tasted for five days — hunger. There was no food to be gotten anywhere in Almería.

Then, as if to mock our hunger, a man appeared on the road from nowhere, pushing a cart of oranges and shouting his wares in a stentorian voice. In the midst of war, flight, death, an ordinary, prosaic street-hawker! I bought the whole cart of oranges, keeping one for myself and distributing the others.

Thus it went, for four days and four nights. By day we worked in clouds of dust, under a hot sun that blistered the skin, our eyes red-rimmed, our bellies rumbling. At night the cold grew unendurable, so that we longed for the tormenting heat once more.

A great silence settled over the refugees. The starving lay in the fields, gripped by torpor, stirring themselves only to nibble at fugitive weeds. The thirsty sat on the rocks, trembling, or staggered about aimlessly, the wild glassy stare of delusion in their eyes. The dead lay indiscriminately among the sick, looking unblinkingly into the sun. Then the planes swept overhead — glinting, silvery Italian fighters and squadrons of German Heinkels. They dived toward the road, as casually as target-practice, their machine guns weaving intricate geometric patterns about the fleeing refugees....

Again I saw the truck return. We piled up as many as we could. This time I got in as well, a child on my lap, moaning, looking at me with hot, feverish eyes. Probably meningitis. After a while, he no longer seemed to be in pain. A bad sign. I hoped we would get him to Almería in time. He was about seven or eight.

I dozed, then awoke to find the truck rolling slowly downgrade. This looked like the last mile. But what a mile! From the Sierras into the city tens of thousands of refugees were fanned out like a funnel with a giant spout and a narrow, twisting stem. They swarmed over the hills, the road, the beaches below, some wading into the sea to get to the city sooner.

Where the highway entered the city the truck could move only as the jam-packed bodies moved, inch by inch, till it seemed we had been stalled for hours. Then the line of refugees in front of us surged forward and we were in Almería at last.

In four days the city had become a vast encampment. The streets were filled with refugees who had nowhere to stay and nowhere to go. Several thousand were quartered on the main square, out in the open. Men and women rose wearily from the pavement to let us through.

At Socorro Rojo we were directed to an old building where a hospital and reception centre for the children had been improvised. We helped the refugees in and put the sick child in a doctor's care. Then I found a cot and collapsed....

I jerked awake with a feeling of discomfort. For a moment I thought I was lying out in the hills, beside the road, but my hand slid over the rough floor and I remembered this was no longer the road but Almería. I wondered at the ringing in my ears. From my stupor I guessed I had slept an hour or so.

It was the wailing of the siren that had awakened me. I scrambled to my feet, and fell on my knees again as the first bomb went off. The explosion was like a giant mailed fist smashing deep into the earth.... I could hear the terrible, frightened screams of the children. In the hallway people were running and shouting. I scrambled up again, the floor still vibrating under my feet. More explosions sounded, some nearby, some distant.

I ran through the dark corridors, jostling against people hurrying in every direction. In the dormitories children were crying with fright. I found my way into the street, and made for the centre of the city, on the run.

The planes kept sweeping in, one after another, the roar of the engines filling the streets till it seemed my eardrums would burst. Then came the bombs, falling up ahead.

I caught a glimpse of one bomber banking gracefully in the moonlight, disdaining the protection of height or darkness. The devils could afford to take their time! The occasional burst of anti-aircraft fire merely prettied up the sky like roman candles.

In a few minutes I reached the densely populated section of the city. Here the streets were no longer dark. Great sheets of flame shot up from the skeletons of buildings, hit by incendiaries. In the glare of the burning buildings, as far as the eye can see, vast crowds of people surged about wildly, running into bombpits, clutching and screaming as they vanished.

There were no sounds of bombing from the direction of the port. The bombers weren't interested in the port! They were after *human* prey. They were after the hundred thousand people who eluded them at Málaga, who had refused to live under the fascists, who were now penned together here in a perfect target. For a week they had let Almería alone. For a week they had prepared. Now that the trek from Málaga was over, now that the refugees were caught in a few city blocks where mass murder required a minimum number of bombs — now Franco was slaking his thirst for revenge. He cared little for the port. A port couldn't think, defy fascism or bleed. Only *people* had brains, hearts, courage. Kill them, maim them, show them the merciless claw of fascism....

I fought my way through the dense crowds, shouting, "*Médico! Médico!*" My voice was lost in the shrieking of the sirens, the explosions, the fearful braying of the donkeys impaling themselves on twisted railings.

Then suddenly the bombing stopped and the roar of the planes faded away in the sky. The flaming buildings lit up the faces of men and women looking numbed, shocked, horror stricken....

The raid was over. My ears ached in the silence. Silence? No. With the bombing over I could hear the voices ... the raid was over, but the dead and dying remained.

I bound the wounds of the injured with strips of cotton torn from their shirts. In a gutted house I found a little girl whimpering beneath a pile of heavy beams. She was perhaps three years old. I pulled the beams away and carried her in my arms till I came across an emergency ambulance. I laid her on the stretcher, thinking it would be kinder if she died, for if the crippled body survived, the light of sanity had gone out of her childish eyes.

In the centre of the city I came to a silent circle of men and women. Inside the circle was a great bomb crater. Inside the crater were twisted drain pipes, torn clothing, a splattered mass of what had once been human beings....

My body felt as heavy as the dead themselves. But empty and hollow. And in my brain there burned a bright flame of hate.

So went the journal of his four nights and days on the Málaga road. He wrote it in a burst of cold fury, during most of the next day and night. When he had finished he stood at a shattered window of the children's reception centre, looking out at the city still smoking in the dawn.

His body ached for sleep, but he stayed at the window a long time, thinking. In Madrid, at the front, he had heard the cry, "Death to fascism!" He had joined in the cry, but now he seemed to understand the taste of the words for the first time, like a deep, passionate judgment that had to be carried out before he would ever know peace and sanity again. Yes, death and damnation to the evil, murderous brood that slaughtered women and children! Infamy and a curse for those who stood by with smirking indifference! And for the deluded, the innocents in all lands still watching the gravediggers without thinking the same grave would some day open wide for *them* — pity, and a warning.

"Into whatsoever house I enter, there I shall heal the sick...."
How jauntily he had once taken the Hippocratic Oath, like thousands of others. But in the house he had now entered death came
from bombs, lies, men who buried whole cities under the banner
of anticommunism. Here in Almería, more than a city lay under
the ruins. Here two worlds had met in bloody collision. In the
memory of Almería, he vowed, he would have to change himself,
to crush all weaknesses and vanities, to live as the soldier lives, to
make himself a man of steel — for only men of steel would be
able to defend the world struggling to be born.

29

In Valencia, a few days later, he prepared a shorter version of his
journal for the government. He called it, *Málaga — the Crime on
the Road*. It was published in booklet form by the government in
English and Spanish editions, illustrated by photos Sise had taken.

In Valencia he heard also that the days of the Caballero government were numbered. The giving up of Málaga without a
fight was viewed by most Loyalists as a staggering mistake to be
laid directly at the door of the administration. Not even rear-
guard fighting, Bethune heard, had been ordered. Málaga had
been handed to the fascists on a platter.

On his return to Madrid he pushed the work of the blood
unit with increased energy. To the other members he seemed
filled with a new tension, an impatience with delays and red tape,
a greater need for action. All lethargy and inefficiency were now
seen through his eyes as "Caballero-ism," with potential Málaga-
like results. In the Institute the least negligence on the part of
Spaniard or Canadian alike provoked his famous rages. But at the
front he continued to work with his cool, smooth efficiency that
never failed to surprise and excite his co-workers.

Between regular trips to the front he brooded over an idea
that had haunted him since Málaga — the thousands of children
orphaned by the war needed help. The hard-pressed government

had taken some measures to cope with the situation, but Bethune decided that a special project was needed that would draw support from the outside world. Barcelona, the northern industrial metropolis, was at the time remote from the fighting. He decided that the Barcelona region would be ideal for a chain of Children's Villages where war orphans could be cared for. He flew to Barcelona and spent five days there in the Catalonian capital discussing his suggestion with government officials. When he won their approval he sent a cable to the Spanish Aid Committee in Toronto proposing that money be raised for the project. The Committee agreed, and the first two Children's Villages, eventually set up north of Barcelona, were financed by friends of Republican Spain in Canada.

Back in Madrid once more Bethune extended the work of the unit to cover the whole of the central front. In early April, when the Loyalists struck hard in the Guadalajara sector, the unit gave transfusions for three days at Brihuega, the centre of the front where 30,000 Italian troops were put to rout.

Guadalajara was the first decisive offensive victory of the Republic. With it a wave of optimism spread through Spain. The taste of victory was sweet, and Bethune, in an easier mood now, begun to think of new experiments with blood and to envisage a further extension of the unit's work throughout the country. But the optimism was short-lived.

One afternoon he received a phone call from Carlos Contreras, who suggested an immediate conference. In his office Contreras got to the point quickly. He had a proposal — that Bethune undertake a trip to America to bring the plight of Spain directly to the people of the United States and Canada.

Contreras put the position before him grimly. Guadalajara, he said, had shown that the Republic could defeat the fascists if it had the weapons to fight with. But it was being denied the weapons. The Soviet Union was too far away, and her unarmed merchant ships were too easily sunk by Italian submarines in the Mediterranean for her aid alone to overcome the fascists' superiority in arms. Britain, France and the United States refused to lift their embargoes. Germany and Italy, on the other hand, continued to pour their men and arms into the country. In this situation aid from America could be decisive. And since the blood transfusion unit was now working efficiently it was felt that Bethune's most significant contribution would be to advocate Spain's cause before the people of North America.

Bethune received the suggestion at first with distaste. The thought of embarking on a lecture tour while the fighting continued filled him with dismay. But he had no answers to the grim facts put before him by the Fifth Regiment leader.

He discussed it with his Canadian colleagues in the unit, who agreed with Contreras that Bethune could help Spain most effectively in the coming months by trying to develop a popular campaign to lift the embargo. Bethune cabled the Committee back home, waited till the Committee sent back its agreement, and brought in a cameraman* from Paris to make a film of the war called *Heart of Spain*, to take with him to America.

Now he had only one piece of unfinished business left. Some weeks earlier he had received a request from a Canadian literary magazine, *New Frontier*,** for an article on Spain. He decided to write it while still in the atmosphere of Madrid.

He called it "An Apology for Not Writing Letters." It was a completely personal piece. He had delayed writing it, he said at the outset, because in Spain at war "I am afraid of the banality of words." He could describe a bombardment, murder in the streets, but it would not be enough. Art alone could transmit the experience of death and horror among which he had lived all these months, art which was "the legitimate and recognizable child of experience."

> The true artist [he continued] lets himself go. He is natural. He "swims easily in the stream of his own temperament." He listens to himself. He respects himself....
>
> He comes into the light of every-day like a great leviathan of the deep, breaking the smooth surface of accepted things, gay, serious, sportive. His appetite for life is enormous. He

---

* Geza Carpathi.

** Now defunct.

enters eagerly into the life of man, all men. He becomes all men in himself.

The function of the artist is to disturb. His duty is to arouse the sleepers, to shake the complacent pillars of the world. He reminds the world of its dark ancestry, shows the world its present, and points the way to its new birth. He is at once the product and the preceptor of his time. After his passage we are troubled and made unsure of our too-easily accepted realities. He makes uneasy the static, the set and the still. In a world terrified of change, he preaches revolution — the principle of life. He is an agitator, a disturber of the peace — quick, impatient, positive, restless and disquieting. He is the creative spirit working in the soul of man.

When his Canadian colleagues in the unit had read the manuscript they found nothing strange in the fact that he, the doctor, should write from the Spanish war about the role of the artist. He was an artist as well as a doctor. But more than that, they understood he was not merely trying to sum up the artist, but to define the emerging outlines of his own life.

On June 6, 1937, he left for home. At the Institute on Principe de Vergara there was a brief ceremony of farewell, attended by all the members of the unit, representatives of the newly organized Sanidad Militar, and government officials. With the blood transfusion methods he had introduced at the fronts, fatalities among the wounded had been drastically reduced, in some sectors as much as 75 percent. That was the eloquent note of oratory on which Spain's spokesmen sent him off on his new mission.

He was going home, with the memory of all he had seen and been and done in Spain, "to rouse the sleepers...."

30

At eight o'clock on the morning of June 18 Bethune arrived in Montreal.

Despite the early hour, thousands of people had gathered in the old Bonaventure Station and the surrounding streets to welcome him. As he stepped off the train from New York a large crowd burst through the gates and streamed down the long platform.

Before he knew what was happening he was surrounded, eager hands clutching his suitcases and he was raised up on the shoulders of the cheering, enthusiastic crowd. Camera bulbs flashed as reporters fought their way closer. In the sea of grinning, unfamiliar faces he caught glimpses of old friends. "*Vive le docteur Bethune!*" voices cried. He was carried through the station and into the street behind a banner reading: LONG LIVE LOYAL- IST SPAIN — WELCOME HOME, DR. BETHUNE!

Outside the station a long line of cars was waiting, decked out with bunting and welcoming banners. Still held aloft he responded to the resounding cheers of the crowd with a few words of thanks, ending: "I wish I could tell you how deeply I appreciate the way in which you have received me this morning. I know this is not a welcome for a mere individual, but a dem- onstration of your support for the cause of Loyalist Spain." The crowd's roars reverberated through the downtown area. Then, with horns honking, banners flying, and Bethune in the leading open car, the motor cavalcade moved up Windsor to St. Cath- erine Street and into the heart of downtown Montreal. On the sidewalks thousands of people waved as they saw the banners. In the tall factory buildings workers leaned out the windows, drop- ping streams of paper.

The cavalcade wound slowly through the French-Canadian East End, back to the centre of the city, and then to a downtown hotel.

From the moment he stepped into his hotel room he was besieged with telephone calls, old friends, doctors' groups, requests for interviews, messages and congratulations from all over the continent. His work had once been reported only in the medical journals; now he found it spread across the newspapers, intertwined with events changing the course of history.

Friends who came to see him during the first two hectic days left with a feeling he had altered in some subtle and elusive manner not apparent on the surface. He was a bit leaner, browner, and gave the appearance of weariness. Yet it was not so much physical weariness as a quality of withdrawal, of private brooding. The least question about Spain could stir him into spirited explanations. But often, when he had ended, he would fall abruptly silent, and his eyes would rover warily over the face of his listeners. Sometimes, in the midst of conversation, he would grow remote, as if listening to his own thoughts, or as if the friends about him had suddenly become strangers whom he was addressing for the first time.

When Frances visited him the reunion was cordial, yet something seemed to be left unsaid between them. "You know," she said suddenly, after he had talked about his life in Spain for a while, "you look no different than when you left. But somehow you feel different. Is it so?"

He smiled. "I hope it is. I damn well sincerely hope it is."

In an address at the Mount Royal Arena, he began his mission to America.

From the moment he had cabled Toronto he was returning to Canada, the Committee to Aid Spanish Democracy had launched preparations for a country-wide speaking tour, opening with a great meeting in Montreal two days after his arrival.

There were bitter divisions in Quebec public opinion abut the relative merits of the Loyalist and Franco cause, and there had been several official moves to deny the public platform to spokesmen for the Loyalist side, but the nature of Bethune's work in Spain had softened many a political antagonist and won him universal respect. When the doors of the Arena opened, the line of people waiting to get in stretched around the block. By the time he arrived with members of the local Spanish Aid Committee, the great building was literally filled to the rafters, with an estimated 15,000 people seated or waiting outside.

The audience was drawn from every walk of life and divergent political faiths. There were groups from every section of Montreal's polyglot minorities, schoolteachers, university professors, trade unionists, doctors, those who shared Bethune's personal views, even some who violently rejected his views but admired the man and his work.

When he stepped to the microphone, after the speeches and eulogies, he was greeted by a tremendous cheer. It was a strange sensation, standing alone, in a pillar of light, while in the darkness surrounding the platform about 15,000 men and women forgot all reserve and raised their voices in a deafening tumult. He waited calmly, lighting the inevitable cigarette and smoking, until the applause died out and he began in an easy, conversational tone.

> Mr. Chairman, ladies and gentlemen. I went to Spain as a matter of honour. I have come back because there are some things that need to be said in reply to those outside of Spain who speak in the name of dishonour.
>
> I am a doctor, a surgeon. My job is to sustain human life, in all its beauty and vigour. I am not a politician. But when I went to Spain because the politicians betrayed Spain and tried to drag the rest of us into their betrayal. With varying accents, and with varying degrees of hypocrisy, the politicians ruled that democratic Spain must die. It was my belief, as it is now my conviction, that democratic Spain must live.

After this opening he spoke of Madrid, the heart of Spanish resistance — the "city in the front lines, working and fighting with the fascists on its doorsteps." In a quiet voice he described the people: the women bombed out of their homes, the mutilated children, the men at the front with little more than courage to hold off German tanks, the spirit of comradeship drawing all patriots together. The people of Spain had a rock-ribbed faith in their ability to defeat the traitors and the invading armies. But they were dismayed by the attitude of the Western power. They had shown at Guadalajara that they could inflict crushing blows on the fascists despite the failure of the Western world to grant them the arms which the fascists received in abundance. But they knew that every day the embargo against them remained in force would mean more Spanish homes destroyed, more lives lost, more cities and towns reduced to ruins.

The audience listened in tense silence so that only the creaking of chairs could be heard behind his quiet voice. He described his visits to the fronts, the refugees on the road from Málaga, the bombing of the evacuees, the people falling by the roadside, and then the attack on Almería, the entombment of the dead and the living, the child he had carried in his arms through the flaming streets. He pictured for them the thousands of children left without homes or bodies or parents, wandering along the road, their minds in a daze, their bodies sick. This was the fruit of Franco's uprising, of the German-Italian invasion, of the supposed non-intervention of the Western powers. "This is the agony of a people which international action condones and sanctions under a guise of 'non-intervention.' But where governments have turned their backs on suffering Spain, decent men everywhere have come to their aid. The International Brigades have come to the defence of Spain, and in the Mackenzie-Papineau Battalion more than one thousand Canadians are upholding the honour of Canada."

There was a sustained burst of hand clapping from all parts of the Arena. Bethune paused, took a last puff at his ever-present cigarette, and ground the stub under his heel. When silence was restored he reported on the work of the blood-transfusion unit and came to his final point:

> To the Spanish people, and to anyone who has seen Spain for himself, the position is clear. So clear, in fact, that Franco and his fascist backers urgently need a diversion to conceal their aggression, just as the Tory bleaters of "non-intervention" need a fig-leaf to dress up the naked shanks of their miserable policy. They have found one, to their mutual relief. It is nothing more than the bastard child of the Austrian

paperhanger and the Italian turncoat. It is — "the menace of Communism!"

Fourteen years ago Mussolini was shipped into Rome in a parlor car and installed in office — to destroy the "the communist menace." He promptly proceeded, in the name of his holy mission, to destroy the living standards of the people and the very right to life, liberty and the pursuit of happiness. More recently, no doubt as part of the same holy mission, he has militarized Italy and brought Abyssinia into the grip of fascism and bloodshed.

Four short years ago, in Germany, Adolf Hitler was installed as Chancellor, also to save Germany from the "communist menace." He proceeded, as you will remember, with even more dispatch than *Il Duce*. In the name of the holy war against Bolshevism he made unholy war against every democratic German grouping, communist or anti-communist, ruined and murdered "non-Aryans," drove out some of the finest minds of the century, filled Germany with the horrors and brutality of the concentration camps, and fastened on the people the most terrible tyranny the world has ever seen. Herr Hitler is still raging against the "menace of communism," but already the guns of his new armies are pointing towards the territories of the leading non-communist governments of Europe.

And now Franco and his Moors and his German and Italian backers announce the same theme: they too are saving Spain from the communist menace. And in Downing Street, and at our own capital, and among learned American senators, it is sagely opined that it is of course deplorable about Spain, but the Reds are back of it, after all, and the present fighting is merely an alleged national reaction to Moscow's connivings.

Now I am not the least bit interested tonight to discuss the merits or demerits of the communist program and philosophy. If the people of Spain wanted communism it would be for them and nobody else to decide when and how they should have it. But I must say that the attempt to paint the invasion of Spain as a crusade to save the country from the "communist menace" is not only a wretched lie, it is a calculated and vicious insanity.

Is it not clear that if this insanity is to prevail, it will strike a mortal blow at all the rights and liberties of non-communists as well as communists? For if you are unfree, as the Spanish people were unfree, and you defend your freedom, you will be struck down as a communist. If you are hungry, as the Spanish people were hungry, you will be overwhelmed with cries of "communist menace" when you ask for bread. If you long for a decent, peaceful life of minimum abundance, again like the Spanish people, you will have to face the vengefulness of those scouring the earth with fixed bayonets for the contamination of communism. Every sincere word, every desire for a better life, every protest against injustice, every plea to improve an imperfect world will be suspect, dangerous, an invitation to reprisals, an act to be put down as the rankest subversion.

There are some who argue, of course, that the Soviet Union is assisting the Loyalist regime, and the communists inside and outside of Spain are supporting the Spanish Government. This argument, presumably, is supposed to prove the existence of the "communist menace" in Spain and thereby to disqualify the Loyalists. I fail to follow the logic. I fail to follow the argument that because the Soviet Union, or the communists elsewhere, approve of something it is thereby necessarily proven bad. I further cannot accept the suggestion that because the fascists and their "neutral" Tory friends everywhere say that something is good, it cannot therefore be quite bad.

Yes, the Soviet Union has sent aid the Spanish Republic. So has Mexico, which is not communist. That is an undeniable fact. Is that to the discredit of Spain? I would reverse the question. I would say that it is to the credit of the Soviet Union and Mexico that they have lived up to their obligations to the Spanish Government, which represents Spain's people. The Soviet Union and Mexico, by according the Spanish Government its legal rights, are aiding the government elected and supported by the people themselves. The Western powers, by embargoing the Loyalists and shutting their eyes to the flow of arms and armies from Italy and Germany to Franco, are supporting the choice of Hitler, Mussolini and the clique of the Spanish financiers and feudalists who mint their wealth out of the poverty of the people.

Let us have done, then, with the miserable deception of anti-communism. It has served Hitler and Mussolini well, but not the enslaved German and Italian peoples. It may have a pleasing sound in Tory ears, and salve the consciences of some spinsterish British labour leaders, but it is rank dishonesty nevertheless. It is the great lie of our decade. It is the last refuge of the reactionary whose patrons' thirst for power is desperate and undiminished. That is one of the lessons of Spain. I hope we will never forget it.

Spain *can* be the tomb of fascism. History will some day take full revenge on those who fail her.

The entire audience rose to its feet in a prolonged ovation.

31

Two days later he left for Toronto where he spoke at another huge meeting. It was the beginning of a long and grueling tour across the continent.

For seven months he shuttled back and forth between the towns and cities of Canada and the United States, showing *Heart of Spain* and lecturing, beginning on the East coast, working his way through southern and northern Ontario, across the prairie provinces, till he reached Vancouver on the west coast and started back through the United States.

The moral and financial response to his lecture tour surpassed all expectations, but a cloud began to gather over his mission. As he travelled from city to city, warning that failure to uphold Loyalist Spain would invite further catastrophes, history overtook his direst predictions. The anticomintern struck again — this time in China.

"In Spain," he declared in one of his speeches, "fascism has attacked 24,000,000 people, with the United States, Britain and France embargoing the Loyalists. Now, in China, the attack has spread against nearly one quarter of the total population of the Earth. If the same treacherous policy of blockading the victims and making arrangements with the aggressors is continued, we may well wonder whether any man, woman or child is safe anywhere in the world."

He watched hopefully for hints of a change in the policies of the Western powers, but none came. In 1931 Japan had invaded Manchuria. There had been some verbal rumpus on the part of the Western powers and paralysis in the Chiang Kai-shek government. Now, the Japanese had launched their open attacks at Peiping in July 1937 and as in Spain, the Japanese anchor of the anticomintern bloc raised a loud hue and cry about suppressing "communism" in Asia.

Bethune read the news from China as he had once followed the communiqués from Madrid. He sounded a new note of urgency in his speeches. He could sense, in the reactions of his audience, a greater receptivity to the things he had to say. There was a growing feeling of uneasiness about Axis moves among wide sections of the public. But it seemed to him that the menace hanging over the world was growing much more quickly than the awareness of the people.

When he read of Japanese bombings of Chinese cities his mind went back to Madrid, to Almería, to the sound of the bombs, the cries of the wounded, the sight of the dead. Canada and the United States had to be awakened! But they were being fed on "supine editorials, the soothing words of political spokesmen, the opiates of Hollywood, the skillfully planted propaganda of powerful business lobbies."

To a friend in Montreal who reminded him in a nostalgic note of pleasant times they had shared before he had gone to Spain, he replied: "No, for me they can't return. No one knows better than I the lure of pleasures, excitements, people....Yes, I know my own vulnerability! But those days are gone for me. I have steeled myself against them. The future looks lonely and dangerous."

To a medical colleague he wrote:

> Today I picked up some Canadian papers between trains. Buried somewhere in the back pages I found an item reporting a demonstration at the Vancouver waterfront against the loading of scrap iron for Japan. Splendid, any decent person would think. But was some cabinet minister there to praise them, to assure them that Canadian materials would not go to make armaments to destroy Chinese lives? No. Only the police were there, to pounce upon and assault the demonstrators. Idiocy! But what bloody and malevolent idiocy! And I keep on *talking*...."

In the face of the "idiocy" he came to a decision. On a train somewhere in the Midwest he wrote a letter to a member of the Spanish Aid Committee in Toronto. He had now spent half a year, he pointed out, lecturing on behalf of Loyalist Spain. He had undertaken the job because he had been convinced of its necessity. But the military situation in Spain had become worse since his return home, and elsewhere the political situation was deteriorating as war spread over the Orient. In these circumstances, when military considerations grew more important in the struggle to defeat reaction, and when he had, in any event, covered most of North America in his tour, he felt his usefulness once again lay in more direct participation.

He now had several meetings to address in Canada as the windup of his tour. He spoke to a McGill students' group then at a rally in Toronto. A week later, at a meeting in Saskatoon, someone in the audience shouted a question at him: "Is it true that you're a communist?" He replied. "Yes, I am communist."

The press carried his avowal throughout the country. Some quarters received the news with surprise; others viewed it as a gesture; but to his closest friends his action had an air of inevitability about it.

When someone, after his Saskatoon meeting, suggested that his communist affiliation might tend to diminish the effectiveness of his work for Spain, he reacted vehemently:

> Oh no! I can't let that go unchallenged! Yes, I am a Communist. That is a matter of my own beliefs, and my own decisions. If I say now that milk is good for children, will anti-Communists therefore suggest that it is *not* good? And if I say that the people need bread, does it mean that they don't, simply because the man who says it considers socialism the most equitable, the highest political and moral form of human society?

At another meeting, when a heckler called him a "Moscow hireling," he replied amiably:

> My poor deluded friend … Why a *Moscow* hireling? Why not a *British* hireling? The theory of socialism was proclaimed in London 60 years before the Russian Revolution. If Russia disappeared from the face of the earth tomorrow, do

you think that would eliminate communism? I am sure that if Christ walked the earth again, preaching the brotherhood of man, He too would have thrown at Him the label of "Moscow hireling."

Now, with his tour completed, his future plans were clear in his mind. In Toronto, after addressing a Spanish Aid conference in a local Protestant church, he discussed his new plans with the Committee to Aid Spanish Democracy. He had been hoping to return to Spain as a surgeon, he announced. But a new group of American doctors had just left for Spain, and events in the Far East were focusing attention on the battle of the Chinese people against invasion. He had no intention of ever again hanging out his shingle in private practice. Spain needed help, but some help was being given. In China doctors were needed even more urgently than in Spain.

In New York, he went on, a China Aid Council had been set up, functioning in co-operation with the China Defence League, headed by Madame Sun Yat-sen, widow of the first president of the Chinese Republic. The Council's program was the sending of medical aid to the guerillas fighting the Japanese in northern China. He had volunteered to take a medical unit to northern China to work with the guerillas. His experiences in Spain, he felt, would be invaluable in China.

He left for New York a few days later to complete arrangements with the China Aid Council. On January 2, 1938, he left Vancouver on the Empress of Japan for Hong Kong, taking with him enough equipment and supplies to outfit a few surgery units.

In the hectic weeks of preparation he had no real time to speculate about what the future might bring. He had seen Frances in Montreal, visited his family in Hamilton* and said goodbye to a few intimate friends. But on ship he felt the need to write a farewell letter to Frances, which he mailed in Hong Kong:

When I saw you in Montreal before leaving for Vancouver I tried to explain why I was going

---

* His mother, sister and brother. His father had died in 1930.

to China. I don't know whether I succeeded....
The fact that I went to Spain doesn't give me,
not could it give anybody else, some special
indulgence to sit quietly on the sidelines now.
Spain is a scar on my heart. Do you understand?
It is a scar that can never heal. The pain will be
with me always, reminding me of the things I
have seen.

I refuse to live in a world that spawns murder and corruption without raising my hand
against them. I refuse to condone, by passivity,
or by default, the wars which greedy men make
against others.... Spain and China are part of the
same battle. I am going to China because I feel
that is where the need is greatest; that is where I
can be most successful,

With best wishes....

BETH

PART FOUR

THE ENEMY —
THOSE WHO MAKE THE WOUNDS

32

For forty years I have devoted myself to the cause of the people's revolution with but one end in view: the elevation of China to a position of freedom and equality among the nations. My experiences during these forty years have convinced me that to attain this goal we must bring about an awakening for our own people and ally ourselves in a common struggle with those peoples of the world who treat us as equals.

—Dr. Sun Yat-sen, President of the Chinese Republic, in his will, 1925.

On January 20, 1938, Bethune reached Hong Kong, the British Crown Colony on the southern China coast. Three days later he flew to Hankow, seat of the National Government headed by Chiang Kai-shek. In Hankow he found himself in another world — the strange, backward, far-flung land of the oldest surviving nation on earth.

In the city where fantastic squalor surrounded dazzling opulence, where political bureaucracy stubbornly resisted the ferment of modern ideas, he interviewed lower government officials, inspected primitive army hospitals, and prepared for his journey to the north.

The initial impact of China was staggering. Here, among the swirling tides of war, nationalism, foreign imperialism, semifeudal reaction, communism, events shaking the foundations of Asia were unfolding. Their origins had to be traced through thousands of years of Chinese history, the rise of modern Europe, the rivalries of the great powers, the dramatic upsurge of the Chinese people.

Civilization had come to China 5,000 years ago. While Europe was still immersed in barbarism, China had already entered the period of feudalism. Her influence on Europe was indirect, but profound. From China, Europe received the printing press and gunpowder. China was then a mecca for European traders, a legendary storehouse for envious eyes in the West. But three centuries before the first cracks were to appear in China's feudalism, the industrial revolution began to topple feudalism in Western Europe. The printed word helped spread the challenge to the old order. Once the capitalist was enthroned, his *new* order went in search of markets and raw materials. He used his gunpowder to seize both on the undeveloped continents of Asia and Africa.

While Europe was forging swiftly ahead of Asia, China was suffering overland invasion, the despotic rule of the foreign Manchus, the indignities of foreign armies on her soil. But it was in the nineteenth century that Western imperialism subjected her to the bitterest humiliations.

It was the century of the "big grab." England seized Hong Kong, forced China to grant her extraterritorial rights and brought opium into the country under the threat of bombarding the coast. Japan took over Korea and Taiwan.* France grabbed Indo-China. Germany helped herself to various mainland cities. Czarist Russia seized key ports in Manchuria. The United States, with its own frontier to develop, arrived on the scene as a "Johnny-come-lately." Finding itself in a special position it devised a special formula. It helped itself to the Philippines and pressed for "equal rights" with the other powers in China. It summed up its policy in the demand for an "open door," which to the Chinese people meant a policy of "me too."

While the imperialist powers profited through their privileged positions in the country, the people were borne down by universal poverty, disease, illiteracy and repression. But the feudal landlord class, which had traditionally allied itself to the ruling dynasties, remained fat and corrupt. When the peasants revolted, they were always crushed by the alliance of their own feudal rulers and foreign armies. But as the Western powers kept cutting into China, more and more Chinese, especially students and intellectuals, came into contact with Western techniques, history and progressive thought.

---

* Formosa.

In the first decade of the twentieth century the movement for national independence found its greatest spokesman, Dr. Sun Yat-sen. Now, too, a new factor entered the situation in the spread of nationalist ideas among the soldiers of the native army the Manchus had formed. In 1911 sections of the army revolted, the Manchu dynasty was overthrown, and the Chinese republic was established under the presidency of Sun Yat-sen at Nanking.

At the beginning the change was little more than a change of outer trappings. The landlords and bureaucrats remained. Vast areas of the country were ruled by local war lords who opposed Sun and joined avidly in conspiracies with foreign powers against him. Dr. Sun still faced the problem of expelling imperialism, of unifying the country, establishing a truly national government, defeating the old feudal clique and introducing reforms overdue for centuries. The World War of 1914–1918 accelerated the process.

The defeat of Germany and Austro-Hungary removed them from the bloc of powers exercising their imperialist sway over China. After the October Revolution in Russia the new socialist state renounced all the Czarist privileges in the country and openly declared its sympathy with the colonial world's aspirations for full independence. Along with the weakening of the bloc of foreign powers holding China in their grip, two new elements now appeared inside the country to strengthen the national independence movement. In the special conditions of the war the first steps towards local manufacture had been taken. This had produced a native class of industrialists and a new working class. The industrialists, irked by the economic disabilities they suffered at the hands of outside powers despoiling China's economy, desired a strong government that would protect their interests. The working class, though still small, was a cohesive element that made itself felt through compact organization, was strongly influenced by the Russian revolution and gave birth to the Chinese Communist Party.

Around Sun there now grew a coalition, first, of workers and peasants, increasingly led by the communists, and second, of the national *bourgeoisie* and the Kuomintang party. The program of the coalition was expressed in Sun's Three People's Principles — national independence, democracy, improvement of the people's living conditions, and in his Three Great Policies — active anti-imperialism, co-operation with Soviet Russia, support of the workers' and peasants' movements.

When Sun Yat-sen died in 1925 conditions were ripe for putting an end to the "era of the war lords." At Canton an army of a new type had been created as a result of the co-operative efforts of the communist and Kuomintang parties. Its officers were trained at the famous Whampoa Military Academy, of which Chiang Kai-shek was president and communist Chou En-lai was dean. There now began what came to be known as the Northern Expedition, the march of the Kuomintang-communist army against the war lords and the strongholds of foreign influence in other parts of the country.

The Expedition roused tremendous popular support among the people. By 1927 the coalition forces were at the gates of Shanghai, chief centre of foreign influence. Between Canton and Shanghai the war lords were overthrown. Britain, France, and the United States brought troops to the country, but found it prudent not to use them. Inside Shanghai the workers, led by Chou En-lai, who stole into the city in disguise, rose up in revolt against the local militarist bureaucrats and seized control before the army entered.

The last will and testament of Sun Yat-sen, it seemed, was on the road to fulfillment. But now the influential industrialists, yesterday's feudal landlords, took fright. In the new power of the people, demonstrated so dramatically at Shanghai, and in their enthusiastic demand for social reform, they saw the possible eclipse of their own economic and political domination. At the suggestion of foreign representatives, and operating through the right wing of the Kuomintang, they quietly cast about for ways and means of halting the popular upsurge and effecting a compromise with the feudal elements and foreign interests that would guarantee their own privileged positions. As their "strong man" they selected Chiang Kai-shek.

Now, without warning, Chiang turned on his working-class and peasant allies, ordered the physical extermination of the Communist Party, had thousands of labour and peasant leaders put to death, disarmed and incarcerated left-wing troops, suppressed every vestige of liberal thought. Sun Yat-sen's Three People's

Principles and Three Great Policies were discarded. The fight against the war lords was shelved. The first stage of the people's united effort to achieve a democratic, independent China was over, betrayed by the Kuomintang in an unparalleled bloodbath.

But it was only the first stage. Though badly mauled, the communists and those who stood by them led their surviving troops to the province of Kiangsi, where they set up a revolutionary base.

In the special setting of semifeudal, semicolonial China, they were a proletarian party leading a peasants' agrarian revolt with an organized army.

Despite Japan's known blueprints for aggression against the Chinese mainland, Chiang raised loans in the United States and launched large-scale military action against the Kiangsi region. Thus began the second stage: the Ten-Year Civil War.

Taking advantage of the civil war, Japan jumped the gun on her imperialist rivals and moved into Manchuria, conquering the vast northern province in short order and setting up a puppet Manchu emperor. Chiang paid little attention. Without even bothering to break off diplomatic relations with Tokyo, he concerned himself solely with wiping out the Kiangsi communists.

In 1932 the Kiangsi communists, staving off all Kuomintang efforts to suppress them, called upon Chiang to stop the Civil War, and urged the people to work for a united, national front against the Japanese aggressor. Chiang replied by sending another military expedition against the communists. Many of Chiang's troops went over to the communists, many others surrendered.

The appeals to Chiang Kai-shek for joint action against the Japanese were based on the thesis that "the greatest oppression suffered by China is national oppression." Therefore, "the Chinese national *bourgeoisie* can, in certain periods and to a certain extent, participate in the struggles against imperialism and the feudal war lords."[*] But Chiang rejected all appeals. From June 1932 to February 1933 he put half a million men into the field against Kiangsi. Again he was badly defeated. But in October 1933, when he used a million troops, he met with some initial successes.

---

[*] Mao Tse-tung.

The outcome of the clash of different opinion in the communist leadership was the famous decision to transfer the communist armies to the northern province of Shensi, where they could better repel Chiang's attacks and take military action against the Japanese.

Thus, in 1934, there began the breathtaking Long March under the leadership of Mao Tse-tung, Chu Teh and others. It was an epic trek on foot 8,000 circuitous miles from Kiangsi to the province of Shensi. Thousands of troops died on the way. The rest were harried by Chiang's armies. But under the leadership of Mao Tse-tung and Chu Teh, 30,000 hardened veterans in 1935 reached Shensi, where the local communists had prepared the way for them. Here, with Yenan as their capital, they set up the first anti-Japanese base in China pledged to resist Japanese aggression.

Now that they had come close to the Japanese, Tokyo threatened Chiang with dire consequences unless the communists were suppressed. Chiang set up a special Pacification Headquarters at Sian and sent another expeditionary force against the new anti-Japanese base. But now the demand for an end to the Civil War and for the defence of China was sweeping the entire country. Not only did the soldiers of Chiang's expeditionary force refuse to fight, but its highest officers negotiated an unofficial truce with the communists. Alarmed, Chiang went to Sian in person to repair the situation, only to be kidnapped by his own officers in the sensational "Sian incident," when his life was saved by the diplomatic intervention of the very communists he had sought to suppress.

Out of the "Sian Incident" came the agreement to end the Civil War and to join the forces of the Chinese people in resistance to Japanese aggression. At Sian, Chiang at last faced the fact that soldier and civilian alike would accept no other course. He submitted to popular demand and reached an agreement with the communists to resist the Japanese. When the Japanese struck again in the summer of 1937, the communist base had spread northwest from Shensi to Ningshsia and west to Kansu. By agreement with the Kuomintang the three provinces were recognized as an autonomous "special district" under the National Administration. The Red Army, now with about 80,000 troops, was renamed the 8th Route National Revolutionary Army, functioning with its own leaders under the National Military Council. Now the third stage had begun: the anti-Japanese war.

As the Japanese drove southwards into the provinces of Shansi, Hopei and Chahar, northeast of the new "special district," the 8th Route Army troops moved into the provinces to contact other Chinese units and to set up a new "military district" known as Chin-Cha-Chi in the Japanese rear. Now, no matter how precariously the revived coalition between the communists and the Kuomintang might develop, a bulwark had been erected in the north against the invader.

It was for this area that Bethune left Hankow by train on February 22. His route lay across mountains, rivers, wild country, roadless valleys. Ten days after he left Hankow, newspaper correspondents cabled the American press that he had been caught and killed in the interior by the Japanese.

33

While inquiries flew thick and fast between New York, Hankow and Yenan concerning his reported death, Bethune was playing cat and mouse with the Japanese armies coming down from the north.

One day out of Hankow he reached Chengchow, a railway centre that had just been bombed. After sleeping overnight on a bench near the railway station he left the ruined city for Tungkwan, where he crossed the Yellow River on a junk and entrained again on the Tung Kou line that ran north into Shansi.

The train chugged slowly along the east bank of the Fen River and into the hollow between two mountain ranges. This was the beginning of China's strange loess country, the low, brownish-ocher mountains that continued for hundreds of miles, in terraces that rose one upon the other like gigantic, man-made staircases.

He passed numerous trains travelling down the line packed with refugees fleeing from the Japanese. On every southbound train they filled the coaches, sat precariously on the carriage roofs, swarmed over the engine, hung onto the steps and the couplings. They went by silently, with the same parched look as the fields about them, too weary to raise their eyes to the thousands of ducks that flew overhead in great, flapping clouds.

Several times, during the day, the train stopped at wayside stations where vendors sold hot millet soup, noodles, tea, fried hare, wheat rolls, steamed buns, hard-boiled eggs. After two days of travel they reached Linfen, only to find they would have to turn back.

The Linfen station, as they pulled in, was jammed with civilians carrying all their possessions, and wounded soldiers, arms, legs and heads wrapped in dusty, red-streaked bandages. The Japanese were a short distance from the city, they were coming on quickly, and the population was being evacuated. In the chaos that was spreading through the streets Bethune tried to locate the headquarters of the local communist troops. But with the Japanese advancing, it had been moved — nobody seemed to know where. All trains, he discovered, were now heading southward only, with as many evacuees as they could carry.

At four in the afternoon the first wave of Japanese bombers came over. Bethune was caught at the station, among flatcars loaded with mules, rice, and munitions. With hundreds of evacuees he sat out the bombardment in trenches that had been dug in the sand. A few hours later, with the fall of the city imminent and all hope of transportation beyond the city obviously impossible, he reluctantly agreed to make the two-day return trip to Tungkwan on the last train to leave.

He got his luggage aboard a boxcar filled with rice bags almost to the roof, climbed in and went to sleep as the train pulled out. At 3 a.m. he awoke to discover that his car had been uncoupled at a town called Goasi, twenty-five miles below Linfen, that he was stranded, and that the Japanese were coming down the railway line from Linfen.

But in the deserted town luck came his way in the person of an 8th Route Army officer, a Major Lee. The major examined the abandoned boxcar, decided the rice was too valuable a prize to be left for the Japanese, organized a corps of volunteer peasants to get it out of the menaced town, and calmly informed Bethune he could get him by mule cart to Yenan. In his diary Bethune recorded the rest of the journey:

February 28: It was as simple as that. To get to Yenan we would have to travel three hundred miles westward. On foot and by mule cart! It would mean crossing the river into Shensi. There would be two more rivers to cross once inside Shensi. (No bridges, of course!) Then would come the range of mountains. But all of this didn't seem unusual to the soldiers of the 8th Route Army.

Waiting for final arrangements I wandered about the deserted town. For food I bought a quarter of a pig in the streets for $1.40. From up the line groups of ten and twenty wounded came straggling in by day and night. The enemy's guns could be heard clearly, but getting out ahead of the Japanese seemed old hat to Major Lee's men.

We left Goasi with a caravan of forty-two carts loaded with sacks of rice, each cart pulled by three mules. It was a fine, brilliant day. I walked ahead of the caravan, enjoying the clear, dry air. Many towns along the way, but because of the news of the advancing Japanese the inhabitants had closed their gates and we were forced to go round the walls in open country and pick up the road on the other side.

Our first brush with the enemy came in mid-afternoon, when we were only four hours out of Goasi. I was walking alongside the leading cart when I saw two bombers going south about two miles on our left. They spotted us at once. Forty-two carts stretched out over a quarter of a mile, with no anti-aircraft guns anywhere about and not a single Chinese pursuit plane in the entire province. We must have simply made their mouths water! We were sitting birds asking to be knocked off, and they proceeded to knock us off to the best of their ability. While one of them stayed high, the other swept over us at a height of about five hundred feet. Our military escort consisted of five men and five boys, armed with a total of five old rifles. With the drivers and our escort I left the carts and lay out on the bare ground. There wasn't a stone or tree to give protection.

As we watched, the first bomber came back, so low I could have hit him with a baseball, and bombed the lead section of the caravan — but missing by about fifty feet! He swept on the rear carts, dropping another four bombs — this time with more effect. This time I could hear the outcry of the wounded.

Our casualties were four men wounded, fifteen mules killed, twelve mules disabled. Major Lee arranged immediate payment to the drivers for all the dead mules — one hundred Mexican dollars for each mule. This, I found, was the set policy of the 8th Route Army. Anything received from the people was paid for.

I treated the wounded and we cut the dead and disabled animals from the wrecked carts. We were now down to twenty carts, less than half the number we had set out with. We travelled all through a dark and overcast night, sleeping on top of the bags of rice, jarred to the bone on the uneven road.

March 1: At five a.m. we reached the bank of River Fen again, where we found a village inn. We got four hours sleep on the inn's *k'angs* with their hard clay tops, rising at nine for a breakfast of sweet fermented rice water, heated, with an egg beaten up in it.

Opposite us on the far bank was the city of Kiangchow. The Japanese, we heard, were coming down the railway at a fast pace from Linfen. We were the rear of the rearguard! We and the walking wounded.

Japanese airplanes flew overhead all morning as we crossed over to Kiangchow. The river was about 200 yards wide at this point, muddy, waist-deep and fast.

Kiangchow lay atop a hill, and as I made my way up I could see two steeples of a Roman Catholic Church of the French style. I made for the Church. Except for some merchants and beggars the city was deserted. I found it interesting that these two classes were all that remained — the relatively wealthy and the beggared. The men of property awaited the coming of the Japanese with some fear and trembling, but their goods were more important than their fears. They preferred to stay with their property under the Japanese rather than take their chances on freedom with their countrymen! Typical the whole world over!

At the Church I found the usual mission compound, now filled with the families of church members seeking refuge. The staff included an apostolic missionary, a Dutch priest and a French priest. They welcomed me cordially, opened a bottle of red wine, gave me a fragrant cigar, and offered me overnight lodging. We had some interesting conversation in a mixture of English and very little French.

They expected the Japanese to arrive in 36 hours. What, I asked, did they intend to do then? A shrug of the shoulder. But hadn't the Japanese been ruthless with Christians as well as Chinese? Did they expect the invader to respect the French flag on the Church spire? They agreed that there had been "unfortunate" atrocities, that some missionaries had already been killed, but they would stay with their parishioners. When I bade them goodbye the next day, thanking them for their hospitality, one of them said: "I hope we meet again on earth. If not, then in heaven."

We started out at 1:30 p.m. after every bag of rice had been carried across the river on the backs of the porters. As we left Kiangchow the news was that the Japanese were twenty-five miles away, and their cavalry even closer. We were relieved to have the river between us and the enemy.

We covered sixty li (twenty miles) by evening, walking all the way, and spent the night at a little village called Chi-Shan.

March 2: We were off early. No soldiers were to be seen — only the walking wounded.

As I walked ahead of the two carts I saw a young lad up the line stopping to rest every once in a while. When I finally came abreast of him I noticed that he was very short of breath. He was a mere child of seventeen. On the front of his faded blue jacket there was a great stain of blood, dark and old. I forced him to stop and examined him. He had been shot through the lung a week before, and had been left with a badly suppurating wound of the upper right anterior chest wall. There was no dressing. The bullet had gone through the lung and come out at the back. There was fluid in the pleural cavity up as high as the third rib in front. The heart was displaced three inches to the left. The boy had been walking in this condition for a week. If I hadn't seen it myself

I wouldn't have believed it possible. I put him up on our cart, where he lay coughing painfully as the mule cart moved slowly over the rough road enveloped in a cloud of dust.

We made only 20 miles that day with nothing in between us and the Japanese following behind. It was a decidedly draughty sensation.

March 3: Today we came to the city of Ho-Chin. It was filled with the provincial troops of General Yen Shi* Shan. We had caught up with the army! We heard that the American Presbyterian Hospital had left the city a month ago. One week after the mission left 500 wounded men arrived from the north. There was no hospital there to give them treatment.

I found the only "doctor" in a "shop." He was a combined doctor, dentist, druggist — in fact, a quack. His shop was filled with wounded waiting for dressings for which he charged a dollar each. He charged me $4 for a small roll of gauze worth 50 cents.

Among the provincial troops there seemed to be no organization. We learned that some refused to obey their officers. There were charges that the old-line officers had cheated soldiers out of their pay, which was little enough — $6 a month with food and uniform. We were told some of the troops hadn't been paid for months....A mess!

March 4: Today is my birthday — my 48th. Last year in Madrid, this year in Ho-Chin, China. I celebrated my birthday by dressing wounded soldiers (arms and hands), finding that the only wounded around had nothing but neglected minor injuries, and that all others had died on the way. I also walked about the town seeing the "sights" — vendors selling live carp in water buckets, black pigs with big, floppy ears, barkless dogs, houses with white paper windows, lousy *k'angs*.

March 5: Today we left Ho-Chin for the village of Shen Chien Shen on the east bank of the Yellow River. We heard before leaving that the Japanese had burnt to the ground the villages we had passed through 36 hours earlier.

We set out late. At 9 p.m., in the pitch dark, we marched down the river bank. There, we came across an unforgettable sight. In the light of a dozen fires 5,000 men were collected,

---

* This is Bethune's spelling. The correct spelling is Hsi.

with trucks, mules, horses, artillery and great piles of stores — all waiting to cross the river into Shensi. The steel, wall-like mountainside rising above the encampment shone with the reflected glow of the fires. The river was a loud, rushing torrent between high cliffs. Ice floes swept by, clashing against each other far out on the dark surface. The whole scene was wild and fantastic.

March 6: We finally slept at midnight, lying on top of the rice bags beside the river. We were up at five in the morning, greeted by a cold, overcast dawn. There were only four junks to carry us over the river. That means it will take at least four days. We hear that the Japanese are now only ten miles away.

March 7: The Chinese officer in charge of the ferrying operations put us on the first junk to leave the bank. It was about fifty feet by twenty-five, with 100 men on board, field artillery, mules, baggage. We were swept swiftly downstream for half a mile, past the spot where about one thousand wounded were being collected, till a naked boy jumped overboard with a pole anchor, slowing us down. Then the men working the junk worked it out of the main current and slowly manoeuvred us to the opposite bank.

The west bank was strongly fortified, with many troops, good trenches and dugouts. I saw several batteries of field guns. The troops looked good. They had a sense of order, discipline and efficiency. They were dressed in dusty, faded uniforms, the colour of the soil which has stained them for months. The equipment looked good too — many automatic rifles, both light and heavy machine guns, stick hand grenades.

We marched to a nearby village and occupied a deserted house. I opened two cans of chipped beef for our midday meal. The last sight I remember was the great red horse belonging to Chu Teh. He had loaned it to Captain Evans Carlson,[*] the U.S. military attaché who had been inspecting the North Shansi front some time ago. Carlson had left it in charge of our commander to be returned to Chu Teh …

We heard the Japanese had reached Ho-Chin one day after we left it. Well, we beat them to it…. However, the river is rising

---

[*] Later, Lieutenant Colonel Carlson, commander of the famed "Carlson's Raiders" of the U.S. Marines.

and I am afraid many men will be captured tomorrow on the east bank when the Japanese reach the river. Ho-Chin is only five miles away. We are expecting a battle on the river bank. It is raining and cold.

March 8: Our fears were well founded. At 4 p.m. yesterday the Japanese cavalry reached the river. I led a party down to the river to get the remainder of our supplies from the beach when the enemy announced his presence on the opposite bank by opening machine gun fire on us. The bullets slapped into the water one hundred yards away. We scrambled up the bank into a trench and from there could plainly see the enemy on the opposite side. We decided on a dash across a piece of open land. Here they fired on us again. We threw ourselves down on the ground, the bullets kicking up dust uncomfortably close. When I looked up I saw to my horror that we were lying directly in front of our own field guns fifty feet away. We scrambled out of the way with remarkably little loss of time. I discovered, in the process, that the Japanese can shoot accurately....

We hear that the force facing us across the river is made up of twenty thousand Japanese, including four or five hundred cavalry, several batteries of field guns, and infantry. I have seen no army doctors. Where are they? I have discovered the medical officer of each division in the Kuomintang army will treat only the men of his own division and not other. Madness!

It is the coldest night so far, with two inches of snow on the ground. We have found ourselves a cave which is snug and warm, but I pity the troops lying outside in the snow without protection. There is nothing to eat in the village but millet.

A little while ago the Japanese artillery arrived on the opposite bank and is now shelling us without let-up. Ours is replying. The noise of the explosions echoes back and forth weirdly between the mountains. A Japanese shell has blown off the top of a house three hundred feet away, but they can't hurt us. Our cave is dug in the side of a hill and goes forty feet underground.

I have found a supply of drugs *abandoned* by some scoundrel of a medical officer — bottles of tincture of Camphor Compound, digitalis, adrenaline, silk sutures, syringes, ampules of cocaine.

March 9: Woke this morning to hear one of our Chinese soldiers singing the Marseillaise. A strange reveille on the banks of the Yellow River. During the morning a child took convulsions and the mother rushed out of the cave, calling the child's name loudly — to bring back his soul which had temporarily, she believed, left his body. Demons and the Marseillaise!

March 10: Today we set out on foot for Sian — two hundred and twenty five miles away. Lee was amazing. Now only thirty-two, he was once a rickshaw man living in Shanghai and was on the Great Trek. He has legs like trees. When we reached Hancheng he was still comparatively fresh.

It was a fine day for marching, and the country looked good, with wheat up about four inches.

We kept the river on the right of our line of march. We passed many students from the University of Linfen. About three thousand of them had scattered south and west before the Japanese. Some had been caught and killed, some had died of cold in the mountains. Many of those we met were eager to make their way to the University of Yenan run by the 8th Route Army.

We reached the city of Hancheng at five in the afternoon, entering through the west gate of the high wall. I, for one, wasn't sorry to make it.

March 22: A hectic time, and not a moment to write! We stayed more than a week in Hancheng, waiting for trucks to arrive from Sian. What a week! I worked among the wounded and was besieged by civilian patients. I treated pulmonary tuberculosis, ovarian cyst, gastric ulcer — everything. After a few days' work at a military base hospital situated in a temple, the chief surgeon and entire nursing staff offered to come up to Yenan with us. Of course we couldn't take them. On March 19th the trucks finally arrived and we set out for Sian, two hundred miles away. We made the trip in two days, and we are here now. I've met Agnes Smedley, a remarkable woman. She has been working hard to get supplies to the hospitals in Yenan. The first thing I did in Sian was go to the bath house. The ineffable bliss of a hot bath — my first in a month!

In four days we leave for Yenan.

34

The truck drove through the pocked hills, came out on a road that twisted sharply downwards, and there, on a pancake plain at the junction of three valleys, Bethune saw the city.

Yenan at last!

Here were the men, still unknown to most of the outside world, who three years ago had been a remnant, a small band cut to pieces, but whose words now resounded throughout China with a prophetic impact. Here, while the outside world still ignored it or wondered, the most complex political development of the twentieth century had unfolded: an autonomous region led by Marxist revolutionaries within the framework of a semi-feudal, semicolonial China.

In the centre of the city a delegation was waiting to receive him. It was headed by a short, merry-looking American who pumped Bethune's hand vigourously. He introduced himself as Dr. Ma Hai-teh. Bethune had heard of him as an American who had come to China a few years ago, had changed his name, married a Chinese, learned to speak the language fluently, and become a medical advisor to the 8th Route Army in Yenan.

At the military and administrative headquarters of the Special Region, word of Bethune's arrival preceded him. He was impressed by the air of expectancy in which Dr. Ma conducted him on a tour of army and government offices.

"We've been worrying our heads off ever since we first got the reports that you were lost after leaving Hong Kong," Dr. Ma told him. "You can't realize how much everyone here has been looking forward to your coming. A surgeon with your background! And your experience in Spain! We've been sending telegrams all over the place, trying to find out what happened to you. By God, how we need you!"

After the first round of interviews, Bethune was taken to his quarters — a cave in the nearby hills. It was the size of a large room in a Canadian home, furnished with a *k'ang* stove-bed and a small table.

His first day in Yenan was a stimulating experience. His diary entry for the day read:

> Although Yenan is one of the oldest towns in all China, it strikes me immediately as one of the best-run. In Hankow I found confusion, indecision, depressing signs of bureaucracy and inefficiency. In Yenan there is a sense of confidence and purpose in administrative circles. In the towns and cities I passed through on my way here I became accustomed to the sights of semi-feudalism — filthy dwellings, polluted streets, people in rags. Here, among the ancient structures, the streets are clean, teeming with people who seem to know where they're going. There is no sewage system, but there is obviously an organized disposal of sewage.
>
> In contrast to the rest of China, the Special Region administration is developing an overall program dovetailing social reform with organization of the Region's capacities to make war against the Japanese. There is a University, attracting thousands of students from other areas. There is a newly created Medical Training School designed to furnish the army with medical personnel. There is a growing hospital, and though medical facilities are primitive, the government here has introduced free medical treatment for all!

With the influx of students and others who had flocked to the support of the anti-Japanese base, the population of Yenan increased from 3,000 to 30,000. The administration had solved the problem by organizing the residents into groups to build comfortable cave homes in the surrounding hills where Bethune now lived. Since the food supply was poor, a ration system had been introduced to portion out available supplies equitably, with soldiers at the front granted twice the civilian ration.

Though the communists were in undisputed leadership,

Kuomintang and other elements were encouraged to join in the administration. Above all, there was an unmistakable sense of combined effort to halt the invaders, untrammeled by the restrictions and intrigues Bethune had observed in the south. The Special Region, it was emphasized everywhere in Yenan, followed a deliberate policy of providing a model to the rest of the country on how to weld all sections of the people into a common front against the enemy.

On the evening of his second day in Yenan Bethune met the man chiefly responsible for the strategy which had culminated in the establishment of the Special Region and new Border Region of Chin-Cha-Chi in the Japanese rear.

That night, at 11 o'clock, he was invited to a conference with Mao Tse-tung, leader of China's communists.

The interview took place in an ordinary house, on a dark street. Besides Bethune and Mao those present were Dr. Chiang, Chief Medical officer of the 8th Route Army, and an interpreter.

As Bethune entered Mao stood up and greeted him cordially. He was tall, well built, with jet-black hair parted in the centre of a leonine head. His handclasp was firm, his smile gentle, his eyes calm and appraising. They stood with clasped hands for a moment, examining each other in the candlelight. At a gesture from Mao they sat down at opposite sides of a table that stood in the centre of the bare room. Apart from the table the only furnishings were half a dozen chairs, the usual *k'ang*, and several well-stocked bookshelves. While Mao exchanged some words with the interpreter Bethune studied him closely. He was surprised to find that the few interviews with Mao published in America had failed to transmit a complete image of the man and had prepared him for something quite different. After the first half hour of conversation this initial feeling deepened. In the flickering candlelight, listening to the soft, low-pitched voice and the searching questions, he received an overwhelming impression of the communist leader as a man of deep culture, a poet who could express himself in sharp political terms, a complex individual in whom a thousand different facets were geared together so smoothly that he thought and spoke with the utmost simplicity.

Mao opened the interview by politely soliciting Bethune's views about Spain. Though he first confined himself to questions, it was soon apparent that he had detailed information on the course of the Spanish war and political trends inside Spain. He knew the names of all the Loyalist political and military leaders, asking about Modesto, Lister, La Pasionaria, Diaz, Negrin and Del Vayo. In the end he expressed the opinion that Hitler and Mussolini could be expected to step up their shipments of men and supplies to Spain in an attempt to bring the protracted war to a quick decision.

From Spain Mao turned the conversation to China and to the medical needs of the front, asking Bethune's opinions in a manner that suggested they would receive the most careful attention.

It seemed to him, Bethune said, that the best way he could help was by setting up mobile operating units to function close to the front and to take care of the seriously wounded.

Mao thought for a moment, then asked if Bethune had brought any equipment of his own.

Yes. He had brought enough equipment for a mobile unit along the lines he had suggested.

Mao rose and began to pace the floor.

"A mobile operating unit," he mused. "Functioning close to the front.... Yes, that would be good. It would be good for our fighters to know they would receive immediate treatment for their wounds."

During his conversation with Dr. Ma earlier in the day Bethune had learned that the army's medical services, in the Western senses, were practically nonexistent because of lack of equipment, medical supplies and personnel. Now he began to question Mao.

Were there any mobile operating units functioning with the 8th Route Army?

The answer was none.

What happened to the seriously wounded?

Unfortunately, Mao replied, too many died, since there were no facilities for treating them.

"But they can be saved," Bethune declared. It could be done, he held, with mobile units, proper equipment and prompt treatment. Dr. Ma had informed him there wasn't a single case of abdominal perforation in any of the base hospitals. To Bethune that indicated not that there weren't such cases at the front, but that they didn't reach the base hospitals. In short, they died before they got there.

Mao nodded.

"I have seen similar examples in Spain," Bethune continued. "From my experiences there I am positive that seventy-five percent of such cases would recover if operated on immediately. That's why I firmly believe in the need for mobile operating units near the front."

Mao looked up with sharp interest. "Seventy-five percent? Where so few now survive you think seventy-five percent can be saved? That is the correct figure?"

"Yes. Seventy-five percent."

Mao's mind seemed to shut like a trap on the figure. It was as if the whole conversation now turned about this single, central fact. "Then it is clear," he said with decision. "You will organize the mobile operating unit at once."

"Good," Bethune said with satisfaction, pleased that his plan had been approved so quickly. He would write to the China Aid Council in New York immediately, he said, to inform them of the decision and ask them to finance the work. Before leaving America he had been assured a steady flow of funds. He would now propose they send at least $1,000 a month.

With the practical question of Bethune's immediate future work agreed upon, the conversation turned back to Spain, to Bethune's work there, the latest developments in blood transfusion, the problem of introducing Bethune's methods in the technically backward areas of the Chinese interior, the possibilities of storing blood without modern refrigeration facilities, the international situation, China's internal politics, the course of the war against Japan. Mao, particularly intrigued by Bethune's experiment in the storing of blood in cold streams behind the front, explored possibilities of using it in China.

As for China, he went on to explain, the communist program for resistance to the Japanese invasion was not based on desperation or mere defiance. Victory was a practical possibility as well as an indispensable condition for internal progress. It was because the communist program clearly indicated the road to victory and corresponded to the needs and desires of the people that it was so easily grasped and was winning needed support. In the Kuomintang regime in Hankow there were still powerful elements which, because of their vested interests, were more inclined to accommodation with the Japanese than to anti-Japanese collaboration with the communists. But the Chinese people, because of the special development of the social and national liberation struggle under Sun Yat-sen and since, were not a helpless people but an armed people. The people's will to resist was powerful enough to isolate the traitorous groups and to prevent capitulation. Even the deep-rooted anti-communist prejudices of the Kuomintang leadership, and certain unfortunate ambiguities in its policies, could not destroy the people's urgent demand for a united, national prosecution of the war. As far as the military situation was concerned, it too was following a discernible pattern. In terms of modern, equipped armies the Japanese were superior. In terms of the larger complex of factors which would ultimately decide the issue, namely, morale, human resources, conscious political understanding, overall potential, national unity, geography, China was superior. At the moment, and for some time to come, the Japanese might win temporary military victories, but in the end China would defeat the invader. The Japanese strategy required a quick war, the Chinese a long one. The Japanese were unable to win a quick decision; in a long war the Chinese people would emerge victorious.

When the interview was over Bethune was astonished to find it was 2 a.m. They had been talking for three hours without interruption and Mao looked as fresh and alert as when they had started.

As Mao escorted him to the door he assured Bethune of the fullest co-operation of the military command and asked that his thanks be conveyed to Bethune's friends in America. Their support, he told him, was a striking example of solidarity, of friendship with the Chinese people. He added that China's fighters would know how to remember their friends, and someday, how to repay them. He paused, clasping Bethune's hand, and said suddenly, as if he wanted the point established beyond all possibility of doubt: "And the cases to which you referred — the seventy-five percent represents the actual proportion than can be saved?"

"At the very least," Bethune said.

Mao squeezed his hand warmly and the interview was over.

It was almost morning when Bethune finished writing in his diary of his meeting with Mao and the agreement that he set up the first mobile operating unit in China. He had returned to his cave directly after the interview, elated, anxious to record the details of his meeting before they slipped from his mind. He sat on the *k'ang*, his typewriter perched on his knees, a candle burning low on a bench beside him, and concluded his account:

> As I sat in the bare room opposite Mao, listening to his calm comments, I thought back to the Long March, to Mao as he and Chu Teh had led the Communists on the great trek from the south — six thousand miles★ to the loess country of the hills. It was their strategy then that made it possible for their strategy *now* to harass the Japanese by guerilla warfare, to nullify the effects of the invader's superior equipment, and to save China. I now know why Mao impresses everyone who meets him the way he does. The man is a giant! He is one of the great men of our world.

35

Bethune spent three weeks in Yenan. During that time his equipment and supplies arrived from Sian, and a fellow Canadian, Dr. Richard Brown, arrived from Hankow. Dr. Brown was a young Canadian doctor attached to the Methodist Mission Hospital in Hankow. Stirred by the news of the guerrilla fighting in the north he had taken a three-month leave of absence from his

---

★ The official Chinese communist version gives the figure as 8,000 circuitous miles.

mission to help the Border Region. He was a skilled surgeon, spoke Chinese fluently, and he and Bethune took to one another immediately. For the work he envisaged ahead of him, Bethune estimated that he needed at least a dozen skilled medical assistants. He was grateful that he at least had Dr. Brown.

On April 24 they set out for a tour of the hospitals at the front two hundred miles north of Yenan. From there, the 8th Route Army had decided, he would move eastward into the military district known as Chin-Cha-Chi. This was the district which covered big sections (100,000 square miles) of the adjoining provinces of Shansi, Chahar and Hopei, where the partisans held the Japanese at bay and a United Front government functioned as an autonomous unit of the Special Border Region. Dr. Ma had considered going along with Bethune, but he was needed at Yenan, and after some discussion it was decided that he should remain as liaison representative between the unit and Yenan.

The first lap of the trip north was made by truck, with a guard of twelve soldiers, over a hard-surfaced dirt road.

> A few hours out of Yenan [Bethune wrote] the
> road banks upward steeply among the hills. At
> a town called Yen Ping we passed two oil wells.
> Further on, running along the road, we saw
> open seams of high grade anthracite coal. Some
> day, this area, industrialized, will become one of
> the richest spots on earth.

One hundred miles north of Yenan, at Suiteh, the road came to an end and they had to continue on foot, transferring their equipment to pack mules. They trekked one hundred and fifty miles to a hospital at Pan Tung, then to a base hospital in Hu Chia Ch'uan. From Hu Chia Ch'uan he sent his first report to the China Aid Council:

> We are now working in Hu Chia Ch'uan, a little
> village of about fifty houses. We are twenty li (6
> 1/4 miles) west of the Yellow River, and about
> seventy-five miles south of the Great Wall. The

country is wild and mountainous. From Mi Shih — the end of the road for trucks — we came on foot, with thirteen mules carrying out supplies. On our best day we covered twenty-five miles. It took us six days in all, mostly through treeless country, except in the bottom of the valleys where a few willows grow.

There are 175 wounded here, scattered among the houses. This is what is meant by a "hospital" here. It would break your heart to see them — lying on the brick *k'angs* with only a little straw beneath them. Some have no coverlets — none have blankets. This country is so cold at night that we fortunate ones in the Unit are glad to have our feather-filled sleeping bags to sleep in.

The wounded are crawling with lice. They all have only one uniform, and that they have on. It is filthy with the accumulated dirt of nine months' fighting. Their bandages have been washed so often they are now nothing but dirty rags. Three men, one with the loss of both feet through frost-bite gangrene, have no clothes at all to wear. There is only a coverlet for them. Their food is boiled millet — that's all. All are anaemic and underfed. Most of them are slowly dying of sepsis and starvation. Many have tuberculosis.

We must help these people. They have fought for the salvation of China and the liberation of Asia. Can we not raise the money to keep our Unit from being an expense to the hard-pressed 8th Route Army? I have calculated the monthly expenses of our Unit to be $1,250 (Chinese dollars) a month. At the last rate of exchange this would be less than $400 (U.S.A.)

In his diary he wrote:

The military situation is bad. Not in this region but in the rest of China. Here in the north it is believed Hankow will be taken within a month or two at the latest.

I have received a cable from the *Manchester Guardian* of England asking me to supply them with some articles. Wonderful! We can use the money for supplies. I don't know when I'll be able to find time to write articles — it seems I can hardly find time to write my reports to Ma and Mao Tse-tung. But I must find the time!

Early in June they were on the move again to other hospitals in Hsing Hsien and Lan Hsing. At the end of the month their tour was completed. It was now six months since Bethune had left Canada, and he had received no word from the China Aid Council.* He sent another cable of inquiry to New York, wrote a final report to Mao Tse-tung on the hospitals he had visited, and set out for Chin-Cha-Chi.

What was Chin-Cha-Chi? How had it developed? How did it manage to survive behind enemy lines? Who were its people? In a long article Bethune recorded his firsthand impressions:**

Here is a region, in the interior of North China, completely surrounded by the Japanese Army, which holds all the railways and main lines comprising its roughly-shaped 100,000 square miles of territory with its population of 13,000,000 people. It has the first United Front Government in China. Because it is the presage of the future development of China, it becomes the greatest importance that its history and the story of its formation be known.

After the Japanese invasion of northern China and the start of the major Sino-Japanese war on July 7, 1937, eastern Hopei

---

* Unknown to Bethune, most of his cables and letters to the China Aid Council were blocked or delayed in transit through Kuomintang China, and similarly with the Council's communications to him. Thus he was never to know the actual extent to which the Council sent aid to northern China.

** This is an abridgment.

province and Peiping were captured. The enemy drive was to the west and south. They were soon in possession of the principal railways of Hopei, Chahar and later of Shansi provinces. The Provincial troops of these provinces were either defeated or retired. The local provincial and municipal government officials soon followed suit. Their authority disappeared. The principal cities on the Peiping–Ta Tung and the Ta Tung–Tai Yuan lines were in possession of the enemy.

The Japanese were confident. They announced a great victory. Their campaign to capture North China seemed successful. They held most of the major cities, all the railway centres, all the highway centres. Garrisons were placed in all the large towns and they continued their drive south, apparently undefeatable. They openly held the Chinese troops in contempt. They swaggered through the captured Chinese towns.

In the fall of 1937, the Chinese troops in Hopei, Shansi and Chahar were composed of widely scattered and independently acting units to a total strength of approximately 25,000 men. There was no central military command. There were no attempts to organize the villagers, to organize partisan warfare on a large scale.

Then a unit of 8th Route Army troops under General Nieh Yung-chen came into eastern Shansi and western Hopei. General Nieh was one of the communists' most brilliant strategists. He established his headquarters in the great Wutai Mountain range, the massive backbone of what is now Chin-Cha-Chi. He sent out his army commanders and political leaders to mobilize the people into partisan detachments, to operate in the rear of the enemy and on his flanks, to co-ordinate their activities with those of the army.

Soon it was possible to deal the Japanese a disastrous blow. Nieh let the Japanese move south, taking towns and railway centres virtually unopposed. Then suddenly the 8th Route Army and the forces it had gathered together struck the enemy from the rear in the vicinity of Ping Hsin, in Shansi. The Japanese were put to rout. It was a Chinese victory of the greatest importance, the first great victory of the war.

Now General Nieh approached the remaining government officials and asked for their co-operation in establishing a stable government for the region. He suggested that the government be a United Front government based on the common aim of the defeat of the Japanese and the improvement of the people's lives.

A representative committee of five was formed on December 29, 1937, to prepare plans for such a government. This committee decided to summon a conference of all people's organizations and of the military forces of the region. (Shansi, Hopei, and Chahar). This now famous conference met at Fu Ping on January 10, 1938.

Here, for the first time in the history of China, there sat down together government officials, both of the provincial government and the Kuomintang; military leaders of the Central Government troops and the 8th Route Army; delegates of workers, mass organizations, Peasants' Union, unions of women and of youth, and representatives of the Communist Party.

There were 146 delegates in all. It was a true democratic parliament. In the old days a handful of men had decided the future of 13,000,000 people. Now the people decided themselves. The peoples' mass organizations represented between them almost three million members.

The Conference elected a nine-man Administrative Committee to govern the region which was then named Chin-Cha-Chi. This Administrative Committee was in reality a cabinet, with ministers of education, internal affairs, agriculture, industry, etc. Its two military representatives were Generals Nieh and Lu. General Nieh was elected supreme military commander. Of the nine Committee members only Nieh and Lu were communists.

How are the partisans and troops of Chin-Cha-Chi supplied with arms? One of the ironies of this war is that the Chinese are fighting the Japanese mainly with Japanese-captured weapons and supplies. My own outfitting is an example. My fur cap, horse, and boots are Japanese.

There are now between 125,000 and 175,000 soldiers of the various armies, partisans and volunteers to arm, clothe, feed and hospitalize when sick and wounded. The cost of government is probably the lowest in the history of Chinese governments. For example, Sung Chao Wen, Chairman of Chin-Cha-Chi (formerly a high Kuomintang official in Shansi) now receives the sum of $20 a month. The pay of the soldier and partisans is $1 a month. General Nieh's salary is $5 a month.... Kuomintang officials receive salaries ranging from $250 to $500 a month (not including the graft which seems to have become an integral part of so many Kuomintang official's lives). In Chin-Cha-Chi there is no graft!

What is a partisan? He is a worker — in uniform. He is usually a peasant farmer. He is strong, tough, accustomed to hardship and little or no food for long intervals. Exposure to all kinds of weather since childhood has made him indifferent to heat or cold. He has been made aware of the danger to his beloved country spread from mouth to mouth through the villages as yet untouched by Japanese planes or guns or bayonets. He is told how he can help. The causes of the war are explained to him. The causes of all wars are explained to him. He us urged to unite with his fellow workers. He joins a mass organization. He is taught to read and write.

He may join the Volunteer Guards and be given an old rifle or rude spear and sent to patrol the roads, to guard bridges and keep a sharp eye open for suspected traitors.

If he joins the Volunteer Guards he may not leave the district in which he lives. He may even carry on part-time work. Or he may go directly into a partisan detachment where he is given military training, a uniform and arms. His attitude to his uniform is the same as all guerrilla fighters. He wears it when he is ordered to. He takes it off when he is ordered to — and may infiltrate the enemy's lines looking like an innocent farmer. His pay is the same as that of a regular soldier although his role is a different one....

The Japanese now hold twenty-five large towns or cities on the fringes of Chin-Cha-Chi. But the partisans have been successful in preventing them from utilizing the resources of the countryside.

Everywhere in Chin-Cha-Chi the people are taught the *meaning* of their struggle in relation to the rest of China and the rest of the world. At every mass organization meeting, at the regular meetings held by the partisans and the 8th Route Army troops, the overall strategy is explained. Chin-Cha-Chi is today the most decisive battle area in China. If the Japanese are bled to death here it will thwart their plans to conquer all of China.

It should be clear that the mass movements of Chin-Cha-Chi have been organized on broad United Front principles. Thus, the co-operation of local governments and the Kuomintang was always appealed to first, before communist organizers entered a district. The three principles of Sun Yat-sen, abandoned by the Kuomintang since 1927, are the basis of the combined Chin-Cha-Chi Kuomintang-communist program. These three principles of democracy, nationalism and improvement in the peoples' livelihood are now being put into practice. The feudal system is being destroyed. Taxes and rents have been lowered. Illiteracy is being liquidated. No effort is made to confiscate property (except in the cases of puppet generals and traitor landlords), no effort to abolish the capitalistic system. The socialist revolution is not a slogan for the moment, but for the future. First, the communists hold, the common enemy must be defeated and feudalism rooted out....

Now the Japanese have decided on a new tactic. They have brought their separate commands in Shansi, Hopei and Chahar under one North China Expeditionary Force headquarters. Having failed by frontal attacks, and by trying to ape partisan methods, they are organizing a complete encirclement of the Wutai Mountain area, the main base of the 8th Route Army in Chin-Cha-Chi.

The Chin-Cha-Chi Region is isolated from the rest of China. Yet here a great flame of determination to resist the Japanese is burning in the hearts of the people, and with that is emerging the vision of a new democratic Chinese Republic. This Region is the hope and presage of the future China, free at last from the grasp of foreign imperialism and domestic corruption and reaction.

36

Bethune had arrived in Chin-Cha-Chi at the beginning of June. "Now," he wrote in one of the many letters never to reach the outside world,* "I am in the centre of the centre of the war. Now I can truly taste the strange, exalted flavour of this stupendous struggle."

---

* Carbon copies of Bethune's letters were among his papers.

The novelty of being inside Japanese lines, yet in free territory, wore off quickly, however. To meet the enemy at the front one day, to sting him and retreat the next, to vanish into the mountains, to attack him suddenly in the rear, to buzz like a wasp about his supply lines, to govern territory a few miles from his advance posts — that was the special character of the war in the north. It was a quality that exhilarated Bethune. Working 18 hours a day, he gave up shaving and let his beard grow.

For three weeks after the unit's arrival at Wu Tai Shan* he divided his time between the subdistrict's three base hospitals at Hopei Tsun, Ho Hsi Tsun and Sheng Yin Kou.

He made the rounds of the base hospitals, checking on all the staffs, methods of treatment, facilities, supplies. In the evenings, after the work of the day was done, he drafted medical charts, studied his notes, wrote detailed reports for General Nieh and Yenan.

His findings, when he pieced them together in his reports, brought him to a chilling conclusion. In the Western sense, there were no real hospital facilities for the 8th Route Army and the guerrillas. The "base hospitals" had a total of three hundred and fifty beds, but the beds weren't really beds and the hospitals weren't really hospitals. The situation was better than he had found it at Hu Chia Ch'uan, but here too the wounded lay on straw-covered, clay-topped k'angs. There were no hospital clothes for patients, so they remained in their dirty uniforms. The staffs did what they could, but there was no adequately trained personnel among them. There were no anesthetics, apart from what he had brought, no regular operating rooms, none of the regular instruments required for surgery. Bandages were washed after use, hung out to dry, then used again. There was only homemade thread for stitching up wounds. Medical supplies consisted mostly of pills of local manufacture and dubious value. Probes were made of wire. For tweezers and pincers pieces of iron were used. There were no training facilities for doctors or medical attendants of any kind.

To care for the wounded of Chin-Cha-Chi there were available, in the final analysis, only the supplies he had brought with

---

* A subdistrict of Chin-Cha-Chi, in the area of the Wutai mountains in Shansi, where General Nieh then had his headquarters.

him, his own equipment, his own technical skill, Dr. Brown, five locally trained doctors, and the volunteer workers who had little or no training but abundant willingness to serve. Then in mid-July Brown's leave of absence ran out and he was forced to leave.

There was a sad leave-taking, both men too moved to say much. They had trekked through the mountains together, warmed themselves at the same *k'ang*, and worked side by side in the crude operating rooms. As he set out on the return trip to his mission at Hankow Brown pledged to do his utmost to help Bethune with supplies.

To replace Brown as an interpreter, General Nieh now sent Bethune a Chinese magistrate who had gone to a university in the United States. His name was Tung Yuen Chian. He was short, young, plump, good-natured. He smiled easily. He had the natural tact of a diplomat. His English was picturesque, his knowledge of Chinese history and politics immense, his admiration for Bethune soon boundless. Within a week Bethune was calling him "my other self."

The day after Brown's departure he sent an urgent cable for help to the New York China Aid Council via Yenan:

> Working for the past month in Chin-Cha-Chi Military District with partisans in rear of Japanese. Averaging ten operations a day. Desperately need money and medical supplies. Cable one thousand dollars gold Mao Tse-tung immediately as supplies can be bought in large cities.

To Dr. Ma in Yenan, now his main contact with the outside world, he sent a request for his X-ray equipment which had been left behind and the query:

> Do you think the New York people are getting any cables? Perhaps you should forward them to Madame Sun Yat-sen. She may get some action. I need help. Brown has left. I shall miss him. He was a wonderful doctor, and wonderful to talk to.

An Associated Press Correspondent by the name of Haladore Hanson has just come through from Peiping and is going south to interview Chu Teh. I told him about our work and the need for supplies. I have written a long article on this entire area and have given it to Hanson to mail when he reaches Hankow.

Nieh has sent me a wonderful interpreter, Tung by name, whose English is rather picturesque but who is indispensible. I've been picking up some of the language. I never learned a foreign language in my life, but it seems I am catching on to Chinese! Can you send me a Chinese dictionary and papers or magazines?

Haven't seen a newspaper or magazine (American or English) for three months. Have any arrived? What's happening in the world? What's happening in Spain? Have you received any news?

I did eight operations today ... I am tired but enormously content ... I see now that I must institute a medical course here from the ground up. I shall have to do something about blood transfusions. Am using a combination of shouts, tears, and smiles to get things done.

I need an assistant! So much for now. We are travelling a road watered with tears and blood.

A few days later he journeyed to General Nieh's headquarters at Chiao Tang Chang in the Wutai mountains for a conference on medial work in the district.

He had looked forward to the meeting with keen interest. He had heard that Nieh had studied engineering in France, attended military school in Russia in the days when Dr. Sun Yat-sen had kept China closely allied to the Soviet Union, taught at the Kuomintang-communist Whampoa Academy in Canton, and then gone over to the Red Army following Chiang Kai-shek's sudden attack upon the communists in 1927. Now only 40, he was already a key military leader in the war against Japan. At Staff

Headquarters in Chiao Tang Chang, Bethune was astonished to find the General looked like 30, with a smooth, youthful face and the manner of a man for whom a moment's idleness was irksome.

He greeted Bethune with an expression of extreme pleasure. "Other men," he said, "might have given up in the face of the conditions you have met here."

He had a proposal to submit to Bethune, he went on, which he thought should be seriously considered. Contact with the American committee supporting Bethune appeared to be a difficult matter. In the meantime, as Bethune had himself indicated in numerous reports, the medical needs of the resistance forces were growing daily more acute. The Army shared Bethune's view that drastic measures had to be taken. He was therefore suggesting that Bethune officially take over the task of instituting a medical system for the regular and partisan troops for the entire Chin-Cha-Chi area. Any financial aid that arrived from Bethune's friends in America would of course be utilized for his work. Now he would operate, if he agreed, not only as a Canadian-American representative, but as the medical chief of the 8th Route Army in Chin-Cha-Chi and as medical adviser to the Chin-Cha-Chi government.

Bethune had his answer ready before Tung finished translating. "I am honoured and feel proud," he wrote to Dr. Ma. "My title now is: Dr. Norman Bethune, Medical Adviser to the Chin-Cha-Chi Military District."

His first act in his new role was to draft plans for the reorganization of one of the primitive base hospitals as a Model Hospital. All the hospitals in the region, he had concluded, were inadequate for the needs of the army and the partisan detachments. With the equipment he had brought in, and with the crude facilities at hand, he felt it possible to set up a hospital with better wards, better trained personnel, better care for the patients. More than anything else, he reasoned, it would demonstrate *by example* how to use existing facilities to improve the army's medical services.

At the end of July, with General Nieh's enthusiastic approval, he called a conference of medical workers. It was held at Hopei Tsun, under the chairmanship of Dr. Yeh, chief of the Sanitary Service. Bethune outlined his plans, the conference approved them, and then it was decided to launch a Five-Weeks Campaign to bring the Model Hospital into being.

37

For many hours they jogged along the road from Hopei Tsun, growing stiff in the saddle. The distance was 90 li (30 miles), but the road was only a mule path, 10 feet wide. It was deeply rutted, sometimes running between high walls of earth and rock, sometimes over rough mountains.

To the north and south the mountains towered steeply above the village. To the west, behind them, the great Wutai Mountain range rose between Shansi and Hopei, with the Great Wall running along its crest. To the east the valley opened towards still another mountain range with its peaks hidden in the clouds.

Soon they reached the village — a collection of mud huts housing two hundred peasants beside a clear-running, green stream. Though accustomed by now to the sudden departures and arrivals of the foreigner with the beard and white hair, the villagers came out into the dusty street to stand by with their grave and dignified air as Bethune and Tung passed. The hospital was the Buddhist Temple on a rocky elevation just above the village, surrounded by willow and pine trees. As they rode up Bethune could hear the doleful drone of a priest's voice intoning the prayer: "Oh Buddha, I have put my trust in thee." The priests had remained on when the Temple was turned into a hospital — "pious and obese," Bethune described them later in his diary, "like the satirical figures of Anatole France's priests in *Penguin Island.*"

> They always give me a feeling of distaste, with their fat faces, their unctuous manners, and their unnecessary servility,
>
> Three times a day they chanted their prayers, accompanied by bells and gongs. I sniffed the air, knowing from the sweet and pungent smell smothering the scent of flowers, that they were burning joss sticks. As I dismounted the soldier's voices were suddenly raised in a patriotic song:

Mayo Chan,	We have no rifles,
Mayo P'ao.	We have no guns.
Dee leng gei	The enemy gives us
Wo men tsao	All we have....

The priests chanted of their trust in Buddha, the soldiers sang of their trust in other gods. I went to the courtyard, delighted as always to see how richly filled it was with flowers in bloom. Huge pink water-lilies, like fat, slightly breathless dowagers over a solid lunch, hung their heavy heads, as big as footballs, over the edges of black earthenware tubs. Geraniums, roses, blue bells and flox surrounded the ornately painted doorways. Small squares of gauze, washed and hung out to dry, were spread out on the low orange trees like crumpled magnolia blossoms. Some convalescing soldiers sat on the temple steps, their bandaged arms and legs in attitudes of awkward repose. Nurses scuttled about, stepping over the occasional sleeping dog or pig. The golden air was filled with the cooing of doves, the murmur of the stream below, the wind in the trees. Opening on the court were the dark wards, formerly in the priests' quarters and guest rooms.

This was the base hospital in the quiet village of Sheng Yin Kou. Tung had said it was "known on no map." But in Bethune's sketches and memoranda it figured as the site of the Model Hospital he had dreamed of, and in five weeks' time it would become a legendry name that Chinese hospitals would write into the long story of China's struggle for liberation.

The Five-Weeks Campaign began with a staff meeting at which specific goals were set, a propaganda meeting for the villagers at which the aim of the campaign was explained, and a message of approval from Mao Tse-tung.

Mao's message came as a telegram to General Nieh which the General forwarded to Sheng Yin Kou. Tung brought it to Bethune in great excitement. He waved it before the other members of staff and finally translated it, with delighted comments, for Bethune. It said:

> Please give Dr. Bethune $100 every month. Dr. Bethune in report to me states that the (Sheng Yin Kou) hospital needs some money for reconstruction. Please instruct the hospital to act according to this program. Agree that Bethune become medical adviser to army and district. Have complete faith in his opinions and ability. Act according as you see fit for the good of our wounded. Mao Tse-tung.

In his reply to Mao Bethune reported further on his project and brushed aside the suggestion that he be paid for his work.

> Mao Tse-tung
> Military Council
> 8th Route Army,
> Yenan, Shensi

> Replying to your telegram. First, I refuse to accept offered $100 a month. I have no need of money for myself, as all food, clothing, etc., is supplied me. If this money has been sent to me personally from America or Canada, make a special Tobacco Fund out of it for tobacco and cigarettes for the wounded. I will draw from headquarters here, from time to time, what little money I need.
>
> Second: The above-the-ordinary expenses authorized by me in the Base Hospitals are approximately $1,500. This is for materials and labour for the reconstruction of the hospital here as a Model Demonstration Hospital for the Chin-Cha-Chi district.... Approximately $1,000 a month will be needed in the future.

Third: Immediate needs are $5,000 worth of medicines. These may be purchased in Peiping.

Fourth: Please inform me of the sums of money coming in from Canada and the United States so that I may know the financial position.

Fifth: All the above does not include the larger projects for the construction of a permanent hospital, which would cost approximately $50,000. These plans for a permanent hospital will soon be submitted to you. What we are doing is reconstructing with the existing materials at hand.

The campaign proceeded at a whirlwind pace. With the help of the villagers Bethune supervised the construction of an operating theatre that was still primitive by Western standards, but effective. It was, in any event, the first real operating theatre the army could boast of in the entire District. He organized "clean-up squads" to enforce disposal of refuse, food and soiled dressings, and to be responsible for maintaining cleanliness in the wards. He introduced a system of sanitation, extending from fly control to incineration. He designed and had built a sterilizer for instruments and dressings. He drafted specific and regular duties for nurses, attendants and doctors. From among the villagers he recruited a number of workers and taught them how to make leg and arm splints, stretcher racks, identification discs for the patients, special pails for the conservation of food, standardized dressing trays.

He selected a plot of ground outside of the hospital, had it leveled, installed comfortable seats, and transformed it into a Patients' Recreation Park. An annex to the temple that had been a cookhouse he turned into a hall for games, lectures, meetings, reading and writing.

Peasant women volunteered to make up 50 sample sets of hospital uniforms, pillows, coverlets and protective oiled cotton sheets. When they were ready he introduced them into a ward which was first prepared for the new regime by a "bee" of cleaning, whitewashing and sterilizing in which everybody lent a hand. Sheng Yin Kou's patients were the first in Chin-Cha-Chi to wear hospital clothes and lie on sheets.

Under the slogan of "learn while you work" he instituted a program of lectures to provide the staff with a basic medical background that had formerly been available only for a limited number of people at the Yenan medical school. The lectures were held in the court between five and six in the afternoon every second day. While the members of the staff sat cross-legged at his feet, following him with concentrated attention, he stood before a blackboard, lecturing on anatomy, the treatment of wounds, physiology and so on, illustrating swiftly on the blackboard.

Alongside the program of compulsory lectures he founded a school, associated with the hospital, for the training of nurses and doctors. He drew up a complete curriculum for the school to follow when he was gone, and since there were no medical textbooks of any kind in all of Chin-Cha-Chi he wrote his own, simplifying it with numerous illustrations. He wrote it at a furious pace, after the day's work was done, and had Tung translate it into Chinese as he went along. When it was published by the Chin-Cha-Chi government it had the distinction of being the first medical handbook for guerrilla warfare published anywhere in the world. In a report to Mao Tse-tung regarding its publication he pointed out that it would be sent to all medical workers in the District and added laconically:

> If it is successful I will write a further series of
> booklets on public health, preventive medicine,
> etc. I am already at work on a fuller and more
> basic medical textbook of 200 pages. I expect to
> complete it in two months.

In the midst of it all, the race against time, the superhuman labours, the satisfaction of helping, creating, leading, he also discovered that there were still things to be learned.

As part of the regular program of the hospital he had initiated weekly staff conferences, held every Sunday afternoon, at which all the nurses and doctors were present and the problems of the week were discussed. The first few conferences had gone well, with criticisms and suggestions made frankly, and the members of the staff, to his gratification, seriously making notes of the proceedings. Now the time came when he felt a full-dress review of the shortcomings of the staff's work would be received in the proper spirit and would result in the necessary improvements.

The conference readily agreed and Bethune dealt with the work of each in turn. Dr. Yo, for example, received commendation for his encouraging technical ability, but criticism for not pressing his sound judgments sufficiently. Dr. Lin, the chief surgeon under Bethune, had good technical ability, led all the others in training, was always eager to operate, but had to learn to do some of the less spectacular routine work in between. Liu, the political director, was very energetic, competent, reliable and performed his political duties with devotion and intelligence.

As Bethune went down the line, they listened attentively, none objecting to the severest criticisms. Then it was their turn to assess Bethune's work.

They spoke easily, like men accustomed to giving and taking criticism impersonally. They had nothing but the warmest praise for Bethune's work, for his leadership, for his skill, for the energy with which he drove them on constantly to better performance. But when they had finished, and Tung had translated, he turned to Bethune with a puzzled frown. "There is one more thing. They all speak the same critical thought of you. But I cannot remember how it can be expressed in English."

"Is it a criticism, you say?"

"Yes."

"Of my work?"

"No, not of your work."

"'Of me personally?"

"Yes. Something — an expression they use ... *chi hsin*.... But in English I cannot find the right word explaining what they mean."

Bethune soon found it. It was: "Irascible."

That night, in the house set aside for him, he recorded the incident in his diary:

> Irascible was the word. My "other self," Tung,
> couldn't find it, but I had no difficulty. I was "iras-
> cible," they said, when things didn't go the way
> they should; when they did things incorrectly;
> when they were inefficient. I was asked by each
> of them to be kinder (in my tone of voice) when

I found that they did something wrong. I promised. Will I ever learn? I promised — and fifteen
minutes later was being extremely icy to a nurse
because of a crude handling of a dressing....

He asked Tung to remind me of my promise.

I answered: "Yes, I remember. But remind
him also that a life is involved when he is sloppy."

I said it quietly, though, and to the nurse I
added: "It is not up to me to forgive you for a
sloppy dressing, but to the wounded soldier."

The soldier (a bad arm wound — shell
splinter) looked up at him and said gravely: "I
forgive you."

The nurse almost cried. I don't think I shall
ever have to be "irascible" with him again. And I
don't think I shall ever want to be.

38

One day a group of 56 wounded was brought across the
mountains from the north. Supervising their admittance Bethune found that most of them, though seriously injured, could
be expected to do well after surgery. Among them was a soldier
who had arrived unconscious and remained inert on his *k'ang*.
Bethune examined his wounds swiftly, laid his hand against the
cold, clammy forehead, and instructed Tung to summon a meeting a meeting of the entire village immediately.

"Is he dead?" one of the nurses asked.

"No. His wounds are not too serious. But he has lost a lot
of blood."

Fifteen minutes later all the villagers were gathered outside
of the temple court. Two hundred men, women and children
stood silently in the clearing among the pine trees. They moved
closer together when Bethune came out, followed by attendants
bearing the unconscious soldier. Bethune directed the attendants

to lower the soldier before the villagers and studied their dark-hued, open faces.

This was the psychological moment for which he had been waiting. Three weeks ago, in the midst of an operation, a patient had hemorrhaged badly and he called for a blood donor from among the nurses. No one in the operating room had volunteered. He had explained that a blood transfusion was in no way dangerous to the donor, but still they had hung back. Then in a towering rage he had cried that the patient's life depended on whether he could get a blood transfusion in the next few minutes. Were they all afraid? Was there no one who would offer a pint of blood to save a soldier's life? "You —" he addressed one of the nurses, a solidly built young man — "What about you?"

The nurse shifted uneasily and hung his head.

Tung, from behind, plucked his sleeve and whispered in a conciliatory voice: "They fail to understand. Perhaps you could take my blood, and later you could explain to them...."

Bethune glared angrily at the nurses and without another word set up the transfusion equipment and withdrew his own blood. Since he was Universal Group O, there was no necessity for typing of the blood of the patient. While the others watched, shamefaced, he administered the transfusion and completed the operation.

That had been three weeks ago. Since then the patient had mended, and he had time to reflect on the reasons for the nurses' failure to volunteer their blood. All of his assistants were men whose personal bravery was unquestioned. They would pass through the Japanese lines if ordered to do so, engage the enemy in the most dangerous raids, or go into occupied territory at the risk of death. Yet they had been afraid. Not of death, not of injury — but of the *unknown*. The enemy was tangible. He had invaded their land and they were prepared to go up against him regardless of the cost. But they had never seen blood transfused. It was something they didn't understand.

> And what we don't understand [he commented
> in the diary], we fear. They and I and all men.
> More than anything else, it is understanding
> and knowledge that defeats fear. When they

saw how I drew my own blood, with no ill
effects to myself, there was no longer anything
mysterious, anything unknown, *anything to fear.*
Then they saw how the patient was saved, saw
the connection and they were ashamed. And
my rage at them had as little basis as their fear
of giving blood. What was it Mao Tse-tung
had said to the writers and intellectuals of
China? "You can teach the people only when
you become their pupil." How profoundly it
fits.... To be a better teacher one must be a
better pupil.

Now, with a friendly smile, he stood before the villagers, and
when there was silence, he said to Tung: "I would like you to
explain to them that I am going to demonstrate a blood transfusion and to translate what I say as we go along." He walked to
the head of the stretcher bearing the wounded soldier, so that he
faced the crowd, and addressed them directly:

Here is a soldier of the 8th Route Army. Yesterday he was wounded at the front. For a day
and a night our tireless comrades carried him
through the mountains, and while they carried
him, the wounds inflicted on him by the enemy
remained open and bleeding. Look at him. He
lies without moving. He seems like the dead,
does he not? If we leave him like this he will
never open his eyes again.

The villagers pushed forward to look at the still form of the
soldier. Their faces grew furrowed with compassion.

Now if I said to any one of you living here in
Sheng Yin Kou that you could save the life of
this soldier by a simple act, what would you
answer? You would answer — "Yes, I will do
it." And that is exactly what I wish to show
you — that you can bring him back to life. His

eyes are closed, he seems hardly to breathe, and
he is dying. He is dying, not merely because of
his wounds, but because through his wounds
he has lost so much blood. Here in the hospital we can cure his wounds, but he cannot live
long enough for us to cure him without blood.
Without seed in the earth, no millet will grow.
Without blood there is no life in the body.
So we must give him back the blood he has
lost. Then we will be able to cure his wounds.
Then he will be able to fight the enemy again.
How shall we get the blood to replace what
he has lost? By taking it from someone else.
When we take some from a healthy person
they remain well, for the healthy body soon
replaces it by itself.

He signalled to one of the attendants who brought up the
transfusion equipment. He sat down on a stretcher beside the
soldier, saying, "I will show you how easily it is done."

As he spoke a figure moved forward hesitantly from the ranks
of the hospital staff lined up behind him. It was the nurse he had
angrily challenged in the operating room three weeks before.
The nurse moved nervously towards Tung and said to the interpreter across the two stretchers: "I beg that the blood be taken
from me. If Pai Chu En *Tungtze* will permit me, I will be honoured to take his place. It is not long since he gave blood, and I
am young and healthy."

Bethune looked up at the nurse with a pleased laugh. "The
wounded soldier will need more than once transfusion. I will
take a liter from myself and then one from you. But we will have
to get your blood type established first."

Bethune unwound the rubber tubing and held up the needle
at the end. "This is how it is done," he continued. "I sterilize my
arm. Then I push the needle into the vein, like this. The needle
is sharp, but hollow, and through the needle the blood flows into
the tubing and then into the bottle."

As the first red spurt of blood stained the bottle held up in the
sight all the all by the attendant there was a gasp of astonishment

from the villagers. Bethune lay back on the stretcher while the bottle filled to 300cc. Then he swiftly removed the needle from his arm, rolled a piece of gauze deftly with one hand and applied it to the affected area of his arm with adhesive.

He rose and faced the villagers again. "As you can see, I am the same as before. Now we will reverse things; now we let the blood flow into the vein of the soldier." With a sureness that had become a reflex action on the battlefields of Spain he inserted the needle into the soldier's forearm, tapped on it securely, and stepped back holding the bottle high.

The villagers pressed closer, murmuring among themselves, then fell silent. They fixed their eyes on the face of the soldier, hardly daring to breathe. They waited in apprehension for something to happen, without knowing what it would be. A flock of birds flapped overhead and wheeled away. The trees swayed gently in the breeze, audible in the stillness like a bemused sighing.

Slowly the blood receded in the bottle. Everyone seemed to lean forward, to be pleading mutely for something to happen. Then the soldier's lips moved, he grunted, he opened his eyes, he raised his head, he looked about him uncertainly, he smiled.

A great shout rose from the crowd; a shout of joy, relief, awe and victory.

An old woman came forward, her face leathery and lined, her back stooped, her eyes shining. "I am old and useless," she said "I will give my blood."

Bethune pressed her arm affectionately and turned to the crowd. "When more wounded come, then we will need it. Many more will be brought from across the mountains. Will you form a volunteer corps of blood donors? Will you give blood so that our soldiers can fight again?"

The villagers surged towards him. "*Wo men gei!*" they shouted. "Yes, we give!"

It was the first Volunteer Blood Donor Corps to be organized in China. It was followed by similar Volunteer Corps in other villages and towns Bethune visited.

39

Now, in the fourth week of the Five-Weeks Campaign, the goals set by the Hopei Tsun conference had been achieved on schedule. The wards had been cleaned up and reconstructed, the responsibilities of doctors and nurses clearly defined, the new facilities completed and put to use. In the old Buddhist temple, what had last month been little more than a crude first-aid station now fulfilled the standards Bethune had set for the Model Hospital.

In one week it was to be officially dedicated. In the meantime Bethune set out for a quick tour of the casualty stations in the area, operating, lecturing, demonstrating surgical techniques.

On the fifth day, on his swing back to Sheng Yin Kou, the caravan stopped at Shiao Tang Chang, where a message was waiting for him to report to General Nieh at once. Expecting some serious news he was surprised to find the General's room prepared for tea with a charming woman present as hostess. She was the General's wife, passing through on her way to a conference of some women's organizations of Chin-Cha-Chi. They spent a pleasant half-hour conversing via Tung.

When Mrs. Nieh left, the General's manner changed. Suddenly his face became stern and he began speaking quickly to Tung, walking back and forth as he spoke. Tung found it hard to keep up with him trying to translate.

"The first point to be discussed," said Nieh, "is Dr. Bethune's total disregard for his health and his safety."

Bethune started to protest but the General waved him to be silent. "No. No. We have heard all about it," Nieh said firmly. "I have received reports from *every* village, from *every* front you have been at. You don't sleep enough. You don't eat enough. And you seem under the impression that no Japanese bullet or shell can come anywhere near you."

Bethune interrupted to say that the reports were highly exaggerated. "I eat as much as I need. I sleep as much as I need. And I take no unnecessary risks."

Tung now departed from the role of translator to agree with his General. "He does *not* eat enough and he does *not* sleep enough and he does the work of ten men."

"That will not do!" Nieh insisted, making Bethune smile with his vain attempts to simulate anger.

When he saw Bethune smile he changed his tack. "Very well. We won't discuss sleeping and eating. The Army Military Council has instructed me to pay you $100 a month. You've refused a salary. Why? You have personal needs. You *must* have money to look after yourself!"

"I have explained it all in my letter to Comrade Mao," Bethune replied.

"But you must live," Nieh insisted. "It is a practical matter. In the army you live at the barest level."

Bethune regarded Nieh ironically. "General Nieh," he asked, "what is your pay as chief of the Chin-Cha-Chi military staff?" He didn't wait for the answer. "Five dollars a month. And what is the pay of the soldier in the ranks? One dollar a month. Now if we take your pay as a basis we find the following: — you are military chief of the entire district, whereas I am only medical adviser. Then you have a family to look after, whereas I have none. By simple arithmetic, that reduces me to a dollar a month of the soldier in the ranks. In fact, his need is even greater than mine, since in many cases he too has a family."

Nieh shifted in his chair. "Well, as you wish. You are a difficult person to deal with sometimes, Comrade Pai Chu En. But there is a matter of principle. The money has to be paid. Since it is your wish, it will be used as a special fund for the patients in your name."

That night, in the house where he and Tung had been quartered, Bethune rose from his *k'ang*, lit a candle, brought out his typewriter and wrote:

> I am tired, but I don't think I have been so happy
> for a long time. I am content. I am doing what
> I want to do. And see what my riches consist of!
> I have vital work that occupies every moment

of my time. I am needed. More than that — to
satisfy my bourgeois vanity — the need for me
is expressed.

I have no money nor the need for it. I have
the inestimable good fortune to be among and
to work among people to whom communism
is a way of life, not merely a way of talking and
thinking. Their communism is simple and profound, reflex as a knee jerk, unconscious as the
movement of their lungs, automatic as the beating of the heart. They are implacable in their
hate; world-embracing in their love.

The stoic Chinese indeed! Here I have found
comrades who belong to the very hierarchy of
humanity. They have seen cruelty, yet know gen-
tleness; they have tasted bitterness, yet know how
to smile; they have endured vast suffering, yet
know patience, optimism, quiet wisdom. I have
come to love them; I know they love me too.

He lay back on his *k'ang*, thinking of Nieh's solicitude, of the
hospital, of the unexpected way one learned while teaching others. In two days, at Sheng Yin Kou, the Model Hospital would be
officially opened and he would make a speech. It would have to
be a meaningful speech.

They would all be proud of the hospital and the work and
he would have to find some way of summing up what had been
accomplished, what they had all learned, what would still have to
be done, and some of the basic truths without which medicine
was nothing.

40

There was a holiday in Sheng Yin Kou. In the mud huts the
women had braided their long black hair. Over two thousand

people had come from surrounding villages to be present for the great event that was to take place up at the old temple. Dr. Yeh had come from Hopei Tsun to represent the Sanitary Service. A delegation of officers had arrived from Wutaishan to represent the 8th Route Army. Another civilian delegation represented the United Front government of Chin-Cha-Chi.

It was the day of the official opening of the first Model Hospital of the district and the 8th Route Army, marking the successful conclusion of the Five-Weeks Campaign. For the soldiers, medical workers, civilians and government administrators it was a day of gay festivities.

The first ceremonies began in the wards in midafternoon. There were brief speeches for the wounded who were confined to bed, with the hospital staff and speakers moving from one ward to the other. Then the staff trooped through the gaily decorated court onto the level ground before the remodeled hospital. Here the nurses, doctors and orderlies, all dressed in spotlessly white gowns, took their places in rows between the speakers' table, the assembled villagers, and the convalescent patients able to get about.

While the speakers' table was arranged and the guests seated themselves on the ground, there was singing by the soldiers. Then Political Director Liu opened the proceedings. He was short, stout, round-faced, with a smiling, good-natured mouth and intelligent eyes. In simple, proud terms he announced the opening of the Model Hospital. He was followed by representatives of the 8th Route Army, the Chin-Cha-Chi administration, the hospital staff and the mass organizations. Then he rose again, with a backward glance at Bethune, who sat alongside Tung on a bench behind the speakers' table, and said:

> Comrades, soldiers, people of Sheng Yin Kou. Today you have seen for yourselves the new hospital we have set up for our wounded in our Five-Weeks Campaign. It is a great achievement for the Chin-Cha-Chi Military District, for all our people. Now our wounded will have a better chance for recovery. Now less fighters will die at the hands of the enemy.

What made this Model Hospital possible? The fact that all of us worked hard at self–improvement, that the District Government gave us the support, that the people helped us in the big job of rebuilding. But there was one more factor; without that factor we would not have the new hospital. That factor is our comrade doctor, Pai Chu En. It was Pai Chu En from whose head came the plan. It was Pai Chu En who guided us, who drove us on, who showed us how the hospital was necessary and how to achieve it. It was he who taught us, who criticized us, who would never let us rest. He set us a tireless example of his own work.

We wish to thank you, Comrade Pai Chu En, for your work and your heroic devotion to our people. But we have nothing to offer anyone except the things we have in plenty: hardship, sacrifices, the determination to make China free. So we have some gifts that we have made ourselves and that we would now like to present to you. We hope they will show you the love and respect that the soldiers and people of our District have for you.

Liu turned and raised his hand in a signal to the courtyard. As the audience rose to its feet to cheer, a procession of nurses, walking wounded and villagers marched from the court, bearing aloft seven red banners. On each of them was an inscription, lettered in Chinese and English by Tung, and sewn into the fabric in gold thread by the village women.

The procession wound its way, singing, round the audience and on to Bethune. As each group approached him they chanted the inscription on the banner and presented it to him:

Dr. Bethune, our teacher.
Dr. Bethune, our fellow fighter.
Dr. Bethune, our medical adviser.
Dr. Bethune, our doctor.

Dr. Bethune, our friend.
Dr. Bethune, our example.
Dr. Bethune, our comrade.

Villagers, hospital staff and visitors roared their approval as Bethune "came slowly to the speakers' table, his eyes dim, Tung at his side grinning with pleasure. For a long time he kept his head lowered, fixing his gaze on the manuscript before him on the table. Then he looked up, smiling fondly, motioned to the audience to be seated, put on his steel-rimmed glasses, and began to speak, pausing after every few paragraphs to permit Tung to translate:

Comrades: I thank you for the beautiful banners you have given to me and for the kind things you have said about me. I feel, as I know you must feel, that today is an important day in our lives and marks a milestone (I should rather say, a li stone), on the path that our hearts and wills are set upon.

The eyes of millions of freedom-loving Canadians, Americans and Englishmen are turned to the East and are fixed with admiration on China in her glorious struggle against Japanese Imperialism. This hospital has been equipped* by your foreign comrades. I have the honour to have been sent as their representative. Do not consider it strange that people like yourself, 30,000 li away, halfway around the globe, are helping you. You and we are internationalists; we recognize no national boundaries to separate and divide us. Japan and the warmongers threaten the peace of the world. They must be defeated. They are obstructing the great historical, progressive movement for a socially organized human society. Because the workers and sympathetic liberals of Canada, England and America know this they are helping China in the defence of this beautiful and beloved country.

It is not too many months since I arrived in the Chin-Cha-Chi military District to work with you in this hospital. I used to think of it as "your" hospital, now I think of it as "our" hospital. For between us we have created it. We have changed each other,

---

* From the equipment Bethune had brought with him.

have we not? We have reacted each to the other in a dialectical way, I might say; modified each other; and the product of our changed relationship is this fine new hospital, the opening of which we are celebrating today. From you I have learnt many valuable lessons. You have shown me a spirit of selflessness, of working co-operatively, of overcoming vast difficulties, and I thank you for those lessons. In return I may have been able to instruct you a little in the matters of technique.

The road to victory is the mastery of technique and the development of leaders. It was the adoption of Western technique that was responsible, in part, for the transformation of Japan from a tenth-rate backward nation into a great world power in less than fifty years. Technique, in the hands of the Dictators of Finance-Capital, has made Japan the enemy of the world. Must China then copy Japan? Yes, in many ways. We must learn from our enemies; we must imitate them in their mastery of technique and surpass them in that mastery. We must use that technique for the happiness and prosperity of the millions and not for the enrichment of the few.

Now the mastery of technique in the Sanitary Service is the learning and the using of the technique of healing our wounded comrades who have fought for us and for whom we, in return, must fight. And the enemies we fight are death, disease, and deformity. Technique will conquer not all, but most of these enemies.

Technique is the term used, in general, to describe the mastery of materials and processes. It is the most improved, the most efficient way of doing things. It means that instead of being controlled by nature, we control her. So we may talk of the technique of sweeping a floor and the technique of an organization of a hospital; the technique of doing a dressing and of an operation, the technique of washing a patient, of lifting him and of making him comfortable. For each of these and a thousand other procedures, there is a right way and a wrong way. The correct way is called "good technique" and the wrong way "bad technique." We must learn the good technique.

Why must we learn the good technique? Because good technique in medicine and surgery means more quickly-cured patients, less pain, less discomfort, less death, less disease and less deformity. And all these things are our job. We have only one reason to offer, one excuse when our fighting comrades at the front ask us: "What are you doing in the anti-Japanese war?" Our answer is, "We are curing your wounds and healing the sick." They may say, "Are you doing it well?" And we say, "As well as we know how." But that last question we must ponder in our minds....."Are we doing it as well as we might?"

What is the duty of a doctor, of a nurse, of an orderly? There is only one duty. What is that duty? It is the duty to make our patients happy, to help them in their fight back to health and strength. You must consider each one as your own brother or father, for he is, in truth, more than either, he is your comrade. He must come first, in all things. If you do not consider him above yourself, there is no place for you in the Sanitary Service. In fact, there is no place for you in the 8th Route Army at all.

There is an old saying in the English hospitals … "A doctor must have the heart of a lion and the hand of a lady." That means he must be bold and courageous, strong, quick and decisive, yet gentle, kind and considerate. That applies to everyone who is engaged in treating the sick and wounded — doctors, nurses, orderlies. So be constantly thinking of your patients, constantly asking yourself — "Can I do more to help them?" Look for ways of improving your work and mastering your technique.

At first you will need instruction and you will need supervision. So you will need leaders. But you must not get into the habit of being supervised constantly. This is only temporary while you are learning. You must finally be able to supervise your own work. So you orderlies — go to your leaders, the Chief orderly, the doctors, the nurses and say to them, "What will I do next? Tell me what to do. Am I doing this correctly?" When you have finished the work you have been given to do, go to him again and say, "Give me more work." And after a while, he will get very tired of your insistence, and to get rid of you he'll make you a nurse. And, when you're a nurse, go to the doctor of your team, to your leader and say, "Show me how to do this. Am I doing this dressing correctly? Is there a better way to do it? What is the reason for this way? Give me more work to do." Then he in his turn will get very tired of you and your insistence, indeed, and to get rid of you, he'll make you a doctor like himself. And, when you're a doctor, go on in the same way making a great nuisance of yourself, creating a big disturbance with your activities, go around eagerly looking for work. Do the work of two or three other doctors, be constantly studying how to improve your technique, be constantly thinking of the comfort and well-being of your patients. If other doctors go and see their patients once a day, or once every other day, you go two or three times a day to see them. Then after a while, General Nieh will hear about you and he'll make you the Chief doctor of one of the military sub-districts. And there you behave as before, constantly discontented with yourself and your work, constantly thinking and planning to improve the conditions of your patients and constantly imparting instruction to others. Then Comrade Mao Tse-tung will hear about you and will want to make you the chief of the Sanitary System of the whole 8th Road Army. Then there will be a friendly fight between Comrade Nieh and Comrade Mao Tse-tung as to who will have you, for Comrade Nieh won't want to let you leave his division!

Now comrades, we need technique and we need leaders to apply that technique. The ideal is the trained, conscientious technical leader. What are the qualities such a leader must possess? He must possess (1) the ability to organize, (2) the ability to instruct, (3) the ability to supervise. Organization means planning — planning as a whole and planning in detail. Instruction means the communication of that plan to others, the teaching of correct technique; supervision means the constant inspection of the progress of the plan, the correction of faults, the modification of theory by practice. And above all — work, work, work.

The army is hungry for leaders. Every department is looking for leaders. It needs leaders more than it needs rifles and food.

One of the tasks of this hospital is to develop leaders. And when I say leaders, you must not consider I am thinking only of generals, colonels, and chairmen of districts. No, I am thinking of the whole army and the whole district from the big leaders at the so-called top, to the little leaders at the so-called bottom. But there is, in truth, no top and no bottom. That is a false conception. Our organization is not like a house — settled, static, and still. It is like a globe — round, fluid, moving and dynamic. It is held together like a drop of water, by the cohesion and cooperation of its individual parts. So, when I think of leadership, I think, principally, of the "little" leader of small units, and not so much of the big leaders of great units. The development of the "little" leaders is the absolute necessity for the revolutionary reorganization of human society into autonomously acting, socially conscious individuals. When that has been accomplished, leaders (like the State itself) will gradually disappear. So, even though you need leaders now, and will for a long time to come, you must begin to learn not to depend upon (I mean not to get into the habit of leaning heavily on) your leaders. Be a leader yourself, though you only lead yourself, for *every leader starts by first leading himself.*

Those of us who are your leaders now because of our experience, are trying hard to be replaced. We are eager for you to take over our jobs and our responsibilities. Then we will be able to sit back and admire you (yes, with friendly envy) for the way you have excelled us.

We need leaders an especially small leaders, to act as germinating centres to penetrate the whole masses of the people and arouse them to realities and show them the way out of poverty, ignorance and misery. It is the lack of small leaders who make dictators possible, and substitute instead so-called "great men," "great heroes," whom we are asked to admire and worship and to be led by them like sheep.

But to return to our particular work. Doctors — instruct and supervise your junior doctors, nurses and orderlies. Lead them; show them an example of energy; of self-disregard; of consideration. Nurses — instruct your orderlies; lead and supervise them; be diligent and quick; don't talk so much and do more work; do not be so apt to give each other advice when you know no better yourselves. Learn to act independently without the help of a half dozen others. Don't ask others to do things you can do yourself.

In regard to conferences, they are necessary and good, but only good if followed by action. Words were invented by man to describe action. Use them for their original purpose.

Today we have accomplished what we set out to do — the fulfillment of our Five-Weeks Plan of making this hospital the best in the 8th Route Army. I think it is the best in the 8th Army and I have seen most of the others. But we must not stop here. We must plan and work to make this hospital the best in the entire

Chinese National Army of which we are a part. That is the goal we must set ourselves. It will take more than five weeks, I assure you! Can it be done? Yes, I am sure it can. How? By the hard work of every comrade. It must be done cooperatively, by energy, by enthusiasm — apply them to that great task. No work is small, no work is unimportant.

If one fails in his duty, all suffer in consequence — *if* one excels in his work, all gain as a result. Yet, one last word of warning. Let us be on our guard, in spite of our success, against wishful thinking; against self-deception; against the confusion between our desires and our actual accomplishments. Let us be ruthless in our criticism, be cruel to personal vanities, be indifferent to age, rank or experience, if those stand in our way. Let all theories be subjected to the bright clear light of practice. Only in this way will our concepts mirror reality.

Let me conclude. I want to thank all who have made this splendid hospital, of which we are so proud. I thank the carpenters who have worked so hard making the buildings, the alterations, the ward furniture; the iron smith for the Thomas splints. I want to praise the doctors, nurses, and orderlies for their splendid work. Especially is it just to praise the volunteer civilian nurses, many of them old in years, whose loving care for the wounded has been, and is, a daily lesson to all of us, in faithfulness and devotion to duty. The civilians of this village, both men and women have been cooperative and cheerful in accommodating such large numbers of wounded and staff in their houses, often to the great inconvenience of themselves. I want to thank the Management Department and Superintendent's Branch. If I would mention names, I might mention a dozen worthy of praise, but I will mention only two. One is Comrade Liu, our political director, for his tireless activity; and Comrade Tung, my other self, assistant and interpreter, without whose patience, good humour, and intelligence, I would be lost.

[When he came to his own name in translating, Tung blushed, and hesitated in embarrassment. Bethune laughed, threw his arms about the interpreter, and the crowd cheered. Then Bethune continued.]

I cannot close without expression my admiration for the courage and uncomplaining spirit of our wounded, both of the 8th Route Army and the Partisan Departments. For these there is nothing we can do, less than to give them the utmost consideration, care and skill, in return for what they have endured and suffered for us. For they have fought, not only for the China of today, but that emerging, great, free, classless, democratic Chinese Republic of tomorrow, which they, and we, may never live to see. Whether they and we will ever live to see that peaceful and prosperous Republic of workers doesn't matter, the important thing is that both they and we, by our actions now, are making that new Republic possible, are assisting in its birth. But whether it will be born or not, depends on your actions today and tomorrow. It is not inevitable; it is not self-generating. It must be created by the blood and the work of all of us who believe in the future; who can believe in man and his glorious man-made destiny. Only in this way is it inevitable. Let us raise our voices so that those who are lying in the wards and cannot move yet, hear us. Comrades, we salute you! We shall repay your suffering with our loving care. Before the graves of those who have fallen, whom we have been unable to save, let us say: We shall remember the sacrifices of the dead. Our goal is the free China for which they did. In their memory, in devotion to our great sacrifice we shall have one purpose, one thought. Then we will be invincible. Then we will know that even if we do not live to see it, some day those who come after us will gather here, as we do today, to celebrate, not merely for the building of a model hospital, but of a great and democratic republic for the liberated people of China.

"Pai Chu En!" a voice shouted. The crowd replied:
"Pai Chu En our doctor!"
"Pai Chu En our teacher!"
"Pai Chu En our friend!"

41

The opening of the Model Hospital was celebrated throughout Chin-Cha-Chi. At Yenan the news was received as a development of major importance. It spread to the front lines, to the free area, to the fighters operating like night shadows in the rear of the Japanese. And with it went word that the man who led the Five-Weeks Campaign to create it was a foreigner, a "Big Nose"★ who had come to help in the war of liberation.

In the mountains of Shanshi, on the Hopei Plain, in the loess country, in mud huts and caves, a strange, melodious name was passed from mouth to mouth: Pai Chu En, White-Seek-Grace, the doctor who turned dying men into soldiers again. Peasant guerrillas who had never seen a large city spoke with pride of the *dai fu*★★ who had come to them from the outside world. Secret propagandists in the Japanese-held territory used his name as an example of international solidarity growing in support of China. In remote villages where no doctor had ever been seen it was said that some day he would come to make the sick healthy. On high mountain trails marching partisans interspersed their songs with accounts of how he led his caravan to wherever there were wounded. Soldiers he had treated, returning to their units, painted a reverent picture for their comrades of his strong-boned, bearded face, his flashing eyes, his strange speech.

A legend began to grow, fanning out to all the north and northwest. He was a man, it was said, who never grew weary. He would travel to the highest mountain peak to tend casualties. He would leave no man's side till there was nothing more to do. He could do the work of many men without rest. He slept only when there was no work to be done — in the open, in village huts, in caves. His anger, when he was delayed, or when he was irked by inefficiency, could shake those about him like a thunderclap. But his eyes shone with love for the soldiers he treated, and for all the wounded his first words in Chinese were: "My son...."

★ "Big Nose" is the colloquial term by the Chinese to designate a Westerner.
★★ Doctor.

As the legend grew, and guerrilla activity against the Japanese flared fiercely around the perimeter of Chin-Cha-Chi, units on many fronts began forwarding resolutions to Yenan asking that he be sent to their areas.

When word of fresh fighting reached him, Bethune was averaging ten operations a day, preparing the equipment for new medical teams and giving them special daily lectures. For the graduate of the Yenan training school who had arrived to take over direction of the hospital he prepared extensive notes for further improvements. While the others slept he worked on his medical textbook for the special requirements of China. In the realistic surroundings of the operating theatre he taught Tung the art of anesthesia. And in the midst of all this activity he prepared his own mobile unit for action in the Wutai mountains, where new Japanese forces had appeared.

The night before the various units were to leave for their respective posts a final conference was held at which he spoke on their new duties. It was at this conference that he laid down a terse formula that was soon to become the official slogan of the guerrilla medical services. "Our watchword must be: Doctors: Go to the wounded. Don't wait for the wounded to come to you!"

Next day, in the chill dawn, there were quick farewells and the medical teams set out towards the mountains. The last to leave was Bethune's mobile unit — a caravan in which every individual, every animal fitted exactly. At the head of the caravan rode Bethune and Tung. The came Drs. Wang and Yo, whom he had selected as assistants and for special training in the field. Behind them came young Chia, a buxom, cheerful nurse, a cook, two orderlies and two grooms. With them went his portable "operating theatre," transported by two mules, consisting of a collapsible operating table, a full set of surgical instruments, anesthetics, antiseptics, leg and arm splints, sterile gauze, and other necessities.

As the caravan descended from the hospital into the village, the main street was lined with people. It had been known for several weeks that Bethune would be leaving for areas closer to the heavy fighting and the villagers had turned out to bid him farewell. The elders bowed gravely as he rode by; the younger ones shouted patriotic slogans. He went down the street with his arm clenched in the Spanish Loyalist salute, a gesture they had come to now as his special comradely greeting.

Heading out into the valley, towards the shadowed mountainsides, he still heard the shouted farewells. It was a proud and satisfying send-off.

They travelled over high mountains and through long valleys. Sometimes the trails were so steep that it was quicker to walk than to ride. They slept in hollows, shielded from the wind but not from the biting night cold. They lay close together in the darkness, and Bethune marveled at the brilliant stream of stars in the night sky. In the morning, before the sun had risen, they were in the saddle and on the move again.

They skirted the town of Po Lan Chin, where there had been fighting, and came to Ho Ku Tsun, the first-aid station for the 5th and 6th Regiments of the 8th Route Army. In six days they attended to 142 patients and performed 105 operations, an average of just under 20 a day.

Then word came that another Japanese force was moving in from Hopei and was being attacked by 8th Route Army men. Bethune's unit turned east and crossed the mountains into the province of Hopei. This was new territory for Bethune, with new casualty stations, new signs of fighting, new place names: Lung Wan Li, Hsia Lung Wang, Hsia Chia Ho — names he could remember only by consulting his medical logbook, villages where the wounded were distributed in the peasant huts.

As soon as the caravan arrived at one of them, the portable operating table was set up, the surgery cases were operated on, then Bethune and his assistants made the rounds of the wounded in the huts. When that had been done he had the local inhabitants brought together, examined the children, administered to the civilian sick, and inspected local sanitary conditions.

In mid-October he headed to Hung Tsi Tien. Now, according to their advance intelligence, there were only a few miles from the Japanese lines. It was an eerie feeling, on the twisting trails, to know that if the mountain were suddenly whisked away they would be in full sight of the enemy. It was as if they were on one side of a stage curtain, the enemy on the other.

271

As they approached Hung Tsi Tien they saw evidence of the recent Japanese advance and retreat: the occasional dead transport mule, an abandoned cart, a spiked Japanese gun. "They came to steal China," Tung said. "The birds will feast on their eyes."

The West Hopei country continued rocky, mountainous, bare, without a living soul to be seen for great stretches. The silent wilderness was disturbed only by small villages clustered along the banks of half a dozen streams, like buds on a willow branch, each village with a population of 50 to 300 families. The villagers met them with curiosity, then with astonishment as they looked for the first time on the stranger with the white hair, the venerable beard of a sage, the tongue of an outlander. They were all ruddy brown, the men quite tall, sometimes six feet in height, the women shorter but sturdy, with handsome faces, often wearing a single thick silver pin in their black, coiled hair, silver bracelets on their wrists and silver rings on their fingers.

In every village there were short ceremonies, speeches, the bringing of the sick for Bethune to attend. The people's hospitality was boundless, but their lives were meager. There was no rice, tea was a luxury, the staple foods were millet and boiled strips of dough like noodles. By knowledge rooted in experience nothing was eaten or drunk unless it had been cooked or boiled. There was no milk, and in every village Bethune saw mothers feeding youngsters of three and four at the breast.

The only tilled land lay about the villages. The farms were mostly tiny plots on the banks of the streams or nestling on terraces built over the centuries up the sides of deeply gouged, treeless mountains. They rode by thousands of such terraces, like rock-buttressed shelves ranging in area from a few feet to half an acre, each an artificial basin full of precious earth.

They reached Hung Tsi Tien on October 18. When they rode into the town it was still acrid with smoke and the smell of watered ashes. This was the furthest point of advance of a Japanese force that had swooped down from Ping Shan, captured the town, then set it on fire before retreating. The town had not been defended, but after the Japanese had begun their withdrawal to close up their lines of communication, the guerrillas had attacked. Casualties of the fighting were waiting for Bethune in the few houses still left standing.

It was in Hung Tsi Tien, while partisan units were still harrying the Japanese rear guard only an hour's ride away, and Bethune was treating the casualties in an improvised operating room, that delegates calmly arrived for an emergency conference of the *hsien* government.

It was 8 o'clock in the morning when the delegates to the Staff Conference gathered at a warehouse that had been left intact by the Japanese and which had been prepared for the meeting.

Except for soldiers and government officials, the town was almost deserted. On the sidewalk of the long, winding, ruined main street half a dozen merchants were selling oil, cigarettes, meat and vegetables. A barber had set up his chair in the roadway and was already at work. Nearby an old man was raking among the ashes of his house. Laughing little boys, completely naked in spite of the cool morning air, played among the piles of scattered bricks.

Outside the government offices a sentry stood stiffly, his uniform patched and yellow green, on his sleeve the badge of the Chin-Cha-Chi Military District. The sling of his old rifle was a dirty piece of bandage, but the new handles of the four hand grenades stuck in his belt were shiny and new. On his bare feet he wrote Sezuan sandals, with woven cloth rag soles and bright red and green wool tops. Over the great toe of each foot they were decorated with green and red wool tassels.

The sun rose up over the mountains, sending its long slanting rays into the blackened, brick-strewn compounds, and playing on the white cement roofs of the houses still standing. As he walked with Tung to the place of assembly Bethune pondered on the sudden fluidity of life in this distant area where for centuries it had gone on without change. Only two weeks ago the Japanese had been here, the townspeople evacuating before them with complete discipline. The Japanese had struck — but there had been nothing to strike at. Now the Japanese were gone, and in a few days the townspeople would be back again, rebuilding their homes, taking up where they left off, ready to retreat once more should the Japanese break through. Tung had once quoted the communist byword, "We are fish swimming in the great ocean of the Chinese people." In the end the great ocean engulfed the exasperated invader, along with his guns and his carefully devised blueprints for victory.

Across the low tops of the few houses still intact Bethune could see a Buddhist temple on a hill outside the town. It was near enough for him to make out, through the open doors, the blackened corridor and the roofless rooms. A flock of pigeons wheeled through it in a gay aerial ballet. He knew that beyond the burnt-out temple, to the east, the Japanese were a mere 17 li (5½ miles) away. Their cavalry could reach the town in an hour. But between Hung Tsi Tien and the enemy the guerrillas were spread over the hills and hidden in the deep mountain valleys. A few hours earlier the sound of machine guns and artillery had been heard in the town as the enemy tried to flush them out of their positions.

When Bethune entered the warehouse with Tung the twenty delegates were already seated about a long line of polished lacquer tables placed end to end. The air of the warehouse was cool and dank, with the faint odour of burning wood still clinging to the stained walls and high ceiling. A place of honour had been left for him at the head of the tables. The meeting was ready to begin. Bethune looked with interest at the faes of the delegates, most of them young, all of them alert and businesslike.

"*Tungtzemen*."* The chairman called the meeting to order. Bethune discovered that the figure standing beside him was a young woman of about 25, dressed in the faded blue jacket and trousers of a partisan, her face broad and serene, her build stocky.

"*Tungtzemen*," she repeated, "this emergency Staff Conference has been called to put before you the work of the past two weeks for criticism and analysis, and to make plans to deal with the new situation that confronts us. The purpose of this Conference is to find methods of stressing the work of mass organizations and to find a way of helping our troops more effectively in the defence of our district. I will call on Comrade Lui to speak."

Bethune's eyes dwelt on her calm face as she sat down. On behalf of 300 villages, he reflected, she had announced an agenda which consisted of an imposing item: the making of war against

---

* Comrades.

the greatest military machine in the east. And she had outlined it n the matter-of-fact tone of a sorority president discussing next week's tea.

Those who followed her spoke with the same simple seriousness. Peasants with bent shoulders, students with bright eyes, women in traditional garb, soldiers in uniform — they addressed the Conference briefly or at length, discussing the intricate problems of occupation and resistance with the air of people for whom such problems were a part of the daily routine of living.

Praise and criticism were voiced with complete objectivity. Here Yenan's military and political program became a focal point for all sections of the people in the *hsien*. Here, through the representatives of each group, it was tested, applied, and flowed down the masses of peasants, the students, teachers, defence bodies, women's organizations, young people in and out of uniform, public officials, the administrative organs at every level.

The first speaker, Lui, was tall, lean, and seemed about 35 years of age. He was dressed in a long, rough, blue cotton robe. His head was shaved, his face was dark brown and lined, the lips thin, the nose large and straight, the eyes serious and intelligent.

He was the leader of the Peasants' Union in the *hsien*. He represented 30,000 small farmers.

He dealt with practical military developments, *Chian Pi Ching Y'eh*, the policy of civilian evacuation and scorched earth, and some of the weaknesses that had shown up in the peasant bodies and other groups during the recent enemy attack. There was still evidence of a feeling in some quarters that there was no point in resisting the well-equipped enemy with flintlock rifles and rusty swords, he said. "But we might fight," he declared, "with the weapons we have, for we are not likely to get others unless we capture them from the enemy."

The chairman rose again. "For a clear understanding of the tasks before us," she said, "we must consider the enemy's objectives and both his weak and strong points."

She proceeded to give an account of the military situation, the chief feature of which was that the Japanese had transferred tree or four divisions from the Yangtze River front for the attack on the Chin-Cha-Chi district:

Now, let us have a look at some of our strong points in this District. We have more weapons and more troops than ever before. Our men have gained much valuable experience in the fighting of the past two weeks, and as a result our casualties are less. Our chief weapon is the hand grenade. That means close fighting. For that we are fitted: our soldiers are brave to the point of recklessness.

The government has given leadership to the people; it has not retired. As a result, the peoples' faith in the government is strong. This faith is shown by the fact that people now don't retire before enemy attacks until the government orders them to do so. The work of the mass organizations in helping the troops has been excellent and the work of the village militia, the People's Guard, is making the invaders' lives a misery. Now, in one village after the other, the village militia takes up the active defence of their village in cases where a Japanese punitive force is relatively small.

What are our duties now? They are to stress our propaganda among the people; to show them the truth about the war. Our staffs must go to the lower leaders to encourage them and to assist them, in mobilizing the people more extensively to join the fight. We must increase the ranks of our partisans. We must widen the scope of our people's armed resistance.

The next speaker was Political Director Liu, of the 4th Sub-district Military Headquarters, who had worked with Bethune at Sheng Yin Kou. He spoke with the snap of a man whose ideas had been clearly defined in his own mind and who was at ease in communicating them to others. He dealt with a single point: unceasing political education as the basis of increasing the *hsien's* military effectiveness.

Two of the speakers who followed were young girls, dressed like the chairman, their faces broad and sunburnt, their black hair cut short. They gave reports on lessons to be learned from *Chian Ping Ching Y'eh* as carried out to date.

It was now noon and the Conference adjourned for lunch. The delegates trooped into the court in front of the warehouse to seat themselves about a long rough table. From an improvised kitchen the women brought great steaming pots of cabbage soup out of which everybody ate communally, to the accompaniment of shouts and laughter. After the soup there were steamed bread rolls, made from unleavened wheat flour. Then the Conference resumed.

For five hours, without interruption, the delegates studied the *hsien's* financial program, food supply programs, the taxation system, the setting up of more mobile co-operative shops, the cutting of retail prices, the building up of reserves of food among the peasants, improved methods of providing collective leadership in all the villages, the training of more political and military leaders, expansion of secret work in the territory held by the enemy. At six o'clock another recess was called. Dusk was slowly settling over the silent town, bringing with it the night cold. Lighted candles were placed on the table, throwing into somber relief the earnest brown faces, and casting on the walls behind them great, wavering shadows. Through the open door Bethune could see the first pale stars.

Now there was no food, for the meal at noon had taken the full day's ration. Instead of food there was singing, beginning with a low hum that soon swelled into full-throated army songs. After a while somebody called for a song from the chairman. At first she demurred, but finally consented, and without rising sang in a good, clear voice:

> We are an oppressed nation,
> We must resist our oppressors.
> Only by resistance can we win our liberation,
> Only by fighting can we continue to exist.
>
> Answer the enemy's furious attack,
> People of China! Arm yourselves — push forward.
> Drive the Japanese out of our territory.
> Only with our blood will we win peace for our
>   land.

Then the delegates turned to Bethune and demanded a song from their doctor. Tung pushed his elbow, whispering, "Something good from the West."

Bethune rose, smiling, his bearded face patriarchal among the youthful delegates, and said:

> As I sat here today, I thought of the millions all over the world fighting for the liberation of mankind from poverty and ignorance. I remembered how many others, like you, yearn for a life of peace and dignity for themselves and their children. And I especially remembered with pride those strong comrades in Spain, fighting with the same courage as their Chinese brothers, in the same great cause. So I will sing you a song from the war in Spain. It is sung by the German anti-Nazis in the International Brigades. It is the song of the Thaelmann Battalion.

First he repeated the words for Tung to translate, then he sang in his light baritone:

> Spanish heavens spread in their brilliant starlight
> High above our trenches in the plain.
> From the distance, morning comes to greet us,
> Calling us to battle once again.

The words were like familiar companions to these youthful veterans of many battles. Even if the melody, in its simple, measured, nostalgic phrasing, seemed to fall pleasantly on their Oriental ears. As he sang, Bethune wondered how normal and even inevitable it seemed to be: he, the Canadian, singing the words of German antifascists, words conceived in the grit and longing of the front outside Madrid, singing them here, clear across the world, to Chinese workers, peasants, soldiers, teachers in the ruins of Hung Tsi Tien:

> Far off is our land,
> Yet ready we stand.

278

We're fighting and winning for you:
FREEDOM!

We'll not yield a foot to the fascists,
Though the bullets may fall like sleet.
Our comrades, stanch men, stand beside us,
And for us there can be no retreat.

Beat the drums. Ready the bayonets!
Forward march. Victory our reward.
Under our banner smash their columns.
Thaelmann Battalion — ready, forward march!

Far off is our land,
Yet ready we stand.
We're fighting and winning for you:
FREEDOM!

From their songs the delegates turned to their work again. For three more hours the discussion went on, in the candlelight that shimmered in ghostly patterns on the lacquered tables.

It was 9:30 when the Conference ended. The delegates separated with quick goodbyes, for the hour was late by the timetable of resistance. Tomorrow some of them would be back in distant villages, bringing the findings of the Conference to local administrative meetings. Some would be at the front. Some would be stealing across Japanese lines to rejoin peasant units or resume secret work in the enemy's rear.

That night Bethune's diary entry read:

> As Tung and I left the other delegates, the stars were shining through a thousand perforations in the dark curtain of the sky. It was cold and clear, with the amazing dead silence of the Chinese night. On the wall of a burnt-out house the flashlights in our hands lit up a slogan written in great black Chinese characters: "Except

by fighting there is no other road to life." It was
a complete description of the day.

42

During the following ten days the mobile unit travelled 175
miles, scaling one of the highest peaks in the region and setting
up its operating theatre in 13 villages housing wounded. By now
the whole unit was attuned to Bethune's pace: up before dawn,
strenuous marches on foot and in the saddle, immediate inspection and surgery on arrival at a casualty station or base hospital, a
brief pause for sleep, then on to the next stop

In the middle of November they travelled to General Nieh's
headquarters in Wu Tai Shan.

While the others rested Bethune conferred with Nieh about
the future work of the unit. Nieh briefed him on two aspects of
the current situation.

The first aspect was the military position. The Japanese
encirclement campaign was being pressed with increasing
vigour. The campaign was forcing a new test on Chin-Cha-Chi.
Among Kuomintang leaders there was speculation as to whether
the region could hold out. The same question had been in the
mind of Lieutenant Colonel Evans Fordyce Carlson when he
had visited the area some months earlier on behalf of American
Intelligence. The British Foreign Office had also made behind-
the-scenes inquiries as to whether the new Japanese drive could
be defeated. Thus, while little news of the fighting found its way
to the public abroad, the strategic importance of Chin-Cha-Chi
was secretly being recognized in a number of capitals.

Against this military background Nieh went on to the second aspect: the internal position in the country. There had been
disturbing signs, Nieh said, that the National Government of
Chiang Kai-shek was moving away from the basic principles
of the communist-Kuomintang alliance. The Japanese, now that
the main cities and transportation centres had been captured,

were cunningly wooing the National Government with peace proposals. To split the nation, they were holding out the propaganda bait that they intended no further military actions anywhere except against the areas where the communists were active. Now an ominous quiet had descended on all the regular fronts where the Kuomintang forces faced the Japanese. Hankow had fallen and the National Government had moved inland to Chungking. At Chungking, away from the powerful pressure of the students, workers and patriotic organizations of the large coastal cities, it had become apparent that the landlord-industrialist-financier groups in the Kuomintang were pressing for a new policy closer to their private interests. It was known that their aim was twofold: first, to restrict military operations and to negotiate some form of compromise with the Japanese; and second, to take whatever military measures were necessary to bottle up the communist-led forces in the north and the new 4th Route Army in Kiangsi.

It was Nieh's conviction that these elements would not be able to force capitulation to the enemy. The Chiang Kai-shek leadership opposed the outright capitulation which it knew the entire nation would never accept. But behind the scenes it was manoeuvering ambiguously. Contacts between Yenan and Chungking were being whittled down. In Kuomintang territory communists and even moderate liberals were being subjected to repressive actions, and military action against the enemy had been reduced to mere "holding operations" on the regular fronts. Most disturbing of all, Kuomintang troops, which should be fighting the Japanese, were being moved into position against the Shensi-Ninghsia-Kansu District and Chin-Cha-Chi. They were clearly setting up a military cordon against the fighting areas of the north, with all the elements of an outright blockade. Attempts were also being made to hem in and even disarm the 4th Route Army in the south.

In this situation, Nieh declared, a new stage of war was developing. If the present situation continued, then the only serious fighting against the Japanese would be that carried by the 8th Route Army and by the partisans of Chin-Cha-Chi. It would mean that Japan would be able to divert many more of her troops from the south and concentrate them against Chin-Cha-Chi.

The Japanese were pinning their strategy on their superiority in manpower and equipment. The 8th Route Army strategy would be to lure them into the mountains, cut their communication, then fall upon them suddenly from every side. But the fighting would be on a new scale, and there would be more wounded than ever. "And that," Nieh concluded "is where you, Pai *tungtze*, will be of strategic importance. Already the knowledge of your presence has in itself done much for the morale of our troops. I have received requests from many units that you be attached to them…."

From Nieh's headquarters the unit returned to Chang Yu. Here, living in a cave, Bethune launched a nurses' training school, tidied up the local base hospital, and found time to bring his diary up to date:

> Word has come through that Dr. Kisch is on his way here to help me. That's wonderful news. But what does it mean for Spain? How is it over there? The news from Spain has been very bad….
>
> Kisch here! And Ma writes that a Dr. Kotnis* (highly trained) is also on his way from India. Ma warns that the Kuomintang blockade is really tight! Clashes have been reported between Chiang's troops and the 4th Route Army to the south.
>
> Ma says Canton fell to the Japanese without a fight, Hankow after bloody bombardments.
>
> When I go back north to work with General Wang's Brigade, Drs. Yo and Wang will go with me. Our supplies are low. Need knives, artery forceps, surgical scissors, catgut and silk ligatures. If no supplies can come through Chiang's blockade, then we'll have to get them through the Japanese blockade! Only bandages,

---

* A distinguished Indian surgeon sent to China by the Indian National Congress, under the patronage of Jawarharlal Nehru.

cotton and gauze supplies are adequate at present. Antiseptics — low. Also anaesthesia. I have constructed a new form of transport for Field Hospital Equipment to carry all necessary material for an operating room, a dressing room and a drug room. All this equipment, sufficient for 100 operations, 500 dressings, and making up 500 prescriptions can be carried on two mules. This includes collapsible operating table, instruments, arm and leg splints, anaesthesia, antiseptics, sterile gauze, etc. I plan to demonstrate its use everywhere I can. This form of equipment should become universally used by all our medical units.

On the day the mobile unit was to depart for the north, in the direction of Lai Yuan, Bethune came out of his cave to find Tung and Drs. Wang, Yo, Yeh, Hsiao and Lin, the whole senior staff of the Sanitary Service, drawn up in line, waiting for him. They were grinning like schoolboys. When Bethune looked inquiringly at Tung, the interpreter stepped forward and said in formal tones:

The directors of the Sanitary Service have wished to give into your hands a letter for you personally, and have inquired of me to render it in English. They wish you this letter on the occasion of your leaving Chang Yu, and I will now read it that you know the thoughts they have of working with you and your leaving.

He held up the sheaf of papers. While the five doctors nodded approval he read gravely:

Dr. Bethune
Medical Adviser to the
Chin-Cha-Chi Military District

DEAR DR. BETHUNE: At first we should thank you for your hard work on the instruction and supervision of our hospitals. You have not only raised the technical standards of our staffs but also well organized our hospitals and given many valuable plans for the improvements of these hospitals, so that a great number of patients can be cured and recovered, and the fighting forces at the front can be increased. We, all the staff members of the Sanitary Service and hospitals, are very glad and earnest to accept your criticism and suggestions.

But we are sorry to say that we have not taken much care about the entertainment of you. So we earnestly beg your pardon. We should never forget your kindness and direction to us.

Next we should also show our most thankfulness to you for you having given our patients a special fund for tobacco and cigarettes with your own salary of $100 a month. This great kindness shows your great consideration for our patients instead of yourself. Not only the patients lying on the *k'angs* would wish to thank you, but also the staff members would like to show their respect to you. You are really one of the saviors of world peace and an internationalist fighting for the peace and democracy of the world.

Now we have bought with your monies many delicious foods and cigarettes for the patients of our hospitals. At the time to distribute these favorable things we hope you come to see them and give them a speech.

We heard that you will travel to the other sub-districts in order to operate on the patients and raise the technical standards of the doctors and nurses. We quite agree with you. But we hope you are returning soon and giving more instructions and training to the staffs of the Sanitary Service and base hospitals here the next time.

With warmest comradely greetings,
DRS. YEH, YO, HSIAO, LIN, WANG

Bethune was silent as Tung ended and pressed the letter, in English and Chinese copies, into his hand. Then he shook hands slowly with each of the doctors in turn.

"You have all been fine and wonderful comrades," he said. "Sometimes I have spoken harshly, but I am happy that you have worked hard, that you are perfecting yourselves as doctors, that you have prepared yourselves for the important work of caring for our wounded." To Doctors Yeh and Hsiao, who were remaining behind, he added: "I shall look forward to being with you again."

"We wish the best for your health," they said, bowing.

"I wish the best for your health," Bethune replied. "And may the wounded fare well under your care...."

43

From Chang Yu they travelled across a long plain towards the distant yellow mountains. In the fields the stubble left from the summer's harvesting was wilted and grey. The frozen road was brittle beneath the horses' hoofs. Following in the rear, Bethune's sprightly young orderly, Shou Yi Ping, amused himself by throwing stones at some passing gulls and sang popular songs:

I look up at the skies ...
An enchantment for my eyes ...

We are all good shots and free ...
Every bullet lays low an enemy....

With the ascent of the first mountain at the end of the plain the air grew colder, the trails more treacherous. Across the crest they descended to another plain.

For five days they continued northward, moving over the endless valleys and mountains. In the valleys the clattering of the horses' hoofs ricocheted from perpendicular cliffs. On the mountainsides they struggled upward on foot, the wind whistling fiercely about them and drying the sweat on their necks. On the peaks their breaths turned to vapour. In the narrow passes, glittering icicles hung over their heads, like poised and deadly weapons.

By the third day they were advancing through blizzards, with the plains lost in a thick white pall and the mountaintops covered by heavy clouds. The snow piled up on Bethune's Japanese fur cap, obliterated the trails, and turned to steam on the dripping flanks of the animals. To keep warm they stamped along on foot, keeping a close grip on the horses' reins. The temperature had dropped 20 degrees since Chang Yu. This was the first cold blast of the dreaded Shansi mountain winter.

At Fu Ping, the town where Tung had formerly been *h'sien* magistrate, they rested overnight, warming themselves on the hot *k'angs* of the townspeople. Then they pushed on again, struggling against the wind, the cold, the sudden snowdrifts. They reached the first casualty station on the evening of November 11, after a final ten-hour march without food or rest. It was the medical post of the 359th Brigade at Ho Chien Tsun.

Their arrival, thanks to the efficient wireless communications systems in the free region, was expected. At the office of the local Health Bureau they were welcomed by the director, Dr. Koo Cheng-chun, and the medical office, Dr. Fong, a tall young man with a long face and a strong peasant body.

They exchanged greetings, removed their damp coats, stamped about on their numbed feet, accepted hot, unsweetened tea, then Bethune asked, "Where are the infirmaries?"

"Food is being prepared," Fong said solicitously. "After you have eaten and rested from your trip we will take you to the infirmaries if you wish to see them tonight."

"I not only wish to see them tonight — I wish to see them now. How long will it be before the food is ready?"

"Oh, it will not be more than twenty minutes," Fong said.

"Then I suggest we go along right now," Bethune said, getting into his greatcoat.

Fong looked apprehensively at Director Koo, then at Tung. When Tung inclined his head silently at Bethune and grimaced in warning, Fong suggested nervously: "But you have had a long trip over the mountains. You have had no food since early morning...."

"Yes," Koo interjected. "It will be good to have some food and rest."

Bethune buttoned his coat. "We have had a long trip, but so have the wounded."

They followed him silently into the night.

The infirmary was in a small temple just outside the town. It was like many another primitive hospital Bethune had seen further south. In a cramped ward some 30 soldiers lay on *k'angs* stretching along the wall. He began immediately at the first *k'ang*, examining the patient swiftly, then moving on to the next. As he completed his examinations he asked questions of Fong, who gave instructions to his assistants, noted those who would need surgery, worked on dressings for the others. Towards the end of the line he was looking at a leg wound when he straightened suddenly. "Who is responsible for this case?"

Fong stepped forward hesitantly. "I am."

Bethune turned, "Prepare this man for surgery at once.... And I shall have something to say to you later."

He completed his examination of the other patients, then strode angrily to the adjoining room where the young soldier had been laid out on a stone table. This was the operating room. White curtains had been strung around the walls, a white sheet covered the ceiling, a buzzing gas lantern hung overhead. Beside the operating table was a stand on which the instruments and antiseptics had been placed. Bethune washed up quickly, and removed the bandage from the soldier's leg as Tung took his place at the head of the table and Dr. Yo stood beside him. The bandage, stiff with pus and blood, was stuck fast to the torn muscles. When it came off a fetid odour filled the room.

Bethune turned to Fong. "You are responsible for this patient?" he spoke coldly once more.

"Yes...."

"You must be punished. You are responsible for the fact that he will lose his leg. Look how the bone sticks out of the flesh like a dog's fang! How could you permit the wound to get into such a state? How is it you failed to use splints?" There was silence in the room. Fong fell back before Bethune's

287

accusations as if he had been whipped. This was Pai Chu En who was castigating him before his comrades; the idol of the army whose arrival he had been waiting with enthusiasm. His simple, honest face twitched with shame. He tried to speak but the words died in his throat. He cast an appealing look at Koo.

The Director shifted uncomfortably. "Perhaps," he began in a placating voice, "it is not so much the negligence of Comrade Fong ..."

"No?" Bethune turned to him icily. "If this isn't negligence, then what is it? Does Dr. Fong know some method of saving the patient's leg at this point? Will he perhaps be able to replace it? It is not only negligence — it is complete disregard for the patient's welfare."

"But there are only ten splints for the whole front hospital and they are all in use. There was no splint for Comrade Fong to use on the patient."

"No splints!" Bethune was choking with rage. "Is that an excuse? Are we to wait till splints are available? Tell me, comrade Koo, do our soldiers always have weapons? Do they stop fighting when they have no weapons? Do they say, 'Well, we will stop the war till we have weapons?' Or do they go out and get them from the enemy? If there were no splints, then it was Dr. Fong's duty to see that some were made, even if he had to make them himself. That is how a true doctor works. That's how we did it at Sheng Yin Kou. I don't understand how we can call ourselves doctors and be so casual about our wounded."

Fong hung his head, Koo remained silent, the others were paralyzed by confusion — all except Tung. From the head of the table where he had been administering anesthetic, he spoke quietly, as if nothing had happened. "Pai *dai fu*, the patient is sleeping ready...."

Bethune turned back to the operating table. For a moment he looked down at the exposed, gangrenous leg of the soldier. Then he began abruptly to explain the operation, his voice no longer harsh with accusation but low and emphatic. Why was amputation indicated? He answered with a description of gangrene, pointed out the shattered, protruding state of the bone, discussed the importance of selecting a suitable site for the amputation, ticked off the muscles, nerves, arteries, bone formation that would have to be severed, sketched the methods of stanching the flow of blood during and after the operation.

The only sounds in the room were his voice, the higher lilt of Tung's translation, the buzzing of the gas lamp overhead. While he talked he began the incision, Wang and Yo moving into their accustomed places on both sides of the table, Fong, Koo, Chia and the other nurses relaxing.

Bethune stopped suddenly, a perplexed look on his face as he held up the tool in his hand. "This," he said, turning to Fong, "is nothing but an ordinary wood saw! *This is for cutting lumber, not human bone!* Do you expect me to amputate with it?"

Fong stuttered: "It … it … is the only saw we have ever had…."

Bethune threw the saw away with distaste. "Dr. Yo, we must get our on set of instruments. Wait, how long would it take? No, it's too late. The mules haven't even been unpacked. There's no time." He picked up the saw again while the others watched apprehensively, twanged it in his hands, cursed, then disinfected it hurriedly and returned to the operating table.

Now he worked with clenched teeth, his lips pressed back above his beard as the saw rasped sickeningly through the bone….

It was midnight when the operation was completed. Doctors and nurses stood in a silent group about the patient. Bethune finished bandaging the raw stump, then turned again to Dr. Fong. "We spend years, working, studying … so that when the time comes we can save a leg, a life … But what if we haven't worked and studied properly? What if we are negligent? Then somebody *pays* with a leg, a life … Tell me, Dr. Fong — what university did you graduate from?"

Fong mumbled something and walked out of the room with downcast eyes.

In the silence that followed Dr. Yo, who only spoke on rare occasions, said placatingly: "The necessity to amputate was most unfortunate. But the poor material conditions we are facing at present … Perhaps since there were not enough splints …"

"Perhaps! Not enough splints! Of what have we enough? When *will* we have enough? No, it was inexcusable. Such cases must be reported to General Nieh. If one of our soldiers should throw away his gun, he would be punished. And if one of our doctors loses the leg of a soldier without reason, then he must be punished too. A gun is something we can replace — but a limb — that we can't replace." Bethune turned away with a gesture to indicate the matter was closed. He made a final check of the patient, issued instructions that a nurse remain constantly at his side, washed up, then glanced briefly at his wrist watch and said to Koo, as if resuming some unfinished business: "What about the other patients?"

At Koo's surprised look he repeated: "The other patients. Isn't there another infirmary? In the telegram asking me to come here it was clearly stated — 'many wounded are waiting.' Here there are only 30. Where are the others?"

"There are others," Koo quickly explained. "But they are at Chu Hui Tse. Our hospital is divided into two sections. This is the rear section — the other is at Chu Hui Tse, further north near the front. The more serious cases are kept there. It was our plan that you inspect the section here, then we could arrange to take you to Chu Hui Tse. We were thinking of your long trip — your expected need for rest.... It is difficult travelling from here...." Koo floundered uncomfortably, as if trying to ward off another outburst.

"It is too many hours' travel," he said earnestly to Tung, whispering so that Bethune missed what he was saying. "Can you not explain? I beg you to cool the fire in the eminent one. He is weary with travel and operating. There will be heavy criticism if we drag him about irresponsibly."

"What was that?" Bethune demanded.

"*Tungtze*," Tung said soothingly. "It is many li to the other section of the hospital. The night is too late now to leave. They must be thinking of preparations for this trip too. Now while we wait we can enjoy some rest. They are thinking of your comfort for the sake of the wounded. And if now we are leaving how will you be efficiently operating the patients?"

Bethune looked at his watch again, wavering. "Well, it's too late to change anything. Can we be ready at 4:30 this morning?" It was more a command than a question. He waited till Koo nodded. "Then it's settled. We'll leave at 4:30 a.m. Dr. Yo — we shall take our full operating equipment with us."

"Perhaps now," Koo queried weakly, "Pai Chu En *tungtze* and all of the *tungtzemen* will honour us by accepting the food that has been prepared?"

They went out into the darkness. They crunched over the snow into the silent village, bending forward against the mountain wind that swept through the street. As Bethune went into the building of the Sanitary Service Koo held Tung back a moment.

"Does he mean seriously that we are to leave at 4:30 in the morning? He will have only two hours' sleep. Does he like only to talk about time, like foreigners do?"

"He is most serious," Tung replied with a smile. "The wounded are to him like iron to a magnet."

Koo looked up at the starless sky, shivering a little in the cold. "He must be like iron himself — white with heat."

They went in hurriedly to the long-delayed dinner.

At 4:00 a.m. Bethune was in the infirmary, examining Shiao, the boy whose leg he had amputated, in the feeble light of an oil lamp beside the soldier's bed. "How do you feel?" he asked in Chinese.

"All right."

"Does it hurt?"

"No."

Bethune put his hand on the soldier's clammy forehead and looked at the strained eyes, the haggard features, the tight lips, the beads of perspiration, like cold dew left by a pain-wracked night. "No, *wo di er*. I know it must hurt now, my son. But you are a brave lad." Tung came quietly into the ward, joining him, and he continued in English: "I am very pleased that you are doing well. For a while the pain will be a part of recovery. I am going to Chu Hui Tse for a few days, but they will look after you, and I shall be back to see you again." To the nurse he said: "Watch over him as if he is your brother...."

At 4:25 Bethune and Tung, mounted, were waiting outside the temple-hospital beneath the statue of a fat Buddha. In a few minutes they were joined by Wang, Yo, Chia, the other attendants and the pack animals. Promptly on the half-hour Koo came hurrying from the village, panting, his face drawn. He climbed heavily onto his waiting horse and whispered to Tung: "May I never spend such a night again. I have never been so fearful that I would fail to awaken in time that I have been walking about my room since I left you, burning the lamp beside my watch to show

291

the time. How does the doctor sleep and rise like a machine?"

They were deep in the mountains when the shadows paled and the first rays of the sun glittered on the snow. Bethune, riding ahead with Tung, shifted his eyes from the trail to his companion's impassive face. "*Tungtze*," he said, "you have said nothing since we started out. You are my other self, you know, and when you are silent it means I am wrapped in silence too."

Tung glanced over his shoulder at the others, strung out several hundred yards behind, and slowed his horse to a walk. "I have been silently giving my thoughts to Fong, *dai fu*."

Bethune cast a swift look at Tung. He knew every expression on his companion's broad and cheerful face. He divined from the innocent look it now wore that Tung had been carefully preparing some method of broaching a delicate subject with his usual diplomatic indirection. "It's a waste of time," he said shortly. "The man's inadequate — he's no doctor. And unable to stand up to criticism, in the bargain."

"Well, that is the matter, of course. That is the reason he has put such sorrow in my thoughts."

"What *matter*?"

"Why, the matter that he is no doctor, that — "

"No, I don't mean that," Bethune interjected. "I mean he is *no good* as a doctor. Hasn't the right approach."

"But he *is* no doctor, ever," Tung continued blandly.

"What sort of nonsense is that?" Bethune was impatient now. "He is a surgeon at Ho Chien Tsun casualty station. And any man fresh out of a university would have handled that leg wound better than he did."

Tung nodded. They tracked on through the snow for a while, then he resumed casually: "Poor Fong. He would have known more well also if some time he had participated in study in a university. He is never in his lifetime a doctor by study. He has learned only through watching and other's mouths. He has operated the wounded only by practice."

Bethune reined in his horse, seized the bit of the other horse, and pulled Tung closer. "How can it be that he never studied to be a doctor? Tung, I can see by your innocent face that you're working me round to something. What's all this nonsense? Are you trying to save him from being punished?

Didn't you see the result of the man's criminal negligence with your own eyes? Would you excuse a thing like that?"

"*Tungtze*," Tung said smoothly, "last night, when you were deeply asleep, I was sitting with Fong for a long time. He gave me a sorrowful picture of his life from his earliest days. That is why all morning I have been wordless. May I direct to you, *tungtze*, the story of Dr. Fong?"

Bethune released Tung's horse and made a wry mouth. They rode their horses at a walk, stirrup to stirrup, while Tung spoke.

"Fong was born in a small village. His family was poor. In the village there was no school, so there was no way for him to learn to read and write. When still in childhood he learned to do the watching of water buffaloes. All his childhood he looked after water buffaloes in the fields. Never did he know the sight of a book. Then one day a detachment of the 8th Route Army was passing in the village. They gave plays to the village and talks about the war, about the happenings in the country. Fong joined with the Army. He taught himself to read and write by asking questions of the others. First he was a guard. When he learned reading and writing he became a nurse. Then a head nurse. Then he began coming to doctors to write out for him the Latin names of medicine in Chinese characters. Some soldiers thought he was making a joke, but he studied the foreign words alone at night ... till he knew them by memory. Then watching the doctors in the operating room he became a surgeon by experience. Now, when we have come to Ho Chien Tsun he has been studying some English words like the Latin medical names so he could better learn from you, Pai Chu En."

Tung finished and folded his hands over the reins on the pommel of his saddle, as if he had been telling an anecdote that no longer interested him.

Bethune eyed him in astonishment. Was it possible? In an unknown village a buffalo tender had caught a breath of the world outside his village. He had been swept up by an army that fought at the front and taught in the rear. By an act of sheer self-discipline he had made himself a surgeon, because war meant wounds, and healed soldiers meant victorious resistance, and in resistance Fong the illiterate became Fong *dai fu*, the doctor, the eminent one, the master of life and learning.

Bethune cursed himself inwardly. Why hadn't he known? Why

hadn't he suspected when Fong said nothing to the question? And how many others were like Fong! Shiao, the partisan who lost his leg and refused to admit pain. The woman chairman of Ping Shan, the *hsien tzu shi*, who shrugged aside a thousand years of servility to lead a country government. The nurse of Sheng Yin Kou, who conquered fear worse than death to give his blood. The young students, trekking without food from the occupied cities to the university at Yenan, stealing through enemy lines, sowing the wisdom of their books from village to village. His own Tung, the educated magistrate, esteemed with civic honours yet going cheerfully into the wilderness beside him. The men and women of a thousand villages, who burned their homes before the advancing enemy, who retreated with a few packs on their backs, joined the guerillas and returned with guns in their hands. Out of the shadows they were rising, the silent, persistent Fongs, the five hundred million, stirred by a giant passion, a hunger as deep as Fong's to learn, to live, to inherit the soil of their own withheld land. And he, Bethune thought, had humiliated one of these! He, who only a few weeks ago had entered the profound Chinese proverb in his diary: "You can teach the people only when you become their pupil!" he had tried to instill the meaning of Mao's words into his address at Sheng Yin Kou. He had thought he understood them. But the road to wisdom had no end. There was always more to understand, to learn, to teach, to live....

He was roused from his reflections by Tug, who suddenly stopped ahead of him and called back: "It is Chu Hui Tse in the valley below."

They had come out of the pass onto a long incline slop-ing down to a glittering plain. In the centre of the plan, dirty brown against the snow-covered fields, stood the collection of compounds that housed the advance casualty station. They dis-mounted, stretched their legs and waited for the others to catch up with them.

Looking down at the village Bethune said: "I am glad you told me about Fong." And then, while Tung eyed him sideways: "You know, in the West, in many books written about China it's always stressed that the Chinese consider a matter of honour never to 'lose face.' Is it still like that among many Chinese? I haven't noticed much of it here in the free regions."

Tung smiled. "Still some people are most sensitive not to lose face. But many things change in China. As you have witnessed, in the 8th Route Army and the organizations in the border regions we teach self-criticism. 'Face' is for the landlords and the rich ones. In fighting there is no time to worry about it." He added with a mischievous note: "Of course, it is everywhere known that you, *dai fu*, give nobody chances to *keep* or *lose* face."

Bethune laughed and put his arm about Tung. "When we get back to Ho Chien Tsun, *tungtze*, I shall go to Fong and I shall see that I 'lose all my face' to him!"

Late the next day they were back at Ho Chien Tsun, making the return trip over the trails still freshly churned by their horses' hoofs. Bethune led Tung into the village at a gallop, far ahead of the rest of the caravan. With Tung still in tow he went directly to Fong's room in the house of one of the villagers.

Fong was lying in the *k'ang* in the evening gloom. "*Haow bu haouw*," he greeted them quickly, rising quickly and lighting an oil lamp.

Bethune sat down beside Fong on the *k'ang*. "Fong *tungtze*," he began without ceremony. "Yesterday Tung told me something of how you became a surgeon."

Fong looked quickly from Bethune to Tung and lowered his eyes.

"It isn't an easy thing, is it — becoming a good surgeon?" Bethune continued evenly. "Now that I know some of the things that happened to you I'd like to tell you a few of the things that happened to me. You know, I was much older than you when I began to practise as a doctor. And as a doctor I suffered from two very difficult diseases."

Fong looked up curiously. He expected that Bethune's arrival meant the beginning of an official inquiry into his work. But Bethune's opening words didn't seem to fit.

"I was only beginning to make my way as a surgeon when I came down with a bad case of tuberculosis. That was — yes, twelve years ago, when many things were still new or unknown in the surgery of tuberculosis. There seemed no possible cure for me. I buried myself in a sanatorium, expecting to die. As it happens, I managed to get myself cured. That's when I decided to become a thoracic surgeon.... For years I have lived with only one thing, but I studied, I did research, I worked under one of the world's great masters in my own country. And in the end I defeated the disease and became a thoracic surgeon."

Bethune paused and lit a cigarette. In the long silence that followed Fong sat still, then raised his head to look at Pai Chu En. He saw an enigmatic smile on the latter's face, a look that prompted him to smile nervously himself. "And your second sickness?" he asked at last, hesitantly.

"My second ... 'sickness' ... well, that wasn't so simple. I caught it from no one — and I caught it from everything. I got it as a boy, as a man, as a doctor. It was much worse than tuberculosis. It was — *my temper* — It wasn't like curing an infection. I couldn't get rid of it with drugs. And many of the things I saw as a doctor made it worse.... Just as I once gave in to tuberculosis, so I once gave in to my temper. But there came a time when I no longer gave in to it. That was after I came to understand that tuberculosis was not merely a disease of the body but a social crime — when I saw in my own country how some were rich and many were poor, when I went to Spain, where the people are fighting like the people in China. I saw men dying because they wanted to live. And now I have been in China over nine months.... I have learned what must be done to cure this second sickness.... But sometimes it breaks out again, and I have to fight with it to keep it under control. Now, it doesn't happen often, but it happened the other night. Do you understand, *tungtze?*"

"Yes," Fong answered softly.

Bethune jumped up briskly. "Well, we are leaving early in the morning and there will be many things to be done before we get to bed. To be a good surgeon, you will have to work hard and face many disappointments, *tungtze*. I would be cheating you if I didn't warn you frankly. You will have to make up for all the things you have missed. You will have to study, to learn — just as our boys have to learn to fight the enemy. I shall ask Dr. Koo to have you assigned to my unit in the near future. You can work under me. I will help you to study. We can use another doctor. And it will give you an opportunity to round out your experience."

"I would be very happy," Fong said, rising. He followed Bethune and Tung to the door, opened his mouth to speak again, thought better of it, then blurted: "Pai Chu En *dai fu* ... I recognize my responsibility in the case of soldier Shiao. I have had to learn everything myself.... It is only a few years since the army helped me to a knowledge of reading and writing. If I can come with you someday I promise to work seriously ... I have a son ... perhaps someday when he grows up the sons of peasants will be able to go to school. I shall do everything to give him the opportunity to study that I have not had. Perhaps he will be a fine doctor to make up for me...."

"Make a fine surgeon of *yourself, tungtze* — that will be the best example for him to follow."

Fong's eyes glowed in his solemn face. "I shall teach him to follow a better example," he said. "The example of our Pai Chu En."

44

The lines of wounded moving back from the front grew longer and the Mobile Unit pushed doggedly through the mountains to meet the increased flow of casualties.

On November 22 Bethune and his caravan reached the village of Chuan Lin Ko, north of Lai Yuan, where General Wang Chen, commander of the 359th Brigade, had established headquarters. Here Bethune was to lose his temper again, but this time without apology.

For three days and three nights the wounded were carried from the front to Chuan Lin Ko. Fighting had been heavy, and there had been heavy casualties. Bethune was ready with his operating theatre when the first 35 casualties were brought in. No sooner had be begun his examinations than his face turned white with anger.

He summoned the litter-bearers, lined them up in the mud building where he had set up his operating theatre, and addressed them angrily:"These wounded have been on their way here from the front for three days. Not a single one of them has received any attention since his wounds were dressed by the regimental doctors. Why? Why is it not a single bandage has been changed? Do you think your job is merely to carry the casualties as it they were so much baggage? You are medical workers, not mules!"

The field men quailed before Bethune's furious look. "From Lai Yuan to this village," one of them attempted to explain feebly, "there are no rest stations ... no first aid units. We could do nothing...."

"That is no excuse! If there are no rest stations, improvise them somewhere. If you have no bandage, use the shirt off your back." Bethune turned to Tung. "I want a messenger sent to General Wang at once. As medical adviser to the Chin-Cha-Chi Military District I am officially requesting that he come here in person to investigate the condition in which the wounded are arriving from the front."

General Wang arrived at the base hospital the next day, in response to Bethune's message, while Bethune was at work in the operating room. He waited till the soldier Bethune had been operating on was taken away, and went in.

"I am Commander Wang," he said. "*Chu yang*, Pai Chu En *dai fu*," I have looked up to your name for a long time."

"I have looked up to *your* name, General Wang," Bethune said. "General Nieh tells me you are one of the bravest and most courageous of his generals. Your Brigade's fighting ability is beyond criticism, but its handling of the wounded is deplorable and impermissible."

Bethune then led Wang through the houses where the wounded were quartered, recounting the manner in which they had been transported without attention for three days. He pointed out infections that could have been avoided, simple wounds that had been neglected, two cases of gangrene resulting from tourniquets that had been left untended.

General Wang listened gravely, then said firmly: "Your criticisms have an edge like a sharp dagger, *dai fu*. But they are justified. We lack equipment and trained people for our medical work, but you have convinced me there must be immediate improvement. I accept personal responsibility to see that every one of your suggestions is carried out. I shall remain here with you till all the wounded are attended. Then we shall decide on the steps to be taken immediately."

For 24 hours General Wang remained in the operating room with Bethune and the others. He watched while Bethune operated. When the morning light filtered in the through the paper-covered window the air in the room was heavy with the smell of blood, sweat, suppurating wounds. With two staggered intervals for food and a five-minute rest the operating continued all through the day. Late in the evening, when the last surgery had been completed, they went outside for a breath of cold air, then returned for a conference on improvements in care of the wounded in the area.

The discussion was brief and incisive. Between the front and the rear a series of first-aid stations would be set up in the villages. In these there would be personnel and equipment to give the wounded provisional attention while they were being transported to the rear.

"The use of the mobile unit directly at the front," Bethune emphasized, "is the most important change we can introduce. I am convinced that it will cut our fatalities drastically."

"Agreed," Wang said. "In one week we are springing a new trap on the enemy. Can you be ready to go into action with us?"

"Give me one day's notice, and we'll be there," Bethune replied. "We are leaving in the morning for the base hospital at Yang Shia Chang, ten miles from here. We will wait there for word from you."

Wang seized Bethune's hand and shook it twice — once up and once down. "We shall be together next week, *dai fu*," he said.

On the night of November 27 a courier arrived at Yang Shia Chang from General Wang's headquarters with a letter for Bethune. With the letter came a gift: a beautiful brown mare which had been captured from the enemy. As a matter of routine the letter went first to Tung for translation. Alone in his quarters Tung read it, glanced at the time, thought for a while, then decided to consult Dr. Yo.

He found Yo in his room, polishing his belt with chicken fat. "*Tungtze*," Tung said with a troubled air, "I would like your opinion as assistant to Pai Chu En ... A message has come from General Wang for the doctor. It says that the attack is to take place in two days ... north of Lin Chu. I wonder whether we should give Pai Chu En the message now or tomorrow morning. What is your opinion?"

"Why not wait till the morning?" Yo asked. About 40 years old, plump, with a good-natured face, he had a reputation for long silences and terse comments. Somebody had once jokingly made a record of the number of words he had spoken on an average day and reported that his total conversation had been ten sentences. Now, having asked the question, he looked inquiringly at Tung.

"He will be very angry," Tung thought out loud. "But in three days he has done 40 serious operations. It is many weeks since he has slept a full night. There will be a long way to travel, but if I tell him in the morning, there will still be enough time. If I tell him now he will want to begin preparations to leave at once.... Again he will have no rest.... General Nieh has personally demanded that we are to take better care of him." Tung wrinkled his face with concern. "But you know how he is when he hears there are wounded somewhere...."

Yo finished polishing his belt and said slowly: "Tonight Pai Chu En can sleep. All the surgery has been completed. If you give him the message in the morning he will be angry, truly, but it will be better for him to be angry than miss his rest. He has lost very much weight. He keeps working faster and longer than anybody, but he is very tired. He is working not with this — "Yo flexed the muscles of his arms — "but with this." He touched a finger to his head and heart. "May I see the message?" It was the longest speech Tung had ever heard from Dr. Yo.

When Yo read the letter he said regretfully: "No, we must give it to him now. It is from Commander Wang himself. It says clearly that the attack will be of great importance. We cannot assume responsibility, in case something should go wrong. We should persuade Pai Chu En that there is enough time to leave tomorrow. But we must mention nothing about taking time for him to rest, for then he will want to leave at once."

In the end Tung agreed. He found Bethune in his room, working by lamplight. From the manuscripts on the table Tung could tell the doctor had been turning out another chapter of his medical textbook.

"There is a message from General Wang," Tung said, translating it then watching Bethune surreptitiously. There was no doubt about it, Tung thought, *dai fu* was in need of a rest. His cotton trousers were baggy. In the turtleneck sweater he still wore in moments of relaxation his shoulders were sharp and thin. His eyes alone seemed to shine with zest and energy, even as he narrowed them behind the preposterous metal-rimmed glasses he used for reading and surgery.

Bethune found a map, flattened it on the table, and calculated distances. "Not too bad. About 200 li to the front."

"The night is already greatly advanced," Tung said judiciously. "For what time should I instruct them to be ready? Some time tomorrow morning?"

Bethune frowned. "It's eleven o'clock now. Say five in the morning. Well, what's the matter with that?"

"From now till five will be the short space of six hours. That means only five hours for sleep and the packing of the animals." Tung was thinking that to leave at five would give Bethune hardly four hours sleep. "Perhaps seven o'clock will be giving more time for the preparations?" he suggested, adding deftly: "It will be giving the others more time for rest before their heavy work."

"Make it six, then," Bethune compromised.

"I shall instruct the others ... Good night...."

Tung went out, highly pleased. To jockey Pai Chu En into an extra hour's sleep, he told himself, was a victory indeed.

45

Early on the morning of November 29, while it was still dark, Bethune set up his mobile operating theatre in a temple near the Kuan Lin-Lin Chu highway. All during the previous day and most of the night he had travelled over 75 miles of mountain country from Yang Shia Chang. He had established liaison with

General Wang, organized relays of stretcher bearers to bring up the wounded, and prepared evacuation teams to transport them to Chu Hui Tse after they had been treated.

The purpose of the action was to cut the Kuan Lin-Lin Chu road, which was of strategic importance to the Japanese in developing their drive southwards towards Chin-Cha-Chi. To do that two groups of General Wang's men were to make surprise attacks on enemy garrisons guarding the road, while other units of the 359th Brigade remained in the rear as reserves. The temple which Bethune had turned into a temporary hospital lay midway between the two attacking units, a mile back of the road.

During the night Japanese tank patrols had passed along the road, noticing nothing unusual in the hills banking their route. The attack began shortly before dawn with the blowing of bugles and the sound of machine gun fire, followed by a few minutes later by the detonations of hand grenades. At 5:15 in the afternoon, exactly seven hours and fifteen minutes after the launching of the attack, the first wounded soldier was brought in. "Not nearly quick enough yet," Bethune commented as the stretcher bearers carried him out of the hills. But 15 minutes later, when the soldier went under anesthesia, an important fact had been established. Never before, on the many fronts of China, had a soldier received full surgery so quickly after falling on the battlefield.

All through the evening and night the fighting continued, the wounded were carried to the temple, Bethune and his assistants kept operating. By eight o'clock the following morning he had performed 25 major operations. While he worked the stretcher bearers brought reports that the battle was growing fiercer.

By midday the rows of casualties on the temple floor had doubled. The unit was now working in a steady, unbroken rhythm: the wounded arrived from the front, the serious cases went into the operating room, those operated on were evacuated by special teams to the base hospital in Chu Hui Tse, about ten miles away.

When a member of General Wang's staff arrived to inquire anxiously whether it would be possible to receive more wounded, Bethune sent back word, without leaving the operating table: "We'll keep operating as long as the wounded keep arriving."

At the fiftieth operation, after standing on his feet and administering anesthetics for 24 hours, Tung's hands began to tremble.

He managed to last out the operation, then sat down on the floor, his eyes glazed, his face suddenly slack.

Bethune helped him to a bench, looked down his throat, took his temperature, and cried: "You blather about *me* not taking care of myself! You've been working a night and a day with an ugly case of tonsillitis and a high fever." He asked Chia to make a bed and gave him some sedatives. Dr. Yo took over the administering of anesthesia and Dr. Wang took his place beside Bethune.

In the evening the wounded were still coming, and the first case of severe shock was brought in. With no one to spare, Dr. Wang volunteered to give blood. Bethune withdrew 300 cc. and Wang returned to the operating table to work for another 12 hours. When another patient hemorrhaged, Dr. Yo and Dr. Fong volunteered their blood. For the next transfusion Chia volunteered, glowing with embarrassed pride at the fond look Bethune gave her.

Then word arrived from the front that Japanese reinforcements were approaching. The issue would soon be decided.

In the early hours of the morning, reserve units of the 359th Brigade stole through the dark mountains till they reached a hill overlooking the highway. Whispered messages passed back and forth, steel clanked against steel, the line spread out, shadowy figures crawled about setting up gun emplacements, then blended into the rocks and hollows.

Fifty yards below, the road was a thin, elliptical line. On the other side the ground sloped steeply upwards again. Sooner or later, according to intelligence reaching General Wang, the Japanese reinforcements would have to pass through this narrow stretch of highway. They were coming, scouts had confirmed, in a convoy of 55 trucks.

For two hours the Chinese soldiers waited, as motionless as the rocks behind which they had burrowed into the earth. Then there was a rumbling sound, and soon a large tank came grinding along the highway, a head peering out of the turret under a peaked cap. Behind the tank came the first group of five trucks. As the tank and lead trucks passed, the next group came into view, then the next. They were travelling slowly, without lights.

They were large, open trucks, packed with Japanese soldiers whose faces were taut and shiny in the moonlight.

On the hill Wang's men silently pulled their rifles to their shoulders, took aim on their machine guns, caressed the grenades hanging on their belts. With the cold-nerved discipline of many battles they waited for the command to open fire. But as the trucks kept passing below and no signal was given, they raised their heads uneasily, their eyes trying to discover the commander in the darkness, the pins of their grenades cold in their mouths. Then, when it seemed at least half the trucks had gone by, the commander's voice suddenly shouted the order. A fusillade of rifle and machine gun fire hit the convoy in the centre, the front and the rear, followed by the shattering detonations of hand grenades.

There were screams of pain from the convoy, hoarse shouts, commands, curses. The lead tank reared up, trying to swing round on the narrow road, then jerked sideways in the blasts of three hand grenades, was lost in smoke, and settled to the ground on crumpled treads. The trucks piled up against each other. Flames leaped from bursting gas tanks. Enemy soldiers jumped and fell on the road. They fired wildly in every direction. Some crawled behind the trucks for cover, others scrambled up the opposite slope in confusion.

With grim precision the guerrillas kept pouring their fire into the stalled vehicles and milling men. Then a captain leaped to a rock, a tall, gaunt figure, swinging a hand grenade. "*Pin-n-n-n ba!*" he cried in a triumphant voice. "*Smash the enemy, comrades! Bethune is here to take care of the wounded!*"

The guerrillas swarmed down the hill.

"*Pin-n-n-n ba!*" the officers roared, running furiously ahead of their men. "*Pai Chu En — tchu tsai — wo men ho mien!*"

The guns blazed point-blank into the shattered ranks of the enemy as they swept down, echoing the rhythmic, victorious shout:

ATTACK! BETHUNE IS HERE TO TAKE
CARE OF THE WOUNDED!
ATTACK! BETHUNE IS WITH US!
ATTACK! BETHUNE IS WITH US!

Up and down the highway and into the hills the strange battle cry pursued the dazed Japanese until dawn came, the last gun was silent, over 500 enemy troops were dead or prisoners, and the victorious soldiers returned to gather up the vast pile of captured equipment.

At ten o'clock in the morning of December 1 Bethune turned wearily away from the operating table and gave the order for the mobile unit to be made ready for departure. He had been operating continuously, without rest, for 40 hours. Since the afternoon when the first casualty had arrived he had performed 71 operations. Tung, still running a fever, was huddled in a blanket in a corner. Wang, after his donation of blood, had finally been forced to stretch out on the floor. Yo was cleaning up, glassy-eyed, falling asleep on his feet. Bethune himself felt an unpleasant ringing in his ears.

Now, with the battle over, and all the wounded evacuated, he found a few hours for sleep. Then he was up again, for at the base hospital at Chu Hui Tse the casualties would need postoperative care and a special check to estimate the results of surgery in the front lines.

At two o'clock, as the mobile unit was ready to begin the trip for Chu Hui Tse, General Wang was arrived to see them off. He took Bethune's hand jubilantly in his and exclaimed: "We have found a new battle cry. Our soldiers go into battle with your name." He sang out: "*Attack! Bethune is with us!* — May the enemy hear it on many fronts!"

On the frozen trails to Chu Hui Tse, swinging gaily on his beautiful mare, Bethune led his tired but cheerful caravan through the snowbound mountains, filled with a happiness he had never known, singing for the others, who followed him, his beloved song of yearning and struggle:

> Far off is our land,
> Yet ready we stand.
> We're fighting and winning for you:
> FREEDOM!

We'll not yield a foot to the fascists,
Though the bullets may fall like sleet.
Our comrades, stanch men, stand beside us,
And for us there can be no retreat.

46

Now, during a few days' lull, Bethune rested and brought his diaries and correspondence up to date:

December 8: Back at Yang Chia Chang.

Tung is better, but all of us are tired. Food hasn't been too good these past few months. We are all a little anaemic. My ears have been giving me some trouble. My teeth are bad and need attention. I think there is a dentist in Sian, but God knows when I'll be near Sian.

Have sent my reports to Mao Tse-tung and General Nieh on the results of the Mobile Unit's work in the front lines with Commander Wang's troops. We have now proved our point. At the Base Hospital at Chu Hui Tse where I checked all the cases that had been operated on at the front, I found: of the 71 wounded who received surgery only one died! Three of the wounded were Japanese whom we've already sent back to their lines. Despite the fact that there were no secondary dressing stations between our unit and the Base Hospital, one-third of the wounded arrived at the hospital without any trace of infection! That is something new here. It is a great advance, but we can do even better. (The Japanese, by the way, used tear and sneeze gas on our men.) It is now clearly established: the time is gone when doctors will wait in the rear for the wounded. The doctor's job now is to be right up at the front.

An important point: two patients, both with identical abdominal perforations, were both given the same surgical treatment. One lived, one died. The reason? The first was operated on eight hours after he was wounded, the second — *eighteen* hours after he was wounded.... The difference between a life and death was ten hours.

During a lull in the fighting the Mobile Units can work at the Base Hospitals. They should go into action at the front when the number of casualties are expected to be greater than the regimental doctor can handle. That is usually the case in any action involving more than two hundred men.

Well, we have come a long way!

December 9:

DEAR MA: I'm getting used to not hearing from you! By God, I've got to! Two months now. The Yenan Medical Unit arrived on November 25.* I had been looking forward to this Unit's arrival, not only because it will be helpful medically, but also because I expected some books, magazines and papers — and some news of the outside world.

What the brought was an X-ray without a dynamo or the upright (iron) so it won't work. They also brought me Canadian cigarettes, chocolate bars, a tin of cocoa and a tube of shaving soap. Since I wear a beard, I won't need the shaving soap. The other things were welcome, but I would have exchanged them all for a single newspaper or magazine or book.

I haven't seen an English language newspaper for over six months, with the exception of the Japan Advertiser, a single issue dated April 18 and left behind by the retreating Japanese in a Shansi village. Without a radio my isolation is complete. If I did not have enough work to fill eighteen hours a day I would feel discontented indeed.

Will you do this for me — just one thing? Send me three books a month, some newspapers and magazines. I would like to know a few facts.... Is Roosevelt still president of the United States? Who is the Prime Minister of England? Is the Popular Front government still in power in France? What's happening in Spain?

Have you been in touch with Madame Sun Yat-sen's China Defence League? Is Canada or the USA sending more doctors

---

* Yenan sent a medical unit to Yang Shia Chang to work under Bethune in Chin-Cha-Chi.

or technicians? What has happened to Dr. Kisch? To Dr. Kotnis? Have they been stopped? Is the blockade that effective?

The supply situation is getting serious. I have exactly 27 tubes of catgut left. After it's gone I'll have to invent something new to use to sew up wounds! I have only half a pound of carbolic acid left. I have only one knife and six artery forceps — the rest I have distributed. I have only two and a half pounds of chloroform. After that is finished we will have to operate without anaesthetics!

It's been a busy month. Travelled 855 li, did 113 operations.... If some of the above seems I am complaining of my lot, I must now protest to the contrary ... Life here is pretty rough and sometimes pretty tough. But I am enjoying it. The country up north reminds me of my early days in the northern Ontario bush. The village here is like all other Chinese villages — mud or stone one-story houses, in groups (families) of compounds. Three or four houses are enclosed in the compounds, facing each other. In the compounds are pigs, donkeys, dogs, etc. Everything was filthy when we arrived — the people, their houses, the children. Our medical unit started cleaning up and today the place wouldn't be recognized by somebody who had been away a few weeks.

I have a house to myself for my stay here. It is made up of a single room, the inevitable k'ang, my cot and table. I have made myself a tin stove in which I burn coal and wood. The single window is covered with white paper. The walls and floor are hard-packed mud.

The country is bare of trees except in the little valleys. The weather has turned mild — about 20 to 30 degrees above freezing-point during the day and 10 degrees above freezing at night. Biting high winds come down from the Gobi desert to the northwest. They blow up great whirling clouds of dust and snow.

We are now 65 li (twenty-two miles) south of Lin Chu. The Japanese are all around us — west on the Tan Tung-Tai Yuan railway, north, east and south. In the south they are putting in a wide-gauge track to replace the old-narrow gauge lines. More work for the partisans!

We are in close contact with the Manchurian troops in Sueiyan province. They are good fighters.

General Nieh believes Japanese plans are to attach south along the Lung Hai Line to Sian and west to Lan Chow in

Kansu province. The northern drive will be west through Suei-yan province and Inner Mongolia, also to Lan Chow or the line from Lan Chow which goes northwest into Turkestan. This is very important for us as all the Russian supplies to China come down this road.

If the Japanese begin their offensive as above, there will be lots of action around these parts.... Where are Kisch and Kotnis?

I shall make an attempt to get into Peiping to buy medical supplies if all other schemes fail. Our people are walking in and out of Peiping, through the Japanese lines, with comparative ease!

Well, I will leave you now. Let me confess that as the Christmas holidays approach I am seized with an attack of home-sickness! Memories of New York, Toronto, Montreal! If I were not so busy I could find reasons enough for a holiday. Am preparing for another tour to get a few more Mobile Units ready, in anticipation of the expected heavy fighting. Don't forget to send me some books and to answer my questions!

BETHUNE

47

At Sheng Yin Kou, while the enemy was advancing from the north and east, the first Model Hospital established by Bethune had been evacuated with all its patients. What was left, a few days later, was destroyed by enemy guns.

What was to happen now to the Model Hospital that had been the pride of the Army, that had set an example for all the medical services, that had demonstrated how modern hospital-ization could be given to the wounded in backward areas?

The peasants of West Hopei gave the answer. They accepted the evacuated patients into their own huts, as so many other vil-lagers of the free region had before. They gave up their warm *k'angs* to the wounded and slept on the bare earth themselves. And early one morning, with the frost on the ground, they marched by the hundreds to the foot of a dusty mountain that sloped towards the sky at an angle of 60 degrees. They marched from their villages in silence, while dawn was breaking, like military formations. Over their shoulders they carried primitive shovels, picks with heads as broad as a hoe, and ordinary sticks. They carried them like weapons of war. They were, in fact, the weapons with which they would defeat the Japanese guns that had demolished the Model Hospital.

While the peasants assembled at the foot of the mountain an advance party scouted the slope, driving stakes into the ground, making mysterious markings, probing the soil. Then there were short speeches, instructions, and the peasants moved up the mountainside in disciplined lines to a distance of more than a hundred feet. Here they began their work.

They dug into the face of the mountain with their picks and shovels, carting the earth away in wheelbarrows. They cut straight downwards through the hard, brush-covered crust. When they reached the firm loess earth, they continued in a perpendicular line.

Day after day they returned to the mountainside, working with bent backs, cutting a long, high ledge into the earth. When at last the ledge was about 25 feet high and ran along the face of the mountain for several hundred yards, they drew a series of semi-circles in the smooth, straight wall, spaced some yards apart and ten feet above the floor of the ledge. These were to be ceilings of caves. To trace them they used stakes attached to a piece of string.

Then began the excavations. Still using only their picks and shovels the peasants began to burrow slowly, deeply, into the side of the mountain, beginning at the ceiling of each cave and working downwards to the floor. As the days passed they disappeared into the holes, digging deeper in the darkness, till each gaping hole had become an airy tunnel, 22 feet long, 10 feet wide, 10 feet high, with a semicircular ceiling that required no support.

Now a further ledge was built into the mountain face some 30 feet below. Here again the peasants gouged down into a perpendicular line, traced out the pattern of the cave openings, and dug into the mountainside like giant ants. When they had finished, there were 100 caves on the two ledges. Then the outfitting of the caves began.

The door of each cave was two-thirds window, covered by

oiled paper. Enough light filtered through the paper windows by day to provide illumination. For the nights there were open oil and wick lamps. In the summer the caves would be cooler than out of doors; in the winter they would be heated by charcoal braziers. The charcoal would be made by members of the hospital staff, who would have to cut the wood and burn it in special caves to be constructed later half a mile away.

To furnish the interiors the peasant diggers became carpenters and masons. In each cave they constructed five simple beds, consisting of two broad boards resting on a stone and a mud trestle. The beds were covered by a grass mattress, two sheets, a cotton quilt and a pillow. Between the beds they built low tables. A number of caves were specially outfitted as kitchens, offices, surgery wards, rest and recreation rooms. Additional caves were dug into the mountainside nearby to house the staff members. The operating room, because of its special nature, consisted of three caves joined together, all with a brick interior. Bethune examined it with the excitement of a man watching a dream come to life. At the foot of the mountain a thick wall was built, with paths leading from the entrance gate to the various levels.

Here, in 100 caves, the Model Hospital was installed again, invisible to enemy planes, immune to bombardment, walled in safely by tons of earth and rock. As the patients were moved into the wards, Bethune wrote jubilantly to Dr. Ma, "With the training school for nurses set up, the hundred-cave hospital built and the Model Hospital running, there is a lot to feel good about!"

He little knew then that the first hospital he had built, now a hospital of caves, would move back and forth across the mountains of the northland another 20 times before it would bear his name on a permanent site.

48

The night was dark and cold. Occasionally a strange sound disturbed the silence of the West Hopei village. Lying on his *k'ang*, fully clothed, Bethune listened and wondered absently which of the wounded it might be.

In the morning there would be any things to do — perhaps some new wounded from the front. But for an hour now he had been lying in his quarters, tired, hungry and unable to sleep. It wasn't easy to sleep, when in every hut the wounded tossed through the night without benefit of morphine, their wounds like flames eating their anguished flesh. And what if more casualties arrived from the front? With patients already quartered in every villager's house, where would the new arrivals be bedded? And with his supplies almost gone, how would he treat them?

He had waited uneasily for word from Yenan that the New York Committee, at last, was sending supplies. But none had come. It was a damnable situation! Down in Chungking Chiang Kai-shek was being most correct in his public utterances about national resistance, but medial supplies weren't getting through the Kuomintang screen to those who were doing the resisting. There was no way out: he would have to see Miss Ho. He would have to convince her to help....

A sharp cry roused him. It was a familiar sound, and even as he rose quickly and went out into the darkness he guessed that it came from the centre of the village. He followed the sudden chatter of voices to a hut where candlelight filtered dimly through a paper window. Inside the single room the owner was holding a candle above the *k'ang*, while his family squatted on the floor on makeshift bedding. On the *k'ang*, a patient was threshing about with his arms, sobbing wildly. He was one of three amputation cases who had been brought in a few days before. Working swiftly, Bethune prepared and administered a morphine injection. While he waited for the morphine to take effect, holding the soldier's arms gently, he said: "The pain will soon be better and you will be able to sleep."

The soldier rolled his eyes, then stretched his hands desperately toward his legless stumps. He had realized for the first time that he had lost his legs.

Bethune waited till the soldier was asleep and went wearily back to his hut. For a long time he sat on his *k'ang* in the darkness, then, with a deep sigh, lit the candle on the rough table, brought out his typewriter, and wrote a personal letter to the China Aid Council.

It was a repetition of the many letters he had sent to Canada and the United States. It had the same theme: men were dying; supplies were almost gone; help was desperately needed....

The next day he went to see Miss Ho. As he made his way briskly along the path that threaded through the hills he thought of Miss Ho and how he would have to approach her. Clearly, it would take an adroit mixture of tact, honesty and persuasiveness. He recalled their first meeting, when she had come with scores of Chinese from the hills to see the first medical unit ever to pass through the area. He had been delighted to find that Ho was only the name by which the villagers knew her, that she was from New Zealand, spoke Chinese as fluently as English, and had for some years headed a nearby Protestant mission. They had talked pleasantly for about an hour and later he had taken advantage of her standing invitation to visit her at her mission. During his last visit he had dropped several careful hints about her work as a missionary and his mission as a doctor, but had pursued the point no further. In some ways, he mused, she reminded him of his mother. She was tall, with an open, strong face, moved with dignity and spoke of her work from a simple sincerity. She had shown him frank and cordial friendship from the beginning, but the test to which he would subject her today would go much deeper than friendship. She had struck him as a woman who would be swayed less by personal considerations than by her beliefs. In fact, if she could be swayed only by personal considerations, she would be of no use to him. No, he would put before her the truth as he saw it; only the truth could persuade her.

The mission was built like a fort on the side of a mountain. In a compound in the centre of the fort stood the chapel, a surprisingly large structure of grey brick with a cross rising high from the steeple. A row of nondescript houses surrounded the compound. He went through the gate, paused, then made for the chapel as the bell began to toll. As he stood in the arched doorway he saw a dozen Chinese kneeling in prayer, led by the missionary. He looked at a portrait of Christ, two silver candlesticks on a table covered with yellow silk, and the light haze of burning incense. It was all familiar, yet somehow incongruous, here in the remote mountains, with the Japanese within marching distance of the image of Jesus. He withdrew silently lest his presence distract the worshippers.

He waited patiently till the services were over and Miss Ho found him on the steps, greeting him with delighted surprise and a firm handshake. "I hope you haven't been waiting very long," she apologized. "Can you stay for breakfast? We'll be able to talk."

She led him to her three-roomed flat at the rear of the chapel. Seated on a large sofa in the living room, he studied her attentively. Though she wore a long, black dress and combed her hair in severe lines, there was a relaxed graciousness about her as she sat opposite him. He guessed that she was in her mid-thirties.

The sun was rising over the hills. Through the window he could see the elongated shadow of the cross falling on the ground outside.

He turned to her and said quietly: "I should like to ask you something, Kathleen. Why did you come to China?"

She regarded him with surprise, as if the answer was self-evident, and shrugged her shoulders. "I was in the service, and there was a mission for me here...."

"No, that isn't what I am asking. Why did you become a missionary? And why in China?"

"Because I wanted to devote my life to God, to spreading the Christian faith. Because there are so many souls to be saved. I entered the mission work to bring salvation to men through God in whatever little way I could."

"I understand," Bethune said. "I come from a family of evangelists. In a way that might seem strange to you, I am something of a missionary myself. You say you are here to serve God. You want to save men's souls that they may have a future life in heaven. I want to save them for life on earth. Wouldn't you agree that no matter where, along the road, one of us might take leave of the other, at least the road we are travelling runs in the same direction? At least, if you are true to the God you believe in, and I am true to what I believe in."

"Yes," she said with interest. "But there is more than that...."

"Of course there is," he interrupted, "but for my purposes, for what I want to talk to you about, that's enough."

"Your purposes?

"Yes." He leaned closer and spoke swiftly. "There is something crying out to be done here, and for the moment you are the only person I can think of to do it. You know how terribly poor we are in supplies. We are blockaded on every side, although it is only here that the real fighting is going on. I have to operate on the wounded without gloves, sometimes without proper drugs and antiseptics. Now our supplies have reached the danger point. We must get drugs and equipment — even if we have to use the most desperate methods. To send to Yenan would be useless — they have none either. We would have to wait weeks and months until arrangements could be made to smuggle them to us in the merest driblets. And while we wait, the wounded will suffer and die needlessly. That's where you can help. As a missionary you can get to Peking without being stopped. I can tell you where to go. As a missionary it will be legitimate for you to buy supplies and bring them back here.... Will you do it?"

Kathleen rose and went to the window. It was obvious she was deeply disturbed. She remained silent for a long time, hiding her face from him, then she said: "I don't know how to tell you what I feel. I cannot take part in a war. I am against killing, I am against war. I cannot do what you ask if only because I am in charge of this mission. I'm supposed to be neutral. But it is more than that. I know how terrible it must seem to you, but I cannot take part in a war."

"I am not asking you to take part in a war. I am asking you to do something that will save men's lives."

She turned abruptly and led him to a small dining room where a Chinese servant was laying out the coffee cups, milk, cakes and a bottle of wine. She ate in awkward silence, avoiding his steady gaze. Then she looked up and smiled. "It is painful to have such words on the Sabbath. You are a most difficult man. Let us sit here peacefully for a while ... without argument...."

The next morning she came to the village to see him. She was dressed in the same black gown. She sat in the chair he offered her, her hands folded in her lap, her manner composed. "I have decided to go to Peking," she said.

"You understand — once again — that it will be dangerous? For yourself — and for your mission?"

"Yes. But hardly as dangerous as what *you* do. I am sure now it is God's will...."

Later, when she had gone, with all the details arranged for her journey through Japanese lines into Peking, Bethune wrote in his diary:

> I have met an angel ... Kathleen H—, of the Anglican Church Mission here....She will go to Peking,* buy up medical supplies, and bring them back to her mission — for us! If she isn't an angel, what does the word mean?

49

Throughout the autumn and early winter the Japanese ring around the Wutai mountains grew tighter. At the North China Expeditionary Headquarters of the Japanese command there was boundless optimism. The new tactic of encirclement, it seemed, was at last pressing in upon the very citadel of Chin-Cha-Chi's resistance. Soon, Tokyo's military commentators predicted, the guerrilla movement would soon be wiped out.

But as Wutai city, deep in the Military District, fell, and the Japanese pulled their noose on the 8th Route Army, they captured — empty air. Their prey was gone. Like fish in the ocean of the people, the partisans had swum through the fisherman's net. While the Japanese had imagined many thousand partisans bottled up inside the encirclement, the partisans had quietly dispersed, filtered through the lines, and once again re-formed in the Japanese rear, still retaining their weapons and their previous formations. And once again the hunter became the hunted.

---

* Peiping is now officially known by its ancient name of Peking, but during the period Bethune was in China he and the others used both names interchangeably. Peiping means "Northern Peace" Peking means "Northern Capital."

The large-scale "seepage" through the Japanese encirclement had taken place with the full knowledge of everybody in
the area but the enemy. The peasants had known of their troops'
stealthy movements, had hidden and kept the secret. When the
full truth dawned on the Japanese military leaders they called
upon their most experienced field commander, General Kishiu
Abe, to devise some way of crushing this troublesome foe who
could neither be caught, nor contained, nor defeated in battle.

General Abe made his preparations thoroughly. Reorganiz-
ing the Japanese forces, he divided them into powerful striking
units of 1,000 men specially trained in assault and every type of
combat. His plan was, not encirclement or the capture of any particular area, but swift and ruthless sorties designed to catch and
annihilate the partisans. And since the partisans' manoeuvrability
was in great part based on the fact they were indeed "fish swimming in the ocean of the people," Abe ordered the systematic
destruction of every inhabited locality in the area of operations.
The 8th Route Army was to be cut to pieces with lightning
thrusts; the population from which it drew its strength and support was to be exterminated.

The new tactic was out into operation early in 1939. The
special Japanese units of 1,000 men struck westwards toward the
partisan stronghold in the Wutai Mountains across the great, flat
plains of Mid-Hopei.

With the main fighting now transferred from Shansi to Mid-
Hopei, Bethune enlarged his mobile unit to 18 people, brought
in Fong from the 459th Brigade as an operating assistant, and
set out for Mid-Hopei. Between the mountains where he had
worked for a year and the plains of Hopei, the Japanese had set up
a blockade line. To get to the battle area it would be necessary to
cross the Japanese-held territory. At the beginning of February, as
the unit made its way eastwards, the mountain passes were piled
high with snow and were lashed by icy winds.

They came out of the mountains on a dismal murky night. On
the last, winding trail, leading their horses. They saw below them
a silvery mist, like a great cloud that had settled over the face of
the earth.

"Here," Tung said, "is the ending of the mountains. Now begin the plains of Mid-Hopei."

On the level ground they mounted their horses again and moved into the mist. Grotesque shapes rose up about them unexpectedly — gnarled, ancient trunks of trees, their bare branches swaying in the wind. The sound of the wind seemed to rise somewhere far away, like a distant whisper that grew to a high-pitched wail and subsided again. In the mountains the cold had turned their faces crimson. Now it began to drizzle.

Up ahead, all but lost in the darkness and mist, a detachment of partisans led the way. Behind Tung and Bethune came Fong, Yo, Lin and the rest of the 18-man unit. Contact with the partisans had been made the night before at a village in the mountains, by arrangement with Staff Headquarters. Their job was to escort the unit through the occupied region, protect it against possible enemy attack, and lead it across the Japanese blockade line. They were gaunt, confident veterans, accustomed to moving about in the vicinity of the enemy and skilled at filtering through his outposts. Heavy packs on their backs, old rifles slung over their shoulders, they were heading warily to a point in the enemy like where they would be least expected.

During the trip through the mountains Tung and Bethune had fallen into long personal discussions. For many hours Tung had questioned Bethune about the latter's life in the West, his family, his work, his early days. Now he guided his horse close to Bethune, wiped his face with his sleeve and asked: "*Tungtze*, you were regretful to leave for Mid-Hopei?"

Bethune, leaning forward in his saddle to peer into the darkness, replied absently. "I should say not. It's high time we did."

"What about Miss Ho?"

"I'm sure she'll get the supplies for us."

"It was in another direction I was thinking," Tung said delicately. "Were you regretful at leaving *her*?"

Bethune twisted in his saddle, then burst into loud laughter that brought a swift whispered warning up ahead. "Tung, you wily dog," he exclaimed, "you've been dreaming up a romance for me!"

Tung joined in the laughter. "People were guessing that you were falling in love with her."

Bethune chuckled to himself, leaning forward as a gust of wind dashed the rain into their faces.

After a while Tung asked: "Is it long since you and your wife had your divorce?"

"Yes, quite a while."

"Are you thinking of getting married again?"

"You're in a strange mood tonight, Tung." Bethune lit a cigarette, protecting it against the rain with cupped hands. In the brief flare of the match Tung watched his face. He was still smiling, as if at some secret joke, but with a rueful nostalgia.

"One feels the need of a comrade," Tung prompted. "Is that not the same with everyone? Miss Ho brought me to thinking … perhaps if you had a wife …" He left the rest unsaid.

"Yes, *tungtze*, I'm sure it *is* the same with all of us. But here at the front? It's hardly the place to find a bride — or to take a wife."

"But perhaps here in China you might find someone?" Tung suggested.

Bethune shrugged his shoulders, and it came to Tung, suddenly, as they jogged along, that his remarks had brought him to an edge of a yawning gulf in the life of the man beside him. With a feeling as if he had somehow suffered bereavement, he thought about the many familiar things Bethune must have left behind him. All of them longed for home, peace, a bit of the dream for which they were fighting. This bearded stranger, who had become his closest comrade — what longings and loneliness *he* probably endured, unsuspected by the others! Tung felt a deep urge to indicate something of his current perception, to say something that would have meaning between comrades who sought out their human frailties the better to subdue them, that would fit the intimacy of the moment and the knowledge that tonight they would be directly under the enemy's guns. But as he started to speak a messenger came running back with the news that they were approaching a village and that a halt had been called while the scouts went forward to reconnoiter.

The cavalcade drew together in silence. In the distance they could make out the faint blur of lights. They waited till word had come back that all was in order, then moved on. In half an hour they passed through the village, a "little devil" running ahead of the partisan detachment, solemnly carrying a banner with the Chinese inscription: "Canadian-American Medical Unit."

An hour later there was another halt, another party of scouts went ahead, and eventually they arrived at the village of Ting Hsien, the last settlement of the free area before they hit the Japanese line. Here they rested, drying their damp clothes on the *k'angs* of the villagers.

When they moved on again it was in close formation. From Ting Hsien to the Peiping–Shih Chia Chuan railway line they were in no man's land. They proceeded warily, knowing that every sound could be an enemy sentry, every blot of darkness an enemy outpost. Smoking and talking were forbidden. The horses' hoofs were muffled with rags, their heads covered with feedbags. In this area, Bethune knew, the villagers had killed all the dogs lest some stray cur bark at partisans passing through and rouse the suspicions of the Japanese.

The mist was now behind them and the night had grown lighter. For Bethune, after a year in the mountains, it was a strange experience to look ahead and see nothing but the dark crust of an endless plain, dotted with trees.

Suddenly an order up ahead stopped the cavalcade. From the partisan vanguard a message was relayed to the rear: "Turn off the road the right, keeping your places in the line."

They left the strip of muddy road in single file, striking out across the untracked plain. From here on Japanese troops manned fortified outposts at scattered points. The partisans knew their exact location, and led the cavalcade in stealthy, winding detours around them. Sometimes they skirted the road, then left it again. After every few hundred yards they stopped, listening, waiting for the scouts to reconnoiter the country ahead.

They had been proceeding in hedgehog fashion for several miles when a scout came running out of the darkness. A terse order passed down the line: "*Dismount, take cover under the trees, don't move, don't talk.*" They moved swiftly into the clumps of trees, dismounted, and squatted close to the earth, keeping short reins on the horses. For five minutes Bethune could hear nothing but the quiet breathing of the men spread out among the trees. Then a powerful searchlight cut into the night, bouncing into the sky and showing a road one hundred yards ahead. This was the highway, patrolled by the Japanese, that crossed the railway. The earth began to tremble, there was the familiar rumbling, and soon an enemy patrol tank lumbered by.

No sooner was it gone than they were alerted for the crossing. They mounted their horses, waited tensely, then at the signal raked their horses' flanks and galloped across the highway, reassembling on the plain on the other side. An hour later they hit the angle of the highway and the railway. This, with spectacular suddenness, was the blockade line running across Hopei.

As the cavalcade halted Bethune could make out nothing, then he saw the gleaming steel bands of the railway, fifty yards ahead. The rendezvous had been perfectly timed. As they dismounted a dark figure appeared on the highway to their left and came rapidly towards them. It was Li Shih, commander of the local garrison of the 8th Route Army. He saluted the commander of the escorting partisans and in low, clipped Chinese reported that everything was in order for the crossing.

All night Le's troops had been deployed in the vicinity, watching for signs of enemy activity and awaiting the arrival of the medical unit. As he conversed with the escort leader two of his men came swiftly out of the darkness and mounted guard at the point where the road crossed the railway. On either side, at a distance of about forty yards, other partisans had set up machine-gun nests. Still others were strung out along the railway, squatting like clumps of bushes.

Straining his eyes Bethune made out a hulking black building several miles away, like an enormous factory. "An enemy fort," Li whispered. "The Japanese garrison is there. And south ..." He pointed in the opposite direction. "That is the railway station." An equal distance away Bethune could see the station clearly, outlined against the horizon by the light coming from its windows.

In a few moments they were in the saddle again, with the unit drawn up along the road. The partisans who had escorted them had spread out along the tracks, facing north and south. Their mission ended at the blockade line. From here on the medical team would proceed with only a guide.

Bethune looked about, making a last check of the unit, saluted the two commanders, and pressed his mare gently forward. They crossed the railway between two lines of partisans and galloped into the night.

They made their first stop at dawn at a peasant settlement that was typical of the ten thousand villages of Mid-Hopei. While their animals were looked after by the villagers, they slept in the usual huts grouped into dusty brown compounds. At night they set out again their destination Ho Chien, headquarters of the fifteen thousand strong 120th division of the 8th Route Army.

For three days they hid in villages along their route; for three nights they made their way along roads that had been dug up to impede the enemy's tanks and vehicles. During the day Japanese planes flew low over the villages, on the lookout for partisans. Twice they were awakened when the Japanese laid down a military barrage from outposts a few miles away. The villagers seemed accustomed to such sudden outbreaks. They waited patiently till the barrage was over, then went about their business again.

On the fourth morning, the unit reached Ho Chien. Here completely encircled by the Japanese, with enemy troops 15 miles away, the found military headquarters and the political adminis-tration functioning calmly, with everything ready for attack or evacuation at a moment's notice.

They were welcomed to Mid-Hopei at a Staff Headquarters banquet presided over by the divisional commander, General Lee. Then the whole village turned out to greet them at a dramatic presentation staged by a local dramatic group that put on propa-ganda skits for the troops at the front.

The play was presented in a large walled-in courtyard. The stage was a wooden platform. The audience sat on rough benches. The play was to be an unusual experience for Bethune.

As it opened, he watched the stylized pantomime with inter-est. Then he gripped Tung's arm. For even without the Chinese he had already learned he would easily have recognized the play's "hero." It was himself. The "hero" wore a beard. He was a doctor. He had come from a distant land. In one of the opening scenes he introduced himself to a guerrilla leader at the front: "I am Doctor Pai Chu En. I have come to take care of the wounded."

The simple but vivid scenes that followed showed the hero-doctor building new hospitals, training guerrillas to be doctors and medical workers, setting up mobile units for action at the front. The last scene was a factual dramatization of the 359th Brigade ambush on the Kuan Lin-Lin Chu road. Bethune was shown setting up the mobile unit near the front and the guerrillas dashing off the stage crying: *"Attack! Bethune is here to take care of the wounded!"*

The little drama was greeted with loud applause. The actors took their bows, beaming, then the make-believe Bethune stepped to the edge of the platform, and announced that the real Bethune was present. The audience, which of course had known all along, rose to its feet, cheering. There were cries of "Pai Chu En! Pai Chu En!" and Tung led the embarrassed Bethune to the stage.

"*Tungtzemen,*" Bethune said slowly in Chinese, pausing occasionally to search for the right word, "I am making my first formal speech in Chinese.... I am proud to be able to help take care of our wounded. In Canada, and in the United States, there are many people who support your struggle against imperialism. I am honoured to work and fight with you. I shall work and fight with you the rest of my life."

It was indeed the first formal speech he had ever made in Chinese, and Tung, with a grin, found it necessary to translate. When he had finished, the audience chanted, "*Tsai hui*, Pai Chu En." It was the respectful greeting reserved for great national leaders: "Ten thousand years to you, Pai Chu En."

In the traditional manner Bethune responded from the platform: "*Tsai hui, tungtzemen....*"

50

Wherever he went now, the stories of his work preceded him.

There was the story of the stone and the wounded, for example. He was leaving one of the base hospitals situated in a temple, it was recounted, when he noticed the last in a series of stone stairs was missing. He jumped over the gap and turned to an attendant following him. "Do you mind jumping?" he asked.

The other answered lightly, "Not at all."

"And the convalescing patients — do *they* mind jumping?"

The attendant's smile vanished. Together they brought up a stone to replace the missing step. The incident went from mouth to mouth in the medical service with Bethune's moral: "Never leave a stone unturned in caring for the wounded."

On another location, at one of the base hospitals of the 120th Division, a famous company commander by the name of Chu Chih-Chieh was brought in on the verge of death, six hours after leading a heroic charge against the enemy. In a long operation Bethune repaired ten perforations of the intestine and gave several blood transfusions. For one week he visited Chu every two hours, permitting no one else to feed him. When the unit left for another front he had Chu taken along on a special stretcher. For twenty-eight days the commander accompanied the unit from one hospital to another, under Bethune's personal care, until Bethune judged him sufficiently recovered to be sent to the rear. On the day he left, Chu clutched Bethune's hand, his gaunt fighter's face covered with emotion, and said, "You are my father, my mother, Pai *dai fu*, You have given me everything. But I can give you nothing in return except to fight the enemy again."

In one of the villages where he was introducing sanitation and public health measures, he came across an old man weeping in the street. "Why are you crying?" he asked.

"Somebody has died," the old man replied.

"Who?"

"My grandson."

"Where?"

"In there." The old man pointed to his home.

In the hut Bethune and Tung found a dead infant, about nine months old, apparently the victim of dysentery. Beside the infant a young woman sat, also weeping, hugging a four-year-old boy to her breast.

"I am sorry for the baby," Bethune said. "But I can fix the other child."

"Fix what?" the old man queried behind him.

Bethune cupped his hand under the child's chin. The round face was marred by a harelip.

"How can that be fixed?" the old man asked. "It has never been known."

"He can do it," Tung said.

"But even if he can, we have no money."

"We ask for no money," Bethune replied gently.

"But medicine will be needed, and we have no money even for medicine."

"We will *give* you the medicine. All medicine is free in the Region," Bethune repeated.

In the end, tearfully, the woman agreed. In his mobile operating room Bethune performed surgery on the child. Weeks later, when he was passing through the village on the way back from the front, he visited the house of the old man and the child again.

The grandfather and the mother greeted him happily, crying, "See how his mouth is greatly cured," and pressing a gift of food on him in gratitude. He examined the child, satisfied himself that the surgery has been successful, and said: "Thank you for your gift. But medical treatment is free for the people."

During a trip to a Hopei village once a local army commander had a banquet prepared in honour of his arrival. When he was led into the banquet room, and saw the steaming dishes of fish and meats, a look of anger darkened his face. In alarm the commander asked whether the food was not to his taste. He replied: "You are treating me like a guest! I am not a guest. I am an 8th Route Army doctor!" Partisans and regulars too pride in telling the story: he was their close kin, not a patronizing distant relative.

At a rear hospital, on another occasion, he found most of the patients suffering from terrible skin eruptions which he had traced to inadequate disinfection. Though he had planned only a one-day inspection visit, he remained on for three days. Each day he ordered the nurses to heat tubfuls of water and had the patients brought out into the courtyard. There, assisted by Dr. Yeh, chief of the Sanitary Service, he bathed them, rubbed their bodies with sulphur ointment, and had their clothes and sheets disinfected. Having taught the untrained personnel how to deal with the skin ailment by example, he organized a unit from among them to tour the other hospitals with the same treatment. "There is no job," he told them, "too menial for the doctor. And there is no job too great for the lowest medical worker to perform some day with work, study and devotion."

The same theme underlay the Practical Work Week movement which he launched as a mass educational program for the medical workers of Chin-Cha-Chi. He held the first Practical Work Week at Chang Yu, with twenty representatives from all the hospitals in the District. Among those taking part were Drs. Fong and Koo and the members of the mobile unit. Though he had infected a finger while operating, and was suffering from tonsillitis, he put them through a grueling routine.

For eight hours a day he lectured on basic problems of surgery and medicine. Another period was spent at the Chang Yu hospital, with doctors and students rotating in various hospital jobs. Thus Fong swept floors and acted as a nurse one day, and assisted at surgery the next. Dr. Koo, though a field medical director, spent one session trimming the fingernails of thirty patients. In the evenings, before retiring, the participants studied their notes of the day. At the end of the week they returned to their hospitals to conduct a similar Practical Work Week for medical workers in their own areas. Thus the technique of caring for the wounded spread from Bethune to the leading personnel, and then to the lowest ranks of nurses and attendants. "What did Pai Chu En teach?" became a watchword of those in the medical services.

Then there was the story — perhaps the best-known story — that General Nieh told of him. The General had become concerned about the reports of Pai Chu En operating right through the night and day without rest, as long as the wounded were brought in. During a battle in Wu Tai Shan, Tung sent a message to Nieh informing him that Pai *dai fu* was working too hard and did not look well. He had not slept for forty hours. While the battle was still in progress Nieh ordered Bethune to come to his headquarters.

Bethune was impatient. "Could this conference not have waited?" he asked Nieh. "We're in the midst of a battle. There are many wounded."

"How long is it since you slept?" The general asked.

"Is that what you took me away from my unit for?" Bethune was angry and abruptly turned to leave.

Nieh simulated anger and assumed a stern expression. "You are under my command," he said, "and I order you to go to sleep!" The general pointed to a door. "In that room is a *k'ang*. You will go to sleep there and not leave until I give you permission. It's an order!"

Bethune stalked past Nieh and went into the other room. Now Nieh was pleased. He sat down, picked up a book, and took up his vigil outside Bethune's door. After half an hour had passed he decided to look in on Bethune to see if he was covered properly. He opened the door carefully and peeked in.

Bethune looked up at him. He was seated on the edge of the *k'ang*, smoking a cigarette, his face grim with anger. "It's no use ordering me to rest when the wounded are waiting," he said.

51

March came with warmer winds, reminders of spring, Bethune's birthday, more battles.

Since the New Year he had been through all the six subdistricts of the Military Area of Mid-Hopei, inspecting the base hospitals. During February he had travelled 400 miles in the mountains of West Hopei and onto the plains of Mid-Hopei. There were now over 2,000 wounded scattered in the hospitals and villages, from 50 to 200 in a village.

His March 1 diary entry read:

> The hospital "staffs" here consist of "doctors" of 19 to 22, not one of whom has had a college education or been in a modern hospital or medical school. The nurses are peasant boys of 14 to 18. Yet this is the only material we possess and we must make the best of it. They are very eager to learn and improve themselves.

They constantly ask for criticism of their work. Although I am often irritable at their ineptitude and lack of medical knowledge, their simplicity, their eagerness to learn, their true spirit of comradeship and selflessness disarm me in the end....

His March 2 diary entry read:

Our worst fears about the National Government seem corroborated. Since the fall of Hankow and the setting up of the government in Chungking the political situation has gone from bad to worse. A virtual dictatorship again exists in the rest of China.

On March 3 the Japanese suddenly made a foray near the Ho Chien base where Bethune was then staying. All through the evening and night the wounded kept arriving. It was the only the next afternoon, when he awakened, that Bethune remembered his birthday had come again. His March 4 diary read:

Today is my 49th birthday. I have the proud distinction of being the oldest soldier at the front. I spent the day in bed. I went to bed at 6 this morning, having operated all night from 7 p.m. yesterday. We did 19 operations amongst 40 seriously wounded. First we dressed the less urgent wounds, then operated on those who needed surgery. Three fractures of the skull were trephined, two amputations of the thigh, two suture perforations of the small intestines, half a dozen bad fractures of arm and legs — and the rest smaller operations. There were two Japanese wounded on whom I operated. There have been several other cases where we gave captured Japanese the same care we give our own wounded. At one base hospital I was photographed with two of them. They wrote to their families in

Japan, telling of the care we had given them and
enclosing the photo.

We defeated the enemy. He left 50 dead on
the field. We captured 40 rifles. We lost 40 men.
A life for a rifle! That is the way we get our guns.

Now the Japanese began their long-awaited offensive. A
week after his birthday Bethune and the unit went into action in
a fierce engagement at Kiu Han. While the fighting there continued for five days, the Japanese pushed into the headquarters
town of Ho Chien. For the next month the fighting flared across
the plains. Bethune travelled across Mid-Hopei, from one danger
spot to another, operating near the front, organizing first-aid stations, carrying out two more Practical Work sessions for doctors
in the rear, setting up mobile units to serve with the troops of
General Ho Lung and the Manchurian general, Lu Cheng-tsao.

At a village called Szu Kung Tsun, where the 8th Route
Army headquarters had been transferred from Ho Chien, and
where he had set up his own base, the enemy suddenly launched
an attack at dawn. Bethune led the unit out of the town's southern gate 10 minutes before 500 Japanese troops entered from
the north.

The drive against Szu Kung Tsun was only one prong of a
Japanese offensive which had as its chief target the town of Chi
Huei five miles away. The unit reached Chi Huei in the midst of
an enemy artillery barrage. In the courtyard of a temple on the
outskirts of the town a score of wounded had been laid out on
the ground. They were the first casualties suffered by the 716th
regiment as it met the Japanese attackers a mile away.

A short, stocky young man by the name of King, field medical director for the 716th, was in charge of the wounded. He was
beside himself with joy at Bethune's arrival. "We shall send word
to the front that you are here," he said at once. "The fighting is
severe and there will be many casualties."

The interior of the temple had been prepared as a makeshift
ward. Strips of white cloth covered the walls. A hissing gas lamp
suspended from the ceiling cast a dull light. The smell of smoke
and explosives from the bombed village filtered in with the salty
smell of blood. The porters' sandals slipped quietly over the tiled

floor as they brought in the operating equipment for assembly under the lamp.

All day the stretcher bearers came up in relays, carrying the wounded from the front. The nurses received the new arrivals, laying them out in the courtyard and attending to their registration. After the nurses came Dr. Lin, to provide provisional aid and to select those requiring surgery first. Inside the temple no one left the operating table except for food or a five-minute pause.

They were still operating in the morning, and the wounded still kept coming. Then a message arrived from General Ho to expect more fighting, and nurse Chia stepped up to the table to stammer something Bethune missed. "What is it?" he asked. An anguished look at on her round, good-natured face, her lips trembling, she said fearfully: "There is no more bandage ... no more antiseptic...."

Bethune held a hurried consultation with King. Was there some way bandages and antiseptic could be found nearby? King shook his head dejectedly.

Bethune resumed his operating without antiseptics, while the nurses gathered up scraps of old bandage and washed them in strong soap.

Night fell again, and still they worked on with no end in sight. At the head of the table Tung kept looking down at the patient's faces with a fixed, hypnotic stare. Lin took over from Yo, while the latter staggered out of the temple to lean against the wall with sick fatigue. No one spoke now, except when Bethune asked for something, his jaw set, pausing occasionally to wipe his clouded glasses and rub his bloodshot eyes.

On the evening of the third day the Japanese began to bombard the village again. For five hours the shells came steadily closer to the temple. As Bethune and his assistants hovered over the operating table the floor trembled constantly under their feet, till they cursed with nausea and frustration. At midnight, at the end of an abdominal operation, a shell landed near the temple wall away from the courtyard. Hot blasts ripped into the temple through the paper-covered windows. The gas lamp blew out, shrapnel crashed dully into the outside wall.

Someone lit the lamp again. Bethune hastily eyed the unconscious patient, looked about at the others and asked: "Is everyone all right?" They stood in frozen attitudes, breathless, then came to life ... everyone but Tung. "Where is Tung?" Bethune asked. "What's happened to him?" Then he spied the interpreter crouching in a corner over the supply cases. "Tung, are you all right?"

Tung rose slowly and turned about, staring with an incredulous look at the gauze and chloroform can in his hands. He walked to the table, looked up at Bethune and said miserably: "It's empty ... The last can ... All the anesthetic is gone ... No more cans left in the supply boxes...."

They looked at him in stunned silence. The shells whined overhead. On the table the patient's breathing was an audible, shallow suction. "Are you sure?" Bethune asked. Tung let the empty can slip from his fingers onto the tiles. "No more," he said.

Bethune walked back to the table, looking thoughtfully at the drawn face of the patient. "We can have him off the table before the anesthesia wears off," he said. "The others won't be so lucky."

He finished quickly and when the patient was being carried out Bethune noticed for the first time that King had been standing directly behind him. "Why are you waiting?" he asked.

"Pai Chu En *dai fu*," King replied gravely, "I am responsible here for your safety. If you are hit by a bomb, and I am beside you, then I will be blown up too. Then I will be blamed correctly for not persuading you to leave, but no one will be able to say that I was in a safe place while you were left in danger."

With a weary smile Bethune put his shoulder affectionately against King. "Stay with me, *tungtze*. I've never yet been blown up."

The next soldier was carried in, a young man in his twenties with shrapnel buried in his leg and thigh. While the others bound him to the table with ropes from the supply cases, Bethune talked to him softly, searching for the right words with which to prepare him for his ordeal. Then he looked warningly at Tung at the head of the table, made sure the others were holding the soldier's limbs firmly, and cut into the thigh. The soldier screamed and fainted. Chia, hardened by many operating rooms, turned her face aside.

Fourteen others followed from the courtyard onto the table. For ten hours Bethune worked on them without anesthesia at a relentless pace, while machine-gun fire came closer and moved away, shells sent tremors through the temple and daylight at last crept in through the shattered windows.

It was midmorning when Bethune splashed cold water on his face and went out, his feet unsteady, his eyes blinking at the sun. The enemy force had been wiped out in the wheat fields a mile away. He had operated during 69 hours on 115 casualties.

He stood for a while in the courtyard, looking down the road at the last of the stretcher-bearing units trekking towards the base hospital further south. To the right, the village of Chi Huei was in ruins. The air was heavy with the smell of seared flesh, powder, smoke. Army carts passed in front of the temple, transporting captured equipment from the battlefield. Another battle was over....

52

The victory at Chi Huei heartened the defenders of Mid-Hopei and threw the Japanese off balance. But once more the Japanese command brought up reinforcements and threw them in a ring around the Hopei plains, moving in again, mile by mile, behind a powerful shield of tanks and planes. One town after another fell to the Japanese, and with them went most of the base hospitals. By July Bethune and the unit fell back to a town called Sung Shia Chuang, where a new base hospital was set up, once again in a Buddhist temple. Here, one night as he was working on his manual of guerrilla medicine, Tung burst into his room and cried: "Miss Ho has come back!"

Bethune rushed to the door, looked out, and came back. "Where? Why don't you bring her in?"

Tung grinned delightedly. "She is not here in her own person. But she has sent supplies with some of our fighters. Here is a letter for you they have brought from her."

Outside there were excited cries as the other doctors gathered around the two pack mules on which special guards had brought the supplies. They unloaded the animals, slapped each other happily on the back as the opened parcels spread drugs, anesthetics, bandages, antiseptics across Bethune's table, then Bethune remembered the letter and opened it eagerly.

It read:

Dear Dr. Bethune:

I left for Peiping the day after I saw you, as planned. Everything went smoothly on the journey. I reached the beautifully ancient Oriental city after two days' travel. I regret that you weren't with me, for I could have acted as your guide and taken you to all the famous places that I am sure you would be delighted to see.

The day after I arrived I went to the big dispensary on Morrison street with your list. Because of the large quantities I wanted they refused to sell me anything. It was obvious the Japanese are working with might and main to prevent anything of military importance, including medicine, from getting out of the occupied areas. I found medical supplies can only be sold on an official permit issued by the enemy authorities. Retail supplies can be bought without the permit, but I found that if I tried to purchase everything retail, I would probably have to spend half a year collecting everything you want.

Fortunately, I have a friend in Peiping who superintends a hospital and is one of our believers. He obtained the permit for me in the name of the hospital. With it I was able to get from the Morrison dispensary whatever I wanted, except for some things that were out of stock.... The latter I obtained the next day at Ha Ta Men★

★ One of the city gates of Peking, near the consulate area.

where there was a branch of Germany's Bayer company.... I can imagine how happy you must be to hear that I procured everything you wanted, and exhausting though it was, I was glad I was able to do it for you.

Later I spent my time transacting some business for our church. I know you will smile at this. I can hear you saying that buying the medical supplies was surely a matter of serving God and the church. I don't object to your saying so. Let us agree that serving you is part of serving the church....

I visited all your friends in the city you asked me to see. When they heard my description of what you were doing in this part of the country they were surprised at first, then delighted, then all expressed a desire to come see you and talk to you. J — even asked whether he could come with me to participate in your noble work. Not knowing what you would think of it, I could only promise that I would bring him back with me on my next trip to Peiping.

The letter went on to describe a brush with the Japanese gendarmes and the puppet police on her return trip, how she succeeded in convincing them the medical supplies were for use at her mission, her stay in occupied towns en route, and finally her rendezvous with representatives of the 8th Route Army after she had made her way back into the free territory. It continued:

I was intercepted by an official from the Third Sub-Area who informed me he had instructions to pick up the supplies from me and forward them to you. That I did, although I would have preferred to hand them over to you personally. However, you travel so extensively that I thought it better to do as asked. So I am sending you this letter with a list of all the items....

I think I have come to an understanding the
significance of your work. Understanding it, I
am anxious to share in it. It is a noble work,
and whatever service I can render it will make
me happy. May God bring swift punishment to
the evil men who have caused all this suffering.
You have said with truth that that would be the
greatest blessing the Lord could bestow upon his
children.

I will pray for you before God tonight.

Yours sincerely,*

KATHLEEN H —

Bethune finished the letter and turned to Tung. "You know,
Tung," he said thoughtfully, "it is said among Christians that there
is rejoicing in heaven whenever a soul is saved. Tonight I rejoice
on earth, for our army has won a wonderful recruit — Miss Ho.
She came to China to convert others to her Christian faith. And
as a Christian she has herself became a convert of our army. Isn't
it an interesting thought," he smiled, "that our troops are bringing heaven and earth closer together?"

A week later the enemy drive reached Sung Chia Chang. A partisan detachment fought a delaying action some miles from the
town, while Bethune operated on the casualties brought to the
temple. Then word came that the troops were falling back, that
the town was to be evacuated, and enemy artillery made a direct
hit on the temple courtyard. One wall of the temple-hospital
crumbled, the roof caved in, but when the dust and smoke cleared
away no one, somehow, was hurt. An hour later the mobile unit
evacuated the town.

Now, with the enemy's armoured units advancing behind
them, they retreated westwards towards the mountains. In the villages they collected the patients who had been transferred from
the base hospitals in abandoned territories to the houses of the

---

* Retranslated form the Chinese.

peasants. In the mountains of West Hopei the wounded would be safe, but before they could be brought to safety they would have to be taken back across the Japanese blockade line over which Bethune had stolen in February.

Those who could walk were disguised as civilians. Those who were incapacitated were hidden in peasant carts, covered with straw. A thousand patients, in all, were smuggled across the blockade like, past Japanese-held towns and fortifications, and into the Wutai mountains. When the last patient was safely over the line, Bethune followed with the mobile unit.

Back in the Wutai mountains, Bethune distributed the patients once more among the peasant villages and prepared his reports on the mobile unit's work since February. It was now July 1939. Six months had passed since the night he had passed the blockade line into Mid-Hopei: six months of battle, forced marches, training courses during lulls in the fighting, heartening victories, and defeat and retreat.

His frustration and fury boiled over into his report to General Nieh:

> Why oh why are we not receiving help from official China and abroad? Think of it: 200,000 troops here, 2,500 wounded always in hospital, over 1,000 battles fought in the past year! And to handle all this, no medical supplies, only five Chinese graduate doctors, 50 Chinese *untrained* "doctors," and one foreigner!

53

In West Hopei, now, Bethune found himself face to face with a grim dilemma.

From Yenan, at last, word came through that the China Aid Council had been sending financial aid for the unit from New York. From the south, Madame Sun Yat-sen had managed to send in a shipment of medical supplies. But the money from

New York was still frequently blocked or delayed in transit, Madame Sun was rumoured to be under house arrest by order of the Chungking authorities, the Kuomintang blockade was turning into an attempt at military encirclement, and word came through that Miss Ho's mission had been burned to the ground by the Japanese.

Where would supplies come from? How would the medical services meet the demands of the new situation? After Chi Huei, the operations without antiseptics or anesthesia, the Japanese advances in Mid-Hopei, their current thrust towards the Wutai Mountains, Bethune found himself forced to a number of conclusions. In August he travelled to General Nieh's headquarters and laid them before the Chin-Cha-Chi military leader.

"In the past six months," he began, "I have convinced myself that we need a complete medical reorganization for Chin-Cha-Chi. We have shown that we can set up model hospitals with the primitive materials available. With our mobile unit we have demonstrated we can operate on the wounded at the front, and can save many lives. But all of that is no longer good enough. We've reached the point where one mobile unit, or half a dozen mobile units, can't do the job we face."

General Nieh, who had been pacing back and forth with his swift, nervous gestures, sat down, his fingers drumming on his table, and regarded Bethune closely.

The war would be a long war, Bethune continued. Years of fighting lay ahead, with increasingly larger army groups involved. A major part of the fighting was already falling upon Chin-Cha-Chi. Could one foreigner, no matter how highly experienced, and five Chinese graduate doctors, continue to do the work that would require thousands of trained men? Obviously, no.

In addition, there was the problem of the Kuomintang blockade, sealing off the aid organized for Chin-Cha-Chi by friends in the rest of China and abroad. It was imperative that the problem of trained medical personnel and supplies be solved as quickly as possible by emergency measures.

"What do you suggest?" Nieh asked, his volatile face attentive.

"I have given it a lot of thought, these past few months," Bethune said. "Especially during the fighting in Mid-Hopei. I have come to the conclusion that we must plan a program covering our immediate and our long-range needs. While continuing to use mobile units at the front, we must establish a new medical training school, with a carefully prepared curriculum, to turn out a whole generation of trained Chinese doctors and nurses. I am completely convinced that the swift training of literally hundreds of skilled doctors will from now on be more important than anything else our mobile unit can do. Do you see my point? We now have 2,500 wounded constantly filling our base hospitals. We have 200,000 troops. We have a civilian population of 13,000,000. A year from now we will have more wounded and more troops. If we don't have trained personnel for our medical service, we won't really have a medical service at all. No matter how many other foreign doctors we might be able to bring in, they can never be a substitute for trained local men.

"In addition, we must break the blockade, find some way of bringing in supplies within the next few months, and establish our own co-operative workshops for the local manufacture of at least some essential equipment and simple medicines."

"The problem," Nieh mused, "is to get the money and the materials to launch such a program."

"There is only one way," Bethune replied. "I must make a flying trip to America. It has become clear to me that I must get the money we will need, the medical supplies and the assistants — by myself ... and bring them in myself. It can be done only by somebody who has worked here, who can give a truthful picture of the situation, and can get in and out. I have drawn up a five-year program for the new hospital, a new medical school and the training of hundreds of doctors and nurses to meet our needs. I have estimated we can set up and maintain these institutions for five years on $50,000. I raised more than that for medical aid to Spain. I am sure I can raise it in America in two months. To me that is the decisive move we must now make."

For a long time Nieh sat silently at the table, thinking. Then he got up and paced the floor. Finally he said, "We will have to discuss it further with Yenan.... It is difficult to bring myself to agree that you leave — even for a few months."

The final decision was made in the next few weeks. The rains had come, pouring down without a letup, flooding the mountains and plains and bringing a lull in the fighting. Bethune was to make his way out of the Border Regions and to the outside world — through Chungking by plane, if the National Government made no trouble, or overland through Indochina. He would spend two months in Canada and the United States, make a public appeal for money and medical aid, and come back to implement the program he had outlined for General Nieh.

But before leaving there were many things to be done. First there were the 1,000 casualties of the Mid-Hopei fighting to be looked after. Then there were new base hospitals to be set up, staffs to be trained, preparations made for the mobile unit's activities during his absence. While the rains continued, and the weather turned hot and stifling, he completed his book, *A Manual of Organization and Technic for Divisional Field Hospitals in Guerrilla War*, followed by a shorter work on the special features of medical work in guerrilla warfare. Then there were the first co-operative workshops to be organized for the manufacture of surgical gauze, splints and artificial legs.

It was the middle of September, and the date of his departure was definitely set for the next month.

54

It happened one evening in the operating room, two weeks before he was to leave, confirming the dread he had long concealed from the others.

He had been working since five in the morning, fighting off exhaustion and a recurring feeling of giddiness. To the others, as the day wore on, he seemed to become strangely inattentive. In the evening he paused often at the operating table, looking about the room with a puzzled expression. Suddenly, as he finished a dressing, he stepped back from the table, put his hands to his ears, shook his head violently, pulled off his white gown, tossed the scalpel away, told Lin to take over, wheeled like a soldier on parade, and marched out.

In the street, heedless of the surprised exclamations that came through the window, he stood rigidly for a moment in the cold night air, tossed his head again like a swimmer coming out of the water, and went to his compound.

He stood for a long time in the centre of the room without lighting the lamp, tasting a strange sensation. In the darkness he seemed lost in a vast and silent void. He pulled his greatcoat off the wall and went out again.

He walked slowly between the huts, filling his lungs with great gulps of cold air. When he reached the edge of the town he continued on into the low hills, raising his hands occasionally to slap them against his ears. He walked with his head stiffly erect, his eyes darting as if searching for something in the night.

In the operating room back in the village Tung and Lin and Fong looked at each other and asked: "What is he doing?" In the hills Bethune kicked the ground with one foot, turned his head back to stare at the thinly starred sky, and listened.

He was listening for the singing of birds, the crunch of earth under his sandal, the sound of the wind. But in his ears there was only a satanic pounding, as if the blood was coursing through his head with the roar of a distant river.

He put up his hand to feel the wind. Yes, it was blowing down as always, but it was voiceless, it carried no echo from the mountainsides, it was a silent, icy breath. He picked up a handful of stones and let the, slip through his fingers. He watched them fall with intense concentration, observing that they hit the frosty ground with no sound.

He leaned wearily against a tree and meditated, the night and the hills silent about him.

He had had warnings enough, he thought — the first feelings of discomfort, the occasional twinges of pain, the ringing in his ears after days and nights without rest, the tonsillitis when the right ear had bothered him, especially. It had begun back in Shansi; it had ended here, today, with the sounds of the world shut out completely.

Would he never, he wondered, hear the miraculous din of life again? Was he to live only in the inner jangling of his own body? No more music? No more voices of friends? No more sounds of fields, galloping hoofs, bugle calls, laughter? Was it infection, creeping infirmity, something that could be turned back? Or thickening bone sealing off the delicate aural mechanism like a rock-fall choking the mouths of magic caves?

He rose, shivering, and went back to the village. From his hut a light shone through the paper-covered window. Inside Tung was waiting for him, dozing in a chair. He shook Tung's shoulder, watched the interpreter's face come alive with concern, followed the lips as they framed hurried inquiries from the other, silent world, and said sadly:

"I can't hear you, *tungtze*. I've gone deaf."

It was a night of loneliness and solitude. Long after Tung had gone — grieved, full of anxious suggestions from which he had turned stonily away — he sat at the table, gazing into the sputtering flame of the lamp, his hands extended before him, ruffling his manuscripts with listless fingers, his thoughts heavy and somber.

He tried to picture his future in a world of silence. How would he continue with his work? They would talk to him, and he would hear nothing. He saw himself in the operating room, like a bird in a cage, Tung and Fong and Lin making signs at him. He saw himself returning to America, exhorting audiences from the vacuum where no one could reach him. He saw his mother, her words stilled for him, her old face tortured with the effort of communicating a mother's welcome. He saw the familiar faces of friends, unfolding like the images of a film without a sound track, strangers suddenly behind their grimaces.

How long since he had become swallowed up in the Chinese interior? More than a year and a half. And how often had he heard in that time from the friends scattered over his wide-ranging life? Five times ... Five letters in 29 months! And the final irony: he had written to Yenan, to Canada, to everyone he could think of, begging for a portable radio to help him feel contact with the outer world once more. Now it would be wasted. Now, even here, in the villages where he had found such contentment, among such splendid comrades, just as he was mastering their own tongue, his isolation would be complete.

How stupid, he reflected grimly, to be caught in the fatal contradiction of flesh and will. "Lao Jen Cha," they had begun to call him. Yesterday, when he had heard even little Shou use the unfamiliar words, he had asked Tung what they meant. "The Old Man," Tung had replied with a grin.

"The Old Man!" He had roared with laughter. "I'm only forty-nine!"

"And more stubborn for work that many of our young fellows," Tung had added cheerfully.

Yesterday he had laughed. Now he rose and crossed the room to a small mirror hanging on the opposite wall. He shut out of his mind the subtle daily changes with which time tricks the eye. He remembered himself as he had once been, and he studied himself as he now was.

The face that looked back at him out of the mirror was the face of a man of about 70, of a stranger he was seeing for the first time — withered by the Hopei sun, roughened by the mountain winds, grooved and scarred and ravaged by hunger, illness, strain, inhuman exertion. It was the face of a patriarch, brooding, intense, the lines of age deep and defiant.

The forehead was higher, narrower, a bony protrusion from the snow-white hair that hung low over his thin, leathery neck. The eyes seemed smaller beneath thickly discoloured brows. They were as bright, as bold as ever, but surrounded by lines of hard-won, bitter wisdom. Under the silvery beard the flesh was gone, the skin falling inwards like a slack pouch. Both cheeks were slashed by deep lines running diagonally from cheekbones to jaw, like wounds that had never healed over. An empty fold of skin hung from his chin to his Adam's apple.

He rubbed his thinned lips. The flashing smile was gone. His gums were shrunken, his teeth stained and cavity-ridden.

He bared his arms and held them out, examining them with calm surprise. They were thin and corded, like the branches of Hopei trees. His chest, shoulders, thighs, the rest of him — all withered, angular, all jutting bones, barely over a hundred pounds, the wreck of a splendid body, of the Bethune who had conquered tuberculosis, climbed Alpine peaks, skied over the Laurentians, marched through the Sierras. He bit his lips, often bluish now with anemia and cold. He coughed, assessing the raspy pull in his chest, hoping it was only the usual 8th Route Army cough, wondering how long his good lung would last.

He went back to the table, leafing through his manuscripts to fasten his mind on something. Then he sat quietly again, thinking of everything he had been and done, of friends far away, of the future like a Shansi peak rising into the clouds. In the mirror he had seen an old man, two decades of his life gone. He remembered the night Tung had talked to him of marriage, the companionship of a wife. That too was gone. But there was more to remember: how he once talked of the doctor going among the people like a monk in sandals, resurrecting the health and vitality of the body; how he had raged against those who made commerce of men's suffering; how he had dreamt of the day when the doctor would be like an artist beautifying the garden of human life.

Once, as Dr. Norman Bethune, he had groped towards the dream. Here, among the plains and mountains, he had found how to live it. Now Norman Bethune was Pai Chu En, heir to many hopes and yearnings, grateful now for all the turbulent years, his life foreshortened but fulfilled, desiring only time, *more time* — for all life was struggle and becoming, all birth was struggle, and the years he had lost would lengthen the future of those who had never heard his name.

Hours later he woke, his head bowed over his arms at the table. The lamp was smoking at his elbow. It was four in the morning by his wrist watch. He rubbed his tired eyes — then he heard the singing of a bird.

He jumped to his feet. Did deaf ears mock the mind with remembered sounds, like the tingling toes of an amputated leg? He rushed to the window, pushing his hand through the paper "glass." The trilling stopped abruptly, but he could faintly hear the beating wings as the startled bird fluttered in the darkness.

He turned away from the window. His head was clearer. The buzzing in his ears was less irksome. He could dimly hear the creaking gates, the muted howling of the wind. Never had the sounds of the night been so sweetly, marvelously wrought.

He turned away from the window and stamped his feet heavily as he walked to the table. He picked up a book, held it high, and let it fall to the earthen floor. He smiled as he heard it slap against the earth with a muffled sound, as if through a blanket wrapped round his head. He unstrapped his watch from his wrist and held it away from his right ear, bringing it slowly closer. Then he did the same with the left.

On the right ear he heard nothing. It remained completely deaf. With the left ear a faint ticking came through when he passed the watch directly against his ear; partial hearing had returned.

He could still hear well enough to function — that was enough! He would turn the right ear to the enemy, the left ear to his comrades, and Tung would do the rest....

Pacing restlessly about the room he looked at his watch. He could still catch an hour's sleep, but he was in no mood to go to bed. He wanted to talk to somebody, to communicate with old friends. Yes, this would be a good time; he would write to Davidson, to Eloesser,★ to J.B., some of the others.

He brought out his typewriter, his precious hoard of carbon paper, and inserted four sheets in the roller. It might be a long time before he could write to them again, and as he often did, he would send them copies of the same letter.

He wrote of his work, his isolation from the world in which they moved, his pride in the young peasant boys and working-men he was turning into nurses and doctors. He wrote of his failing health in guarded terms, described the difficult conditions in which he functioned, but added:

> I find I can operate as well in a dirty Buddhist temple, with a 20 foot statue of the impassive-faced god staring over my shoulder, as in a modern operating room with running water, nice green-glazed walls, electric lamps and a thousand other accessories.

On the progress of the war he spoke with confidence. The areas occupied by the Japanese signified nothing from the standpoint of the final outcome. They were hanging onto the conquered territories like a man hanging onto the tail of a tiger. "In my opinion the Japanese can never conquer China. I think it

---

★ Dr. Louis Davidson and Dr. Leo Eloesser are prominent thoracic surgeons.

is a physical impossibility. The country is too big, the people too numerous, the feeling among the people too intense…."
Then he spoke more personally:

> It seems such a long time since we last met, and so much must have happened to you. It certainly has happened to me. These past months — soon two years — have been very full, so full that I hardly know what to describe. But I am anxious that you should receive one letter at least of those I have written you … I am supposing you have never received them….
>
> The mails are very irregular. It takes at least five months for letters to reach me *after* they have arrived in China. I calculate that I get only one out of 25 letters. I have come to accept that, more or less resignedly, as part of my life.
>
> I sometimes dream of coffee, rare roast beef, of apple pie and ice cream. Mirages of heavenly food! Books … Are books still being written? Is music still being played? Do you dance, drink beer, look at pictures? What do clean sheets feel like in a soft bed? Do women still love to be loved?
>
> How sad that all such things can be easily accepted without wonder and amazement….
>
> I am planning a short trip home, and expect to arrive in Canada by the end of the year. I want to come back from America with $50,000, which should keep all our services (hospitals, schools, etc.) going for five years. They need me here. This is my region. These are my people. Goodbye for the present, dear friend.
>
> Aye,
> BETH

Tung awakened with a start, rising up on his *k'ang*. It seemed he had just fallen asleep. Was he imagining he had heard someone? He called out in Chinese: "Who is it?"

Laughter filled the room, and from the darkness outside the window a familiar voice cried: "Lao Jen Cha.... It's the Old Man of Chin-Cha-Chi! The one-eared rooster crowing you awake. Up, lad, and rub the sleep out of your eyes. It's five o'clock of a busy day!"

55

October came, and he was scheduled to leave. But with the new base hospitals he had set up in Western Hopei there were now 20 in the district, and he wrote to General Nieh: "I am postponing my departure again in order to make an inspection tour of the hospitals. Some of them are new, and some I haven't inspected for some time. It is impossible to leave before doing so. The inspection tour will take a good part of October. I plan on leaving at the beginning of November."

With the other members of the unit he now set out on his last inspection tour. Then on October 20, when the unit was reaching the end of the tour, the Japanese suddenly threw 50,000 troops against Chin-Cha-Chi, spearheaded by the biggest concentration of tanks and planes since the start of the fighting in the Border Regions. From Staff Headquarters General Nieh sent word that the attack was the beginning of a massive drive to wipe out Chinese resistance in all Chin-Cha-Chi. From General Lu Cheng-tsao, West Hopei commander of the 8th Route Army, there came a request for the mobile unit to join his troops, who were bearing the brunt of the attack.

"But if we go to the front for the fighting," Tung said, "it will be impossible again for you to leave at the beginning of November."

Bethune studied a map of the north, recalling what General Nieh had said of the Japanese plan to overcome Chin-Cha-Chi. If Nieh's calculations were correct, the battles now developing would affect the whole future course of the war. For the Japanese the conquest of China was impossible as long as the Border Regions barred their path. And in their plans for an extension of the war in the Pacific, it was known, they looked upon northern China as a military base and a manpower reservoir.

"There will be no point to my trip," Bethune said, "if Chin-Cha-Chi falls. I shall leave when the present fighting is over."

During the last week in October the mobile unit set out for the north, where the main battle was developing on the Lai Yuen-Mo Tien Ling front. On November 2 they reached a small village near Mo Tien Ling, Sky-Kissing Peak.

The unit reached its destination under cover of darkness. Hurried preparations were made for a system of communications between the medical unit and field headquarters and General Lu placed a field telephone at Bethune's disposal.

Word spread quickly through the ranks that Pai Chu En had arrived. Most of Lu's troops were hardened Manchurian veterans who had become part of the 8th Route Army when the Chin-Cha-Chi Military District had been established. Some of Lu's exploits against the Japanese had become legendary. He was known to be a man without fear, who fought beside his men, had a volatile temperament and when the occasion permitted, was a consummate storyteller. When he and Bethune had met they had taken to each other like long-lost brothers. Bethune had not yet mastered the Manchurian dialect and Lu knew no English, but the joke had gone the rounds that they spoke volubly for thirty minutes, patting each other on the back and laughing at each other's jokes as if each understood the other's every word.

The mobile unit established itself in the village, at the southern end of a long valley, as the fighting approached a climax around Sky-Kissing Peak some miles away.

The operating room was the stage of the village theatre, a wooden platform looking out on an empty lot, surrounded by a mud wall but without floor, roof, or benches. The soldiers were brought in from Sky-Kissing Peak on stretchers improvised from doors and laid out on the bare earth. The stage was screened from the wounded by sheets of white cotton.

On the second afternoon of the attack one of the sentinels entered the operating room to report suspicious activity in the mountains to the north of the village. Yo, who had spent his whole adult life with the army, went out to investigate.

From the terrace behind the theatre he could see across two hills to a high mountain directly north of the village. There was no doubt about it: a score of people were descending the mountainside. They seemed to be dressed like Chinese civilians. Where were they coming from? And why? As he kept watch, he soon knew the answer. Behind the strange assembly more people came on, and as these too were lost from sight behind the intervening hills there were flashes of light on the crest of the mountain. It was a trick Yo had seen in many battles. The civilians were a handful of Chinese puppet troops, followed by an enemy vanguard disguised as civilians, with the main enemy force half a mile behind, in full uniform, the sun flashing on their shining helmets.

He left the guard behind and burst into the operating room. "The enemy!" he shouted. "They are coming down on us from our rear. There is hardly time to retreat!"

The nurses jumped to gather up the instruments. From the head of the table where he was administering anesthesia Tung echoed in bewilderment: "The rear! How can they be behind us?" Outside voices cried in confusion: "The enemy!" "We are being attacked! Sound the alarm!" From the open-air auditorium an orderly jumped to the stage, swept aside the curtain and panted, "What shall we do with the wounded?"

"Wait a minute!" Bethune's curt voice pierced the hubbub. They turned to him, silenced by the flashing eyes in the pale, thin face. Without removing his hands from the patient he asked: "Where were they coming from, Yo?"

"Down the northern mountain."

"How many?"

You gestured excitedly. "First a screen of traitors. Then others disguised as civilians. Behind them a regular force with weapons and uniforms."

Bethune, still stopped, looked about. "Fong — how many wounded left out there who haven't been operated on yet?"

"Ten, mostly light wounds...."

Bethune issued rapid orders. "Fong — have those already operated on evacuated at once. Yo — set up two more operating tables in here immediately. Lin — have the attendants bring in the wounded three at a time. Tung — take sixty seconds to station our guard north of the theatre. Also send one of the guardsmen to the porters with instructions the caravan is to be prepared to leave at a moment's notice."

The others were looking at each other dubiously. In complete confusion Yo exclaimed: "But what about the enemy, *tungtze!* They are cutting in from behind us from Wang-an-chen! They are close enough for us to see their uniforms!"

"Yo," Bethune said tersely, "have you estimated the distance from the northern mountain to the village?"

"No more than ten li ..."

"And how long will it take them, over the hills?"

"Forty minutes at a fast march!"

"Then we have exactly thirty minutes left to operate. If we work on three patients at a time we'll get out ahead of them."

The nurses waited nervously, still clutching the implements they had gathered up. Yo and Lin and Fong looked to Tung as their spokesman.

"We are all ready to stay, if necessary," Tung said slowly. "Am I right, *tungtzemen?*" The others nodded. "But we are thinking it is too much risk for *you* to take chances." Bethune shook his head impatiently, but Tung persisted. "It is not like the situation at Chi Huei or Sung Chia Chuang, Pai *dai fu*. Here the enemy *are coming with nothing to stop them.* If one of us captured it is no great importance. But you are the leader and teacher of our whole medical work, and —"

"*And* nothing!" Bethune interrupted. "What will we do with those not yet operated on if we leave now?

"We can take them with us."

"It's not as if we haven't time! We will operate — and *then* leave."

Bethune strode to the edge of the stage, pulled up the hanging sheets aside and shouted to the attendants: "Bring up the wounded three at a time!"

Without another word Tung went out and came back, Yo arranged two more tables beside Bethune, the nurses returned to work, Yo, Lin and Fong began to operate on two more wounded.

They worked swiftly, in complete silence. Suddenly, the field telephone rang. Lin answered it. He listened, saying "Yes, yes," hung up and reported: "Field headquarters. They say our troops coming down from the north are seven li away. Some of our men will be sent to try to hold them up. They order us to retreat at once." He washed his hands in disinfectant and rejoined Yo.

Five minutes later the guard who had first given the alarm ran in. He stopped in stupefaction as he saw everyone quietly at work, them burst out: "At least seven hundred enemy troops have come over the mountain!"

Bethune waved him away.

"But we have only nine guns between all the guardsmen!"

"All the better. You'll have less to carry when you leave."

The soldier withdrew, his mouth hanging open in perplexity.

The first rifle volley clattered suddenly across the valley. "Some of our men must be approaching the enemy," Tung guessed.

"Damnation!" Everyone whirled about as Bethune cursed loudly. But he motioned them back to work with a gesture of irritation. "It's nothing. I just cut my finger. Where in hell are we going to get some rubber gloves!" He held up his bare left hand, plunged it into iodine solution beside him, and went back to work.

Fifteen minutes later the last three wounded were brought in. Two of them were flesh wounds which Fong and Yo handled quickly by themselves. On Bethune's table the patient was a boy with a mangled leg.

Bethune prepared him quickly for surgery, assisted by Tung and Chia. The others, their work finished, went in and out on the run, helping the porters load the pack animals.

Rifle fire broke out again, at closer range, echoing rhythmically through the valley. Lin hurried in, followed by the guardsman. "Pai Chu En, you cannot delay a moment longer," Lin urged. The guardsman, his broad peasant face covered with dismay, said in a choked voice: "The enemy has reached the second hill." Without looking up Bethune answered calmly: "I am operating. Leave at once — we will follow in a few minutes."

"Pai Chu En," Lin pleaded. "*Tungtze*...."

"Everyone must leave at once." Bethune said harshly. "We will follow." He swabbed the blood-encrusted leg.

"No," Lin said with sudden resolve. He seized Bethune's arm. "I will not leave. *I* will operate. If anyone must stay I am the one. I

350

will take over.... I will not permit you to continue operating...."

"I am in command, Lin *tungtze*. It is my order that everyone except Tung and myself and the stretcher bearers leave at once. Take Chia with you. Anyone who disobeys will be cited to General Nieh for disciplining."

The boy on the table raised his head with a beseeching look. "I do not want you to stay because of me, *dai fu*." Bethune forced his head back gently.

"Then you will have to cite me to General Nieh," Lin said. "If you will not leave I will stay and assist."

"Please, *dai fu*," the soldier begged. "It is not a bad wound. Take me with you, or leave me, but please go before the enemy comes."

"It will only take a minute," Bethune said. "If I spend a few minutes on it now I will be able to heal it later. If I leave it you will lose your leg." Somewhere in the hills machine-gun fire suddenly cut across the approaching rifle volleys.

None of them remembered later how long the operation lasted. But when it was over the stretcher bearers were standing by, the soldier was borne away, still unconscious, and Bethune yelled, "Take only what you can carry!" A minute later they were galloping along a narrow path from the village to the southern mountain.

At the top of the mountain they paused for a moment to make sure the stretcher bearers were coming up safely behind them.

Down in the valley the enemy vanguard was entering the deserted village.

Late at night they reached a village on the Tang River to which the wounded were now brought from the front. They operated all night, rested the next day, then the unit split up. One group, headed by Yo and Lin, was to continue the inspection tour of the remaining hospitals. The other, with Bethune, Fong and Tung, was to work behind the shifting front.

With this division of duty it would be possible for Bethune to leave immediately after a decision on the fighting. "If things go well," he said to Tung, "I might still be able to get away in time to spend Christmas with my mother."

"I hope there will be no other reason now to delay your leaving," Tung said. "But what is the matter with your finger?"

"Another of those damned infections ... Cut it in the mad rush ... the other day when we were attacked from the rear.... Nothing to it."

After the day's work Bethune spent the evening in bed, soaking the infected finger in saline solution. In the morning, when he appeared in the operating room, it was badly swollen. "Nothing to it," he repeated, when he saw the others looking at it. But they noticed that he operated with less speed, holding the injured finger straight out, awkwardly. Once, when he knocked it against the table, he cried out sharply and then mumbled, "That was stupid, wasn't it?"

"I think," Fong suggested, "it would be better if you stopped operating until it healed. I can do the operations while you rest." "Nonsense," Bethune replied, "I've had infected fingers before. We'll finish up here today and move on to the next station in the morning."

They didn't leave in the morning. Hours after the animals had been loaded, Tung and Fong stood over Bethune as he lay on his *k'ang*, "I felt a little tired, *tungtzemen*. I'm sorry I've held things up."

He looked at them apologetically. His eyes were dull. He kept moistening his dry lips with his tongue. Fever burned in the sunken hollows of his face. His hand was now like an immense polyp ready to burst. "Are we ready?" he asked.

"You are very ill, *dai fu*," Fong said in a low voice, putting his hand on the hot forehead. "The infection is worse. It has given you fever. I think I should incise the swelling immediately to drain the infection. Do you agree?"

Bethune thought a while, his eyes closed. "It might be a good idea," he said at length. "Yes, do that. That's all it needs. Then we will leave."

They brought the instruments to the room, Chia was summoned to assist, and outside the hut the other members of the unit gathered in heavy silence. As Fong made the cross-incision Chia, holding the instrument pan, began to weep. Bethune looked up at her wonderingly. "Why are you crying? It's only a nasty little infection. When it's over we'll leave, and tomorrow you'll be assisting me again in Silver Town."

All day Tung and Fong stayed in the little room, while Bethune slept fitfully. His face grew more flushed, the wound suppurated, the infection crept into the forearm. In the evening Chang the cook called Fong to the door. "I have seen how he made the dead live with his blood," he whispered solemnly. "I offer my blood to help him." Fong shook his head. "It is not that kind of illness...."

"What is it?" Bethune asked.

Fong tiptoed back into the room. "Nothing...."

"Well, it's too late now to leave," Bethune said vaguely. "We'll have to wait till the morning again." He turned painfully and dozed off.

During the night troops passed through the village, reporting the enemy had taken Silver Town to the north. They were on the way to the front to counterattack, they said. After they had gone Tung issued a warning to the unit: Bethune was not to be told of the fighting.

The next day dawned grey and cold. Rain fell fitfully on the village. Bethune awakened slowly, listening for a long time to the wind whirling through the courtyard. As he listened, he thought his ears were playing him strange tricks again, for in the distance he seemed to hear the booming of cannon.

"Do you hear the sound of artillery?" he asked Tung and Fong when they came to see him. "Is there any fighting going on?" They looked at each other, and shook their heads. He dozed, awoke at noon and heard the sounds of airplanes overhead.

He pushed himself from the k'ang, got into his padded cotton uniform, opened the window, and shouted loudly for Tung.

He was buttoning his jacket when Tung and Fong came running. He swayed slightly, an angry look on his flushed face. "What sort of lies are you feeding me!" he blazed. "Do you consider me an idiot? Who is responsible for tricking me? Never mind — we'll discuss it later. There's fighting north of here, that's clear. Get the men ready to leave as quickly as possible. Why do you keep me here, like an invalid? I have an infected finger, nothing more. Fools! You should use me like a machine gun ... I want the whole unit to be ready to leave at once!"

56

They rode towards the front through drizzling rain. They had pleaded with Bethune, promising to bring the wounded to the village, using every stratagem they could think of, but he had mounted his mare and waited for the others to follow, repeating stubbornly: "My hand is all right."

He rode ahead of the others in silence, slouching precariously in the saddle, his bad arm tucked into his coat. At the foot of the mountain, when the trail became a muddy bog, he walked on foot holding onto the saddle with his right arm.

On the other side of the mountain they crossed more hills, slipping and falling in the mud. In a long wood they broke branches from the trees to serve as walking sticks. When they came out of the forest they mounted again and rode into a blizzard. They camped for the night at the very centre of the howling snowstorm, with only the trees for shelter. While the others ate their meager rations, Bethune pushed himself painfully into his sleeping bag without food. He fell into a deep sleep on the wet ground.

In the morning they set out again, riding steadily till they had covered 70 li and reached the vicinity of the fighting. In a vast, sandy valley they found a casualty centre with no doctors, nurses, or first-aid facilities. Without dismounting Bethune issued for instructions for the wounded to be taken to Wang Chia Chuang, ten li away, commanded the rest of the unit to follow him there, and galloped off.

At Wang Chia Chuang he led the way to the regimental medical office, and fainted in the saddle. When he came to he was lying on a *k'ang* in the office, Tung and Fong and the regimental officers standing over him anxiously. "Telephone all commanders in the field," he said to Tung, "that we have arrived. Notify them all wounded should be sent directly to Wang Chia Chuang. If you can't reach them by phone, send special messengers. As soon as the first wounded arrive I shall be ready to operate. I'll be all right after I get some rest." He closed his eyes, and it was difficult to tell whether he was awake or asleep.

Fong took his temperature, whispering to Tung: "He has a fever. He is in greater danger than many of the wounded will be."

During the afternoon Bethune lay quietly, sometimes sleeping, sometimes with his eyes open, staring unblinkingly at the ceiling. He no longer tried to hide the pain stabbing through his arm. Late in the afternoon he asked for drugs for a severe headache. In the evening his temperature rose above 40° C. He began to talk incoherently.

"Have the wounded arrived, Fong? I will be ready when they arrive ... You do the arms and legs. Be sure to call me for the chest, stomach and head wounds. Why are they taking so long with the wounded? They must hurry ... I have to leave for America ... I have a terrible headache ... My finger is all right ... What's an infected finger? ... Use me like a machine gun ... I shall try to bring back money and supplies from America ... Let them try to stop me in Chungking, let them try ... I'll make a fuss that will be heard around the world ... Hurry, lads, bring the next patient ... No time to waste, lads ... Bring them in three at a time...."

During the night his head cleared and he insisted on taking his place in the operating theatre but was forcibly restrained by Fong and Tung. In the morning he was worse again: now the spreading infection had engulfed the elbow. Fong, who had worked all night in his place, incised his arm in the hope that the pus will drain. This time he felt some relief, but word came from field headquarters that the Japanese were moving towards the village from Wu Mi Ti, and it was necessary to evacuate again.

At first Bethune refused to go. "In a few hours I shall be able to operate again," he said to all their pleas. It was only when the field commander, a Colonel Chi, arrived in person to order him evacuated, that he finally agreed.

Now the trek began southwards through the mountains and valleys, away from the Mo Tien Ling front, with Bethune in a stretcher, Fong and Shou riding beside him, and Tung leading the way on the Japanese mare....

57

In Yellow Stone Village, in the house of Yu, the landlord, Bethune lay trembling on the *k'ang*. "Why is it so cold, Tung?" he kept asking. "Is there no fire in the stove? I am terribly cold." All day he had asked for more heat, his teeth chattering though he was covered with fur rags and the stove cast a cheery glow in the room. Now Tung threw another rug over him, but still he said feebly, "I am cold."

For a day and night they had come through the mountains to Yellow Stone Village from Wang Chia Chuang. Here, yesterday, among the great peaks, the villagers had gathered round the stretcher, pain and disbelief on their faces. Here a partisan detachment, on their way to Sky-Kissing Peak, had adopted a resolution of self-sacrifice in his name. Here a courier had come from General Nieh with the message that Bethune was to be brought safely out of the menaced area at all costs.

Day and night Tung and Fong stayed in the room, spelling each other off only for short naps. Bethune lay restlessly on the *k'ang*, retching often, shrinking visibly under their watchful eyes. Fong incised, cauterized, used the few meager drugs that might counteract the infection, but nothing arrested the blood poisoning discolouring the arm. In the end, despairingly, he suggested amputation.

Bethune shook his head. "No, Fong," he said in a feeble voice. "I'd give both my arms to live, *tungtze*. But it is no longer a matter of the arm. It's in the blood. Septicemia. Nothing can help me."

"But let me try," Fong begged. "Perhaps ..."

"It would do no good." Bethune stared at his assistant. "You have become a fine surgeon, Fong. Your skill is greater than many who have been trained in the best universities ... I'm proud of you ... it would be fitting for you to do it if it could help. But I know the condition well ... too well. In Europe and America new drugs are being found that might help. But we have so little even of the old drugs ... Thank you, Fong ... It would be useless...." He seemed to doze. Then he said in a voice little more than a whisper: "You can leave me alone for a while. I'd like to be alone." Fong and Tung looked at each other uncertainly. "I shall call you when I want you."

They went out silently, avoiding each other's eyes. In the street the villagers looked at them questioningly, but they said nothing. They walked to the village gate, then Tung said, "We should not leave him alone."

"No," Fong said.

They retraced their steps back to Yu's compound and sat on the bench under the window of Bethune's room. The sun moved slowly across the valley as they kept their vigil. The men finished their work in the fields and gathered outside the compound wall, standing in attentive rows as if waiting for a village meeting to begin. Then it was night, and in the darkness the villagers looked over the wall at Tung and Fong, as they sat stiffly before the window, staring with dilated eyes into the room where Bethune lay stretched on the *k'ang*.

"I look at him," Fong said at length, "and I feel he has even counted up the hours he has left ... of all men in the world, how lonely he must be! He must not die!"

Tung began to weep, quietly, without shame, with head erect. "Forgive my weak tears," he said. "They are a spring that will soon run dry. It is more bitter for him than for all the others I have seen. If he dies he will be dying the second time. And he is only 49 years old. Do you understand? Every man dies — so many of our own died — but all of us have one life and one passing, and he has had many lives and this will be his second death. Did you know? This is the second time he is dying, and there will not be enough tears in all China to mourn his second passing...."

"Not in all China," Fong said. "No, *tungtze*, not in all the world will there be enough tears."

Through the window they watched Bethune raise himself slowly on the *k'ang*, holding his left arm as if it were being stabbed by a thousand needles. Dragging it carefully he stood up, lit the lamp beside the *k'ang* and knelt beside the chest in which he kept his papers. He swayed dizzily for a moment, but the spell seemed to pass. With his right hand he extracted the papers he wanted, laid them on the *k'ang* and crawled back into bed.

For a long time he lay with his head back, breathing heavily. Then he forced himself into a sitting position, with his head back against the wall, drew his fountain pen from a breast pocket, and began to write, holding the paper against his knees with his right arm as he wrote. From time to time he let his arm fall and leaned his head against the wall till his strength returned.

He was writing his last will and testament to Staff Headquarters:

DEAR GENERAL NIEH:

I am fatally ill. I am going to die. I have some last favours to ask of you.

Please inform T.B., Toronto, Canada, of my fate … and also the China Aid Council (of New York). Tell them I have been happy here, and my only regret is that I shall not be able to do more.

To B — (New York) I send my Japanese and Chinese swords.…

All my photographs, diaries, narratives and all the motion pictures of our army are to be turned over to T.B. Inform him that a motion picture will be completed soon.*

I should like you to ask the China Aid Council to remit some money to my divorced wife, on my behalf — perhaps in instalments. My responsibility to her is undeniable, and I cannot leave her cut off simply because I myself have no money. Tell her that I have been very happy.

My two cots are for you and Mrs. Nieh. My two pairs of English shoes also go to you. My riding boots and trousers I should like to give to General Lu. Division Commander Ho can select what he pleases from among my things as a memento from me.

---

* No motion picture ever arrived.

My two cases should be given to the director of Sanitary Service of our army area. Dr. Yo is to have eight of my surgical instruments, Dr. Lin eight and Dr. Fong eight. Dr. Chiang, the principal of the medical school, may choose two as souvenirs.

I would like to give a blanket each to Shou, my attendant, and Chang, my cook. A pair of Japanese shoes should also go to Shou.

We need 250 pounds of quinine and 300 pounds of iron compounds each year. These are for the malaria and anemia patients. Never buy medicine in such cities as Paoting, Tientsin and Peiping again. The prices there are twice as much as in Shanghai and Hong Kong. Express my warmest thanks to Miss Ho for the assistance she has rendered us.

Give my everlasting love to T.B. and all my Canadian and American friends. Tell them I have been very happy. My only regret is that I shall now be unable to do more.

The last two years of my life have been the most significant, the most meaningful years of my life. Sometimes it has been lonely, but I have found my highest fulfillment here among my beloved comrades.

I have no strength now to write more … To you and to all my comrades, a thousand thanks. ★

NORMAN BETHUNE

When he finished writing he fell back in exhaustion, letting the sheets fall to the floor.

★ Retranslated from the Chinese.

58

Another day passed. Urgent inquiries came from General Nieh, from Yenan, from the Chin-Cha-Chi government, from the troops in the field. Tung and Fong continued their vigil, hoping against hope. Now Bethune could keep nothing on his stomach, but in his eyes there burned a light that was more than fever.

Possessed by some strange last burst of energy he dictated a list of recommendations to Tung on the future of medical services, slept till evening, awakened suddenly and asked: "How is the fighting going, *tungtzemen?*"

"Many troops are engaged at Mo Tien Ling," Tung said softly. "The enemy is throwing large forces into the mountains, but we are leading them into a trap. General Lu has troops waiting to fall on them from the rear."

"Then it will be as General Nieh predicted," Bethune whispered. After a long silence, his face turned up towards the ceiling, he added: "There will be many wounded ... We should send a courier to have *tungtzemen* Yo and Lin lead the other unit to the front...."

Night closed in on Yellow Stone village. Bethune shivered on the *k'ang*, his teeth clenched. In the light of the candle his eyes became dark hollows.

Early in the morning he seemed to rouse himself. In an unusually vibrant voice he said: "Tung, my papers on the chest — would you give them to me?" When Tung hesitated he said again: "*My papers* ... I need them, Tung." There was a note in his voice that moved Tung to comply.

Bethune pawed awkwardly through scores of manuscripts, letters, reports, diaries, raising his hand painfully, till he found what he wanted. He let the other papers fall to the floor and tried to read it, but the effort was too exhausting. He held it out to Tung with his good arm and said: "My letter to General Nieh, and this ... Everything I have to say is in them."

Tung took the manuscript from his trembling fingers. It was something Bethune had written in Shansi. It was titled, "Wounds":

The kerosene lamp overhead makes a steady, buzzing sound like an incandescent hive of bees. Mud walls. Mud floor. Mud bed. White paper windows. Smell of blood and chloroform. Cold. Three o'clock in the morning, winter, North China, near Linchu, with the Eighth Route Army.

Men with wounds....

Old filthy bandages stuck to the skin with blood-glue. Careful. Better moisten first. Through the thigh. Pick the leg up. Why, its like a bag, a long loose red stocking. What kind of stocking? *A Christmas stocking.*

Where's that fine strong rod of bone now? In a dozen pieces. Pick them out with your fingers; white as a dog's teeth, sharp and jagged. Now feel. Any more left? Yes, here. Is this muscle dead? Pinch it. Yes, it's dead. Cut it out. How can that heal? How can those muscles, once so strong, now so torn, so devastated, so ruined, resume their proud tension?

Gangrene is a cunning, creeping fellow. Is this one alive? Yes he lives. Technically speaking, he is alive. Give him saline intravenously. Perhaps the innumerable tiny cells of his body will remember. They may remember the hot salty sea, their ancestral home, their first food. With the memory of a million years, they may remember other tides, other oceans, and life being born of the sea and the sun.

And this one. Will he run along the road beside his mule at another harvest, with cries of happiness? No, that one will never run again. How can you run with one leg? What will he do? Why, he'll sit and watch the other boys run. What will he think? He'll think what you and I would think. Don't pity him — pity would diminish his sacrifice. He did this for the defence of China.

How beautiful the body is; how perfect in parts; with what precision it moves; how obedient, proud and strong; how terrible when torn. The little flame of life sinks lower and lower, and with a flicker goes out. It goes out like a candle, quietly and gently. It makes its protest at extinction, then submits. It has its say, then is silent.

Any more? Four Japanese prisoners. Bring them in. In this community of pain there are no enemies. Cut away the bloodstained uniform. Stop that hemorrhage. Lay them beside the others. Why, they're alike as brothers!

Are these professional man-killers? No, these are amateurs-in-arms. Workman's hands. These are workers in uniform.

No more. Six in the morning. God, it's cold in this room. Open the door. Over the distant, dark-blue mountains, a pale, faint line of light appears in the east. In an hour the sun will be up. To bed and sleep.

But sleep will not come. What is the cause of this cruelty, this stupidity? A million workmen come from Japan to kill or mutilate a million Chinese workmen. Why should the Japanese worker attack his brother worker, who is forced merely to defend himself? Will the Japanese worker benefit by the death of the Chinese? No, how can he gain? Then in God's name, who will gain? Who is responsible for sending these Japanese workmen on this murderous mission? *Who will profit from it?*

Is it possible that a few rich reactionary men, a small class of men, have persuaded a million men to attack and attempt to destroy another million men as poor as they? So that these rich may be richer still? Terrible thought! How did they persuade these poor men to come to China? By telling them the truth? *No, they would never have come if they had known the truth.*

Did they dare tell these workmen that they only wanted cheaper raw materials, more markets and more profit? No, they told them that this brutal war was "The Destiny of the Race," it was for the "Glory of the Emperor," it was for the "Honor of the State."

False, false as hell!

Are wars of aggression, wars for the conquest of colonies, then just big business? Yes, it would seem so, however much the perpetrators of such national crimes seek to hide their true purpose under the banner of high-sounding abstractions and ideals. They make war to capture markets by murder; raw materials by rape. They find it cheaper to steal than to exchange; easier to butcher than to buy.

Behind all this stands that implacable god of business and blood whose name is profit. Money, like an insatiable Moloch, demands its interest, its return, and will stop at nothing, not even the murder of millions to satisfy its greed. Behind the army, stand the militarists. Behind the militarists, stand finance capital and the capitalists. Brothers in blood; companions in crime.

What do the enemies of the human race look like? Do they wear on their foreheads a sign so that they may be told, shunned and condemned as criminals? No. On the contrary, they are the respectable ones. They are honoured. They call themselves and are called, gentlemen. They are the pillars of the state, of the church, of society. They support private and public charity out of the excesses of their wealth. In their private lives they are kind and considerate. But ... threaten a reduction on the profit of their money and they become ruthless as savages, brutal as madmen, remorseless as executioners ... There can be no permanent peace in the world while they live. Such an organization of human society as permits them to exist must be abolished.

These men make the wounds.

That morning, as the men were trooping out of the village for the day's labour in the fields, they saw Tung standing in the doorway of Yu's house. They stopped at the courtyard wall and inquired after Pai Chu En.

"He is dead," Tung said.

It was twenty minutes after five, November 13, 1939.

59

They carried him through the mountains, a funeral cortege of fighters and comrades. Under cover of darkness they wound slowly westwards, moving from village to village for five nights, hiding the body in peasants' huts during the day.

In the villages where he healed the sick and the wounded they stopped for brief ceremonies. They lowered the stretcher on which he lay; Tung spoke of his life and death; the people filed by to see him for the last time, weeping. Then they went on again under the starry skies. They buried him in a valley in East Shansi, leaving a simple marking over his grave.

The news spread over the 8th Route Army wireless system, leaving those who heard it staring and silent. At his headquarters in the Wutai Mountains General Nieh wept while his staff sat about him with bowed heads.

In a message to the people of Canada Dr. Richard Brown said, "Norman Bethune boasted he was a communist. I say he was a saint of God."

At the front the troops swooped out of the mountains crying "Pai Chu En!" as they closed the trap on the Japanese force, killing General Abe, his entire staff and every enemy soldier with him.

In caves, in the hospitals and schools he had established, in the myriad villages where he had brought medicine and modern hygiene for the first time, the people mourned. "We mourn more than the passing of a man," Mao Tse-tung told his countrymen:

> Dr. Bethune's devotion to the common people is a lesson for all. The manner in which we commemorate his death indicates how deep an imprint his personality has made on us. All of us should emulate his unselfish spirit. It should become a starting point for us to become individuals useful to the people. An individual may have great or little ability, but with such a spirit he can become a man of importance, of integrity, of virtue who forsakes self-interest for the interest of the people.

At Yenan the troops of the 8th Route Army gathered in a mighty memorial. Row upon row they stood, filling a vast corner of the valley between the honeycombed cliffs. From an improvised tribunal, before a great picture of Bethune, Chu Teh, the Commander in Chief of all the communist armies, spoke to them:

> The death of Comrade Bethune is a great bereavement. We have suffered a tremendous loss that fills every comrade of the 8th Route Army with pain. With his great love, his sympathy, his courage in struggle he achieved the highest standards of evolutionary virtue.
>
> He dedicated his life to the cause of China's national emancipation. The Chinese nation will recall him with love and admiration, and some day all progressive mankind will cherish his memory.
>
> Our fighting men and leaders will commemorate his sacrifice with tears of grief, and with courage multiplied a hundredfold by his example.

"*Down with the invaders!*" the vast throng chanted. "*Remember Dr. Bethune!*"

"Everything for the struggle! *Remember Dr. Bethune!*"

"Long live free China! *Remember Dr. Bethune!*"

"Peace for the world! *Remember Dr. Bethune!*"

EPILOGUE

The guerrilla detachments, the patriots, the steel-sheathed troops of the invaders, surged back and forth over his grave, while the war he had fought to prevent engulfed the world.

The men who make the wounds seized one country after another. In faraway cities on three continents they plundered the peoples' treasures and murdered whole populations. In East Shansi, they turned the valley where he was buried into a shooting-range.

"I swear," General Nieh said, "that I shall never return to the valley until the desecration has been repaired."

Nine years later he was able to return. Now no foreign armies remained on the Chinese mainland. Now Bethune's comrades were the rulers of ancient China. Now, at last, the desecration could be repaired — and they carried his remains to rest forever in the Mausoleum of Martyrs, in the city of Shih Cha Chuang, southeast of Peking.

Since then, many years have passed. New controversies have diminished the renown of some men and increased that of others, but Bethune's fame has continued to grow unchallenged. From every corner of China and from all over the world, people come to lay flowers at his grave; to once more hear the stories of those incredible battles in which he shared; to remind themselves of this man's personal Odyssey, of the Long March he himself had chosen to take from the irresponsible world of bohemia to the battlefields of Spain and China.

From all over the world the people come to the sun-drenched streets of Shih Cha Chuang. They drive past the Bethune International Peace Hospital and the Bethune Medical School. Reaching the Mausoleum they pass through one of two large iron gates into what appears to be an immense and beautiful park. They walk between the trees, past the graves of peasants and patriots, whose names have now passed into history. And then, deep within the seemingly endless vistas of the park, they are sudden confronted with the vivid symbol of China's struggle for freedom. Two partisans, frozen in stone on a dazzling white base, faced by two women guerrillas with their rifles slung over their granite shoulders. Behind the monument rise the grey, square stones and the simple lines of the museum itself.

The chamber within is quiet and cool. Along one wall hang the portraits of China's best-known heroes. In death as in life, Bethune is among them, his face bearded, his brows furrowed fiercely as if he is still challenging the world. On the opposite wall, in a special niche, stands a three-quarter-life-size statue of him. He holds a stethoscope in one hand and is gazing off into the future for which he fought to lay the groundwork. Nearby is a plaque to his memory which is always banked by flowers: the roses brought by Westerners, and the everlasting brilliance of the superbly wrought paper flowers, brought by the Chinese.

The visitors come out again into the bright sunlight. Now the guide leads them to a large circular clearing. In its centre is a catafalque surmounted by a cross. Behind it, on the left, is Bethune's grave, topped by a long slab of chiselled granite, with a simple upright column at its head, and a stone plaque bearing his name in English and Chinese. Parallel to it, and on the right, is the grave of Dr. Kotnis of India, who died during the attempt to penetrate to Chin-Cha-Chi, in the hope of being able to take over Bethune's work.

The setting and the design of the graves have been created by an artist who has felt the heartbeat of the world. Here, in this lovely park, in a quiet disturbed only by the soft wind in the trees, in death as in battle, the two men once more state the brotherhood of black and white, of Asian and American, of all who yearn for a better world, who have set out to destroy the power of those who make the wounds.

The myriad visitors to Bethune's grave include peasants and men of renown, famous names and anonymous workers. They stand with equal reverence before it, and they leave it feeling an equal gratitude. For, in the memory of Bethune's life, the great are reminded of people from whom they draw their strength, and the people are reminded of the road that everyone can travel to greatness.